Effects of Your Genetics on Pain
Why You Hurt More than Others

William Edward Ackerman III MD
Pain Management Specialist

Effects of Your Genetics on Pain

Copyright © 2016 by William Edward Ackerman III MD

All rights reserved. No part of this book may be reproduced or transmitted in any form or by any means without written permission of the author.

This book is dedicated to my significant other who encouraged me to adopt a healthy lifestyle to decrease my own aches and pains as well as exercising on a daily basis.

Acknowledgments

I wish to recognize my oldest son William E. Ackerman IV MD, a genetic engineer and MD, and researcher who tweaked my interest in genetics and its effects on more common disease states. I furthermore, wish to acknowledge my office staff who are constantly wanting to learn new information about pain treatments. Lastly I want to acknowledge my patients who have changed to a healthier life style to decrease their pain.

Foreword

When one is young, body cells grow and replicate which is dependent on telomeres in the chromosomes. This process slows down when one becomes an adult and gets progressively slower with age. Some cells like those in the brain and nerves do not continue to grow. Bodies reflect the genetic capacity to adapt and repair, as well as tolerate the cumulative damage from disease processes. With advancing age, all of the body systems eventually demonstrate reduced efficiency, slowed building and replacement and actual loss of tissue. There is a gradual loss of bone tissue and the reduced tissue loss may be permanent. When a person is born, cells in the body duplicate rapidly which enables growth resiliency.

A chromosome is a cell with a long strand of DNA in it. At the end of a chromosome is a telomere, which acts like a bookend. Telomeres keep chromosomes protected and prevent them from binding with other DNA. Many cells in the body need to replicate to keep the body healthy. When the telomeres fail one's health is affected and this failure is related to aging and chronic pain perception.

Table of Contents

1. Aging effect on telomere length 1
2. Elderly patients are like old cars 9
3. Pain concepts 17
4. Pain is common in the elderly 25
5. Pain Assessment 35
6. Psychological assessment 43
7. Physical therapy 55
8. Alternative medicine 61
9. Chiropractic 71
10. Nutrition 81
11. Opioids 91
12. Addiction 101
13. Anti-inflammatory medications 107
14. Anticonvulsants 117
15. TENS unit 127
16. Spinal fluid opioid therapy 133
17. Topical analgesics 137
18. Acute post-surgical pain 151
19. Injection therapy 157
20. Cervical spine pain 167
21. Whiplash injuries 177
22. Joint pain 187
23. Myofascial pain 195
24. Headaches 205

25. Spinal deterioration and back pain 213
26. Fibromyalgia 221
27. Reflex sympathetic dystrophy 231
28. Shingles 243
29. Peripheral neuropathy 255
30. Cancer pain 265
31. Chest pain 275
32. Facial neuropathy and neuralgia 287
33. Osteoporosis 299
34. HIV/AIDS 315
35. Arthritis 329
36. Abdominal Pain 341
37. Diagnostic tests 353
38. Telomere length and health outcomes 361
39. Palliative care 367
40. Who pays for elderly care? 373

1. Aging effect on telomere length

When a person is born, cells in the body duplicate rapidly which enables growth. This process slows down when one becomes an adult and gets progressively slower with age. Some cells like those in the brain and nerves do not continue to grow. Our bodies reflect our genetic capacity to adapt and repair, as well as tolerate the cumulative damage from disease processes. With advancing age, all of the body systems eventually demonstrate reduced efficiency, slowed building & replacement and actual loss of tissue. There is a gradual loss of bone tissue and the reduced resiliency of blood vessels.

A chromosome in a cell contains a long strand of DNA. At the end of a chromosome is a telomere, which acts like a bookend. Telomeres keep chromosomes protected and prevent them from binding with other DNA. Many cells in the body need to replicate to keep the body healthy. For example when the skin cells stop replicating, an individual will have "wrinkled skin'. The telomeres get shorter each time a cell divides. Cells stop replicating when telomeres are short. This is why a body "falls apart" when cells stop dividing. In older individuals many cells have stopped dividing. Every cell in a body has the genetic code to make telomerase, but only certain cells need to produce this enzyme. White blood cells are the most studied cells to date.

Aging is an inevitable biological phenomenon. The incidence of age related disorders (ARDs) such as cardiovascular diseases, cancer, arthritis, dementia, osteoporosis, diabetes, neurodegenerative diseases increase rapidly with aging. ARDs are becoming a key social and economic trouble for the world's elderly population (above 60 years), which is expected to reach 2 billion by 2050.[1] Aging involves cellular changes that occur over the course of one's life. Individuals look for what distinguishes normal aging from disease processes.

On occasion abnormal aging could be a sign of disease. However the rate of cellular aging can vary from person to person aging affects the cells of every major organ at some time. Body cells also referred to as 'somatic, cells are the most common cells in the body. These include cells in our skin, hair, and muscles and the cell reproduction used for these types of cells are mitosis.

Cell reproduction is important for the growth of the body. The body undergoes different stages in cell growth and cell reproduction plays a vital role in its development. Cells reproduce due to various reasons and some of them are to help repair damage cells and promote continuous growth to the body. There are two types of cell reproduction and these are done by mitosis and meiosis.

Mitosis is the process when a cell divides into an exact replica of the other. This helps repair the damage cells and promotes growth and development. Some cells are reproduced continuously like the nails and our hair, while some stop at a certain period of time like the brain and nervous system when we reach adulthood. Meiosis on the other hand is much more complicated than Mitosis. The human reproductive organs (human sex organs) undergo Meiosis in cell reproduction. Mitosis creates 2 cells from a parent cell. But cell reproduction in Meiosis differs from men and women.

Cell reproduction of multicellular organisms is complicated that much is true. In fact, there are still a few questions involving cell reproductions. Cell reproduction is important in our daily life, whether we are in our growing years or in our older years. Without it, growth and development will not be even possible. Imagine a little cell when combined forms tissues, tissues combined become organs, organs become a part of a system that helps monitor and regulate the body.

Without cell reproduction there wouldn't be anything, No life on earth or anywhere in the universe would even exist. All cells are derived from preexisting cells. Some tissues must be repaired often such as the lining of gut, white blood cells, and skin cells with a short lifespan. Other cells do not divide at all after birth such as muscle & nerve.

Most human cells are frequently reproduced and replaced during the life of an individual. However, the process varies with the kind of cell. Somatic, or body cells, such as those that make up skin, hair, and muscle, are duplicated by mitosis. The sex cells, sperm and ova, are produced by meiosis in special tissues of male testes and female ovaries. Since the vast majority of our cells are somatic, mitosis is the most common form of cell replication.

The cell division process that produces new cells for growth, repair, and the general replacement of older cells is called mitosis. In this process, a somatic cell divides into two complete new cells that are identical to the original one. Human somatic cells go through the 6 phases of mitosis in 1/2 to 1 1/2 hours, depending on the kind of tissue being duplicated.

Some human somatic cells are frequently replaced by new ones and other cells are rarely duplicated. Hair, skin, fingernails, taste buds, and the stomach's protective lining are replaced constantly and at a rapid rate throughout our lives. In contrast, brain and nerve cells in the central nervous system are rarely produced after we are a few months old. Subsequently, if they are destroyed later, the loss is usually permanent, as in the case of paraplegics.

Liver cells usually do not reproduce after an individual has finished growing and are not replaced except when there is an injury. Red blood cells are also somewhat of an exception. While they are being constantly produced in our bone marrow, the specialized cells from which they come do not have nuclei nor do the red blood cells themselves.

The discovery of a common regulatory pathway in both kinds of stem cells supports the idea that cancer stem cells and normal stem cells share fundamental properties. Mitosis and meiosis are similar processes in that they both result in the separation of existing cells into new ones. They differ, however, in their specific processes as well as in their products. The reason for these differences lies in the difference in the class of cells that each process creates. Mitosis is responsible for reproducing somatic cells and meiosis is responsible for reproducing germ cells.

Many of the changes that occur with aging are not considered pathologic and do not negatively affect overall wellness or quality of life. Ruling out disease is essential, however, when attempting to determine whether an aged individual can be considered 'healthy'. The aging process doesn't discriminate. It starts early and it affects every major organ in the body. "Aging" refers to the biological process of growing older in a harmful sense. Aging is one of the most complex biological processes. Aging has been defined as the collection of changes that render human beings progressively more likely to die.

Cell death is needed to destroy cells that represent a threat to the integrity of the organism. Cells age based on the number of times they have replicated. A cell can replicate about 50 times before the genetic material is no longer able to be copied accurately, which is due to shortened telomeres. The more damage done to cells by free radicals and other factors, the more cells need to replicate.

Accumulated damage is all external. Exposure to toxins, the sun, harmful foods, pollution and smoke takes a toll on the body. Over time, these external factors can lead to tissue damage and the body cannot maintain and repair cells, tissues and organs. The process of cells metabolizing and creating energy results in damage to the body over time. Some believe that slowing down the metabolic process through practices such as calorie restriction may slow aging in humans. Cells in the body may be killed by injurious agents. Mechanical damage may occur by exposure to toxic chemicals.

Aging is universal, but each individual experiences it in different ways. Aging may be inevitable, but the rate of aging is not. Healthy living delays many of the body changes that aging brings. Aging is primarily the result of environmental damage to our cells. Free radicals are produced as part of the millions of chemical reactions the body performs to sustain life. The body makes them in response to environmental toxins such as excessive amounts of unprotected sunlight and cigarette smoke.

Free radicals destroy or alter DNA, the cell's genetic blueprint, and disrupt many other cell functions. Free radicals may kill cells or they may give rise to mutant cells that can lead to chronic conditions including cancer and heart disease. Fortunately, the body maintains a sophisticated defense system against free radicals. Unfortunately, our defenses wane with time, and cell damage ensues. A poor diet, too much alcohol, and cigarette smoking are thought to accelerate natural wear and tear from free radicals.

Aging is a biological process that affects most cells, organisms and species. Telomeres on chromosomes have been postulated as a universal biological clock that shortens in parallel with aging in cells.[2] Inside the nucleus of a cell, our genes are arranged along twisted, double-stranded molecules of DNA called chromosomes.

As mentioned previously, at the ends of the chromosomes are stretches of DNA called telomeres, which protect genetic data, make it possible for cells to divide. Telomeres are protein complexes that cap and protect the ends of chromosomes. Each time a cell divides, the telomeres get shorter. When a cell becomes too short, the cell can no longer divide; it becomes inactive or it dies. This shortening process is associated with aging, cancer, and a higher risk of death.

Telomeres are gene sequences present at chromosomal ends and are responsible for maintaining genome integrity. Telomere length is at a maximum at birth and decreases progressively with advancing age and thus is considered as a biomarker of chronological aging. This age associated decrease in the length of telomere is linked to various ageing associated diseases like diabetes, hypertension, Alzheimer's disease, cancer etc. and their associated complications.[3]

Telomere length is a result of combined effect of oxidative stress, inflammation and repeated cell replication on it, and thus forming an association between telomere length and chronological aging and related diseases. Considered a marker for biological aging linked to increased risk for morbidity and mortality, shortened leukocyte telomere length now has been associated with pain in the central nervous system and effects fibromyalgia patients. Investigators have found that shortened telomere length was directly related to evoked pain sensitivity and altered brain structure, suggesting that pain may accelerate cellular aging.

Leukocyte telomere length (LTL) has been regarded as a potential marker of biologic aging because it usually shortens in a predictable way with age. Recently, a growing interest in cardiovascular aging has led to a number of new epidemiologic studies investigating LTL in various disease conditions.[4] Telomere length is possibly a reliable marker of biological age, shorter telomeres reflecting more advanced age. The initial telomere length of a person is mainly determined by genetic factors. Moreover, the telomere length shortens with each cell division, and exposition to harmful environmental factors also results in shorter telomeres. Leukocytes of patients with atherosclerosis and heart failure display remarkably shorter telomeres compared to leukocytes of healthy subjects of similar age.[5]

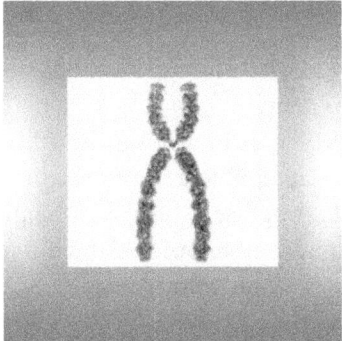

Figure 1. Telomeres are on the four ends of the chromosome.

When telomeres reach a critical length the cell will not further undergo cell divisions and become senescent or otherwise dysfunctional.[2] Telomere length was reported to be shorter in aortic tissues which presented atherosclerotic lesions compared to corresponding tissues without atherosclerotic lesions.[6] Chronic psychological stress is a risk factor for multiple diseases of aging. Accelerated cellular aging as indexed by short telomere length has emerged as a potential common biological mechanism linking various forms of psychological stress and diseases of aging.[7]

Telomere length is shortened in Systemic Lupus patients compared to controls and does not appear to be a reflection of disease activity or immune cell turnover.[8] Obesity and smoking are important risk factors for many age-related diseases. Both are states of heightened oxidative stress, which increases the rate of telomere erosion per replication, and inflammation, which enhances white blood cell turnover.[9] A dose-dependent relation with smoking was recorded and each pack-year smoked was equivalent to telomere length lost. These results emphasize the pro-ageing effects of obesity and cigarette smoking.

The association between leukocyte telomere length and mortality differs by race/ethnicity and cause of death.[10] Processed meat intake furthermore, has shown an expected inverse association with telomere length, but other diet features did not show their expected associations.[11] Subsequent chapters will discuss common pain disorders in seniors as well as the role of telomeres in these syndromes. Body composition and dietary factors are related to leukocyte telomere length, which is a potential biomarker of chronic disease risk.[12]

Improving telomerase activation in stem cells and potentially in other cells by diet and lifestyle interventions may represent an intriguing way to promote health-span in humans.[13] Greater adherence to the Mediterranean diet was reported to be associated with longer telomeres. These results further support the benefits of adherence to the Mediterranean diet for promoting health and longevity.

The 2009 Nobel Prize in Physiology and Medicine was awarded to three scientists for their pioneer research on telomeres and the enzyme that forms them which is the telomerase. Their work highlighted the considerable connection between the length of telomeres and intensive changes in lifestyle and nutrition as well as behavioral and psychological factors.[1]

References

1. Srivastava I, Thukral N, Hasija Y. Genetics of Human Age Related Disorders. Adv Gerontol. 2015;28(2):228-247.

2. Oeseburg H, de Boer RA, van Gilst WH, van der Harst P. Telomere biology in healthy aging and disease. Pflugers Arch. 2010;459(2):259-268.

3. Rizvi S, Raza ST, Mahdi F. Telomere length variations in aging and age-related diseases. Curr Aging Sci. 2014;7(3):161-167.

4. Nilsson PM, Tufvesson H, Leosdottir M, Melander O. Telomeres and cardiovascular disease risk: an update 2013. Transl Res. 2013;162(6):371-380.

5. Huzen J, van Veldhuisen DJ, van Gilst WH, van der Harst P. [Telomeres and biological ageing in cardiovascular disease]. Ned Tijdschr Geneeskd. 2008;152(22):1265-1270.

6. Nzietchueng R, Elfarra M, Nloga J, et al. Telomere length in vascular tissues from patients with atherosclerotic disease. J Nutr Health Aging. 2011;15(2):153-156.

7. O'Donovan A, Tomiyama AJ, Lin J, et al. Stress appraisals and cellular aging: a key role for anticipatory threat in the relationship between psychological stress and telomere length. Brain Behav Immun. 2012;26(4):573-579.

8. Haque S, Rakieh C, Marriage F, et al. Shortened telomere length in patients with systemic lupus erythematosus. Arthritis Rheum. 2013;65(5):1319-1323.

9. Valdes AM, Andrew T, Gardner JP, et al. Obesity, cigarette smoking, and telomere length in women. Lancet. 2005;366(9486):662-664.

10. Needham BL, Rehkopf D, Adler N, et al. Leukocyte telomere length and mortality in the National Health and Nutrition Examination Survey, 1999-2002. Epidemiology. 2015;26(4):528-535.

11. Nettleton JA, Diez-Roux A, Jenny NS, Fitzpatrick AL, Jacobs DR, Jr. Dietary patterns, food groups, and telomere length in the Multi-Ethnic Study of Atherosclerosis (MESA). Am J Clin Nutr. 2008;88(5):1405-1412.

12. Cassidy A, De Vivo I, Liu Y, et al. Associations between diet, lifestyle factors, and telomere length in women. Am J Clin Nutr. 2010;91(5):1273-1280.

13. Boccardi V, Paolisso G, Mecocci P. Nutrition and lifestyle in healthy aging: the telomerase challenge. Aging (Albany NY). 2016;8(1):12-15.

2. Elderly patients are like old cars

Elderly people are like old cars; over time they fall apart. Older individuals are those who are over 65 years of age. Because of the baby boomer generation, between the years 2010 and 2030, the population of the United States over 65 years of age will increase to 73%. One out of every five Americans will be over 65 years old. The majority of these individuals will require life time medical care including pain management. Pain can result from a variety of sources, including arthritis, surgery, cancer, trauma, poor blood circulation, cramps, or chronic disease.

Over time as a patient ages, one's cells lose the ability to repair themselves. In essence, the cells in the body essentially wear out. Consequently, the joints become arthritic, the muscle mass decreases; their hair becomes thin, the bones fracture easily, etc. A patient's genetic makeup (DNA) determines when the body begins to wear out. Almost everyone experiences pain at some time, but elderly individual experience the most pain. Pain can be a natural response to injury and disease.

The etiology of aging is important to understand, but it is equally important to differentiate the normal physiological changes from those associated with diseases. The clinician's inability to recognize these differences may result in unnecessary testing, misdiagnoses and mismanagement of the elderly person. An individual may experience these changes differently as the level of decline may be rapid and dramatic while in others, the changes are much less significant. The research field that emerged from the analysis of the aging process is known as gerontology.

Suffering is how patients are affected. With the advent of pain management as a medical specialty, elderly patients no longer need to suffer. Patients who suffer have significant reductions in the normal joys of their lives. They cannot enjoy their families or enjoy recreational activities, etc. Their pain affects them emotionally.

Elderly individuals who are unable to care for themselves have more pain than independent elderly patients. Depression is more common in the elderly population and depression makes your pain worse. Chronic pain on the other hand, can worsen your depression.

Pain management in elderly patients can be a challenge. The reason is that physiologic changes occur in an aging patient's bodies that include: the heart, lungs, kidneys, brain and sensation. A patient's heart rate may eventually decrease making it hard for a patient's tissues to get oxygen while he/ or she exercises. Lack of tissue oxygen can cause pain.

A patient's lungs may not be able to ventilate like they did when he or she was younger. The progressive loss of elastic recoil within lung tissue, the chest wall becomes stiff, and there is a decrease in alveolar surface area. These changes diminish the efficiency of gas exchange and make it more difficult to exercise.

A patient may get short of breath with exercise. A patient's kidneys become smaller with aging making it hard for a patient to excrete some drugs. As the body ages, muscular activity becomes less efficient and requires more effort to accomplish a given task.

A patient's liver size decreases, which can make it difficult for a patient to metabolize some drugs. A patient's decreased acid production in their stomach can cause a decrease in drug absorption from the stomach.

In other words, when a patient takes a medication, it may not be absorbed from the stomach into the blood stream. As a result, a patient will not derive any benefit from the medication. A patient's brain will shrink as well. A patient's ability to hear, smell and see will also decrease with aging.

Liver size and liver blood flow decrease after age 50. As a result, liver function can be compromised in elderly patients. This decreased function can affect the breakdown of many drugs that need to be excreted by their body. As a result, an elderly patient's blood level for a particular drug can be increased. This increase could cause drug toxicity which means that a patient may have too much drug in the body which could result in a drug overdose.

Aging is characterized by a progressive decline of cellular functions. The aging liver appears to preserve its function relatively well. Aging is associated in human liver with morphological changes such as decrease in size attributable to decreased hepatic blood flow.[1]

Cardiac output of healthy exercising elders can usually be maintained, allowing moderate continued physical activity throughout their lives. The cardiovascular function of a resting healthy elder is usually adequate to meet the body's needs. Old age is accompanied by a generalized reduction in hormone production and activity. Water, mineral, electrolyte, carbohydrate, protein, lipid and vitamin disorders are all more common in the elderly.

Diabetes is common in the elderly because of the inability of skeletal muscle to absorb glucose and because skeletal muscle becomes less responsive to insulin. There is generalized atrophy of all muscles accompanied by a replacement of some muscle tissue by fat deposits. Calcium is lost from the body and the bones become less dense. This can result in osteoporosis and a reduction of weight bearing capacity.

When a patient takes a dose of a drug, the drug is distributed through the various body tissues. If a patient is emaciated, the body mass is decreased and as a consequence, a dose of the drug that a patient takes will remain in the blood stream instead of being distributed throughout the body. As a result, the concentration of drug in a patient's blood stream may be higher than expected.

Decreased saliva noted in some older patients may interfere with swallowing medicines. Drugs prescribed by mouth may be absorbed differently than younger persons because of changes in stomach acid levels in older patients.

Pain management in aging patients can be a challenge. The reason is that physiologic changes occur in an elderly patient's bodies that include: the heart, lungs, kidneys, brain and sensation. A patient's heart rate may eventually decrease making it hard for tissues to get oxygen with exertion. A patient's lungs may not be able to ventilate effectively. A patient may get short of breath with exercise. A patient's kidneys become smaller with aging making it hard to excrete some drugs.

A patient's liver size decreases, which can make it hard for a patient to metabolize some drugs. A patient can have decreased acid production in their stomach. This can cause a decrease in drug absorption from the stomach. In other words, when you take a medication, it may not be absorbed from your stomach into your blood. As a result, you will not derive any benefit from the medication.

A patient's ability to hear, smell and see will also decrease with age. Elderly patients can be taking many different medications, prescribed by many physicians. Some of these drugs can adversely interact with some pain medications and do not allow the pain medication to be effective. This action is called a drug-drug interaction.

Senile patients may forget to take their medications as prescribed. Their kidneys may not function as well as in younger patients. Your kidneys are responsible for eliminating drugs. As a result, drugs like morphine can accumulate within an elderly patient's body which could cause a drug overdose. A patient's liver metabolizes (breaks down drugs). Liver size and liver blood flow decrease after age 50. Liver function can also be compromised in elderly patients.

This decreased liver function can affect the breakdown of many drugs. As a result, the patient's blood level for a particular drug can be increased. With aging, the kidney function decreases. The kidneys excrete drugs. If a patient cannot excrete a drug or its by products, the individual you could possibly be overdosed by the drug. Morphine by-products are excreted by their kidneys.

If a patient has too much of a morphine breakdown product in the body, he or she may experience an overdose. Understanding how the upper gastrointestinal tract changes with advancing age could allow interventions that lead to more appropriate prescribing for older people, potentially reduce adverse effects, increase compliance with treatment regimens, and may allow older people to take medications that they would not otherwise tolerate.[2]

An elderly patient's physical examination by his or her doctor should focus on the musculoskeletal system and include palpation for trigger points, evaluation for joint swelling and inflammation, and evaluation for pain with passive range of motion. Pain is suggested by facial grimacing, frowning, or repetitive eye blinking. In the elderly, pain often has multiple causes (bone, muscles, tendons, etc.) and no single predominant cause is usually identified.

Many of the risk factors for cognitive aging are modifiable such as hypertension, diabetes, and levels of physical, mental and social activity.[3] At a population level, primary prevention or reduction of cognitive aging is possible through addressing modifiable risk factors. This in turn may reduce population levels of dementia.

Poor pain management decreases the patient's quality of life and may contribute to suicide. The elderly are more likely than younger patients to experience adverse effects of analgesics. Drug dosing should be done starting low and going upward slowly. Oral analgesic administration is usually preferred because it is convenient and results in relatively steady blood levels.

Pain medications must be prescribed with prudence in aging patients. For example, elderly patients can lose the ability for the stomach to repair itself after taking a drug that could cause ulcers (i.e. aspirin, ibuprofen, etc.).

For thousands of years, doctors have been helping to relieve their patients' pain with a variety of medications and treatments. Like other areas of medicine, new subsets of doctors have become specialists in treating pain. In most instances, nothing will completely stop an elderly patient's pain.

If a patient's pain is acute such as post-surgical pain, or after a fall on, a patient should expect to receive significant pain relief from a physician. Chronic pain, on the other hand, is that pain that persists after one's body has healed. Chronic pain is more difficult to treat. The goal of treatment is to decrease pain. Nothing will totally eliminate this type of pain.

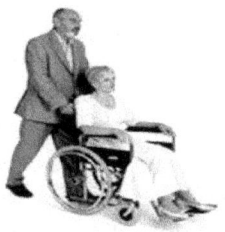

Figure 1. The goal of pain management in elderly patients is to try and maintain many Activities of Daily Living.

If a patient has chronic pain the goal should be to decrease the pain to a tolerable level. Pain management is expensive. Because nothing will completely alleviate chronic pain, a patient will need to follow up frequently with the pain care provider. Different treatments will be tried until a patient beginsto have a reduction in the pain intensity.

Geriatric pain management can be a challenge, and the patient must have a pain management physician well versed in elderly pain treatment. Individuals must be aware that in many instances, elderly pain is not adequately treated in the United States. This includes both acute and chronic pain.

Acute pain in the elderly is most likely to occur as a symptom of disease or injury (e.g., fracture from a fall). Medical and surgical treatments also contribute to pain in the elderly. It has been shown that older adults do not receive adequate pain management during hospitalization and commonly are given significantly fewer postoperative pain relievers than younger patients with the same diagnosis. This practice is particularly troublesome in light of research that demonstrates better patient outcomes, reduced length of stay, and reduced resource use as a result of aggressive pain control and improved mobility.

The following diseases are more familiar in the elderly population: arthritis, cancer, blood pressure elevation and heart disease, strokes, dementia, depression, diabetes, falls and fractures, gastrointestinal disorders, hearing impairment, memory loss, nutrition problems, osteoporosis, Parkinson's disease, respiratory disease, skin ulcers, sleep problems, thyroid disease, urinary disorders and visual impairment.

Some diseases that are common in aged patients are associated with pain. Arthritis, for example, can cause joint pain. Diabetes and thyroid disease can cause a neuropathy. Osteoporosis may be associated with bone pain. Depression can elevate a patient's pain perception. Chondrocytes differ from other somatic cells as articular cartilage is an avascular tissue.

Chondrocytes manufacture cartilage to cushion joints. When the cartilage is gone, a patient experiences joint pain. Taken together, oxidative stress considerably accelerated telomere shortening and cellular aging in chondrocytes. This is why individuals develop joint pain.[4] Recent findings indicate that reduced telomere length is also associated with chronic psychological stress and mood disorders.[5]

Unanswered is whether elimination of intrinsic instigators driving age-associated degeneration can reverse, as opposed to simply arrest, various afflictions of the aged.[6] Accumulating evidence implicating telomere damage as a driver of age-associated organ decline and disease risk and the marked reversal of systemic degenerative phenotypes in adult mice observed here support the development of regenerative strategies designed to restore telomere integrity.

Pain management in elderly patients must be tailored to each patient needs with attention to each patient's overall medical condition. There must not be a "one size fits all" mentality when treating an elderly patient. It is a patient's choice as to which pain management modalities or methods could work best for a particular patient with respect to pain treatments.

The presence of oxidative stress induces telomere genomic instability, replicative senescence and dysfunction of chondrocytes in OA cartilage, suggesting that oxidative stress, leading to chondrocyte senescence and cartilage ageing, might be responsible for the development of osteoarthritis. New efforts to prevent the development and progression of osteoarthritis may include strategies and interventions aimed at reducing oxidative damage in articular cartilage.[7] The rate of bone formation is largely determined by the number of osteoblasts. Transplantation of osteoblasts to correct bone loss or osteopenia in age-related osteoporotic diseases may be accomplished in the future.[7,8]

A patient's genetic inheritance has an impact on how long one lives. Each of us has a biological clock set to go off at a particular time. When that clock goes off it signals the body first to age and then to die. There is also the telomerase theory of aging. Telomeres are sequences of nucleic acids extending from the ends of chromosomes. Telomeres act to maintain the integrity of our chromosomes.

Aging is a universal, intrinsic, progressive and deleterious process. Understanding it is of major interest to scientist, physicians as well as to the general population. More than 300 theories have been postulated.[9] The free radical theory of aging is one of the most prominent and well-studied. The free radical theory is supported by direct experimental observations of mitochondrial aging.

Shorter telomeres have been associated with poor health behaviors, age-related diseases, and early mortality. Telomere length is regulated by the enzyme telomerase, and is linked to exposure to proinflammatory cytokines and oxidative stress. The triad of inflammation, oxidative stress, and immune cell aging represents important pre-disease mechanisms that may be ameliorated through nutritional interventions.[10]

Every time cells divide telomeres are shortened, leading to cellular damage and cellular death associated with aging. The key process in aging involves reduced expression of a number of genes. Silencing of genes has a complex mechanism, which involves methylation of DNA, histone modification and chromatin remodeling.[11]

Geriatric pain management can be challenging. However, medical science still has limited knowledge of aging. Years ago, Voltaire summarized the medical situation of his time with respect to the practice of medicine: "Doctors pour drugs, of which they know little, for a disease, of which they know less, into patients, of which they know nothing". Pain management physicians must have training in elderly pain management. A link between premature cellular aging and chronic pain exists.[12] Preliminary data imply that chronic pain is a more serious condition than has typically been recognized in terms of bodily aging.

References

1. Anantharaju A, Feller A, Chedid A. Aging Liver. A review. Gerontology. 2002;48(6):343-353.

2. Newton JL. Effect of age-related changes in gastric physiology on tolerability of medications for older people. Drugs Aging. 2005;22(8):655-661.

3. Anstey KJ, Low LF. Normal cognitive changes in aging. Aust Fam Physician. 2004;33(10):783-787.

4. Brandl A, Hartmann A, Bechmann V, Graf B, Nerlich M, Angele P. Oxidative stress induces senescence in chondrocytes. J Orthop Res. 2011;29(7):1114-1120.

5. Choi J, Fauce SR, Effros RB. Reduced telomerase activity in human T lymphocytes exposed to cortisol. Brain Behav Immun. 2008;22(4):600-605.

6. Jaskelioff M, Muller FL, Paik JH, et al. Telomerase reactivation reverses tissue degeneration in aged telomerase-deficient mice. Nature. 2011;469(7328):102-106.

7. Yudoh K, Nguyen v T, Nakamura H, Hongo-Masuko K, Kato T, Nishioka K. Potential involvement of oxidative stress in cartilage

senescence and development of osteoarthritis: oxidative stress induces chondrocyte telomere instability and downregulation of chondrocyte function. Arthritis Res Ther. 2005;7(2):R380-391.

8. Yudoh K, Matsuno H, Nakazawa F, Katayama R, Kimura T. Reconstituting telomerase activity using the telomerase catalytic subunit prevents the telomere shorting and replicative senescence in human osteoblasts. J Bone Miner Res. 2001;16(8):1453-1464.

9. Vina J, Borras C, Miquel J. Theories of ageing. IUBMB Life. 2007;59(4-5):249-254.

10. Kiecolt-Glaser JK, Epel ES, Belury MA, et al. Omega-3 fatty acids, oxidative stress, and leukocyte telomere length: A randomized controlled trial. Brain Behav Immun. 2013;28:16-24.

11. Burzynski SR. Aging: gene silencing or gene activation? Med Hypotheses. 2005;64(1):201-208.

12. Hassett AL, Epel E, Clauw DJ, et al. Pain is associated with short leukocyte telomere length in women with fibromyalgia. J Pain. 2012;13(10):959-969.

3. Pain concepts

The word "pain" is derived from the Latin word poena that means punishment. St. Augustine wrote in the 5th century that all diseases afflicting Christians were derived from demons. Ancient tribal concepts of pain were based on beliefs that evil spirits were sent as punishment from their gods to invade one's body and cause severe pain.

In the book of Genesis, Eve was condemned to pain during childbirth as a result of her encounter with the devil in the Garden of Eden. It has been reported that a shaman could suck an evil spirit from a wound to decrease one's pain. The ancient Greeks such as Aristotle were the first individuals who believed that pain was derived from various nerves in the body. The exact cause of pain was unknown to them.

Unfortunately, not unlike ancient times, the diagnosis and treatment of many chronic painful conditions today remain mostly guesswork in both young and elderly patients. Pain medicine is, for the most part, subjectively based, because pain is a subjective symptom while other medical specialties are based upon objective curative evidence. Pain in general is not bad.

Pain is a protective mechanism that warns a patient that the body has something wrong in some location. The International Association for the Study of Pain defines pain as" an unpleasant sensory and emotional experience associated with tissue injury as a result of trauma (e.g. bone fracture) or disease (e.g. cancer, shingles).

Pain has psychological effects in some instances especially when pain is severe. Pain may cause anxiety and depression. Acute pain is associated with injury, bone fractures, surgery or sprains and strains. Once these entities have healed sometimes, the pain continues. Arthritis is another example of chronic pain. Arthritic pain is caused by continuous joint destruction. However, once the pain becomes chronic, your pain it becomes a problem. Not only does pain become a personal problem but pain can become a social problem with creation of family problems, loss of self-esteem and lost wages. Fibromyalgia patients have alterations in CNS anatomy, physiology, and chemistry that potentially contribute to the symptoms experienced by these patients.

A study was done that investigated the impact of age and gender on (1) experimental pressure pain detection thresholds and pressure pain tolerance thresholds and (2) participants' self-reports of pain intensity and unpleasantness at supra threshold and subthreshold levels.[1] The intensity and unpleasantness of the pain stimulus were significantly rated lower in the elderly as compared with the young. No gender differences were observed in the report of intensity and unpleasantness of the stimulations. The elderly appraise pain experiences using different psychological strategies.

Pain impulses are, in essence, electrical signals that travel from various areas of the body such as the extremities, heart, appendix, etc. to the spinal cord and eventually reach the brain where the pain signals are processed like data in a computer. The brain is like a computer hard drive, which stores painful experiences that ultimately result in the suffering associated with chronic pain.

Pain is produced by unpleasant stimuli to nerve endings throughout the body which include chemical, extreme heat cold and mechanical injury. These nerve endings are silent until mechanical, heat or cold injures tissue. In order to experience pain, we need these pain receptors and the nerve fibers that transmit pain to the spinal cord and then to your brain.

As people age, they become more motivated to maximize positive emotions and minimize negative ones. The results highlight the importance of studying the mechanisms older adults use to successfully cope with pain.2

Nerves, which conduct pain impulses to the spinal cord, are composed of neurons (nerve cells) that make up nerve fibers that form neurons. Two common pain fibers are the C fibers and the A-delta fibers. A-delta fibers conduct fast onset sharp pain impulses. The C fibers conduct slow onset dull, aching or burning pain.

Other types of fibers that transmit touch and vibration do not cause pain in most instances. However, these fibers can become hypersensitive and may contribute to your total pain experience. A neuron is an electrically excitable cell in the nervous system that processes and transmits information. Neurons are the significant core components of the brain and spinal cord as well as peripheral nerves.

Neurons are typically composed of a cell body, a dendrite and an axon. Neurons receive input from dendrites and transmit output via the axon. Neurons are the building blocks of nerves. In other words, multitudes of neurons are necessary to form a nerve. Nerves that exist outside of your central nervous system are called a ganglion. The stellate ganglion in the neck is an example. An injection into this ganglion may relieve pain associated with Reflex Sympathetic Dystrophy (now called Complex Regional Pain Syndrome). Various ganglia may form a plexus. An example of a plexus is your celiac plexus. Sometimes this plexus is blocked with numbing medicine, phenol or alcohol to relieve severe abdominal pain.

Dendrites

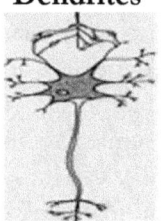

Axon

Figure 1. A nerve is composed of neurons. A neuron has one axon that takes nerve signals away from the neuron. The long end of the axon communicates with multiple dendrites.

Action potentials generated by the neuron initiate pain signals. If the skin is pinched a mechanical pain receptor begins and action potential. An action potential begins after a depolarization (a change in the electrical activity within the neuron) such that it could cause a membrane transitory modification, turning prevalently permeable to sodium ions more than to potassium ions. Sodium permeability can cause an action potential.

A neuropathy generates a local accumulation of sodium channels, with a consequent increase of density. This model seems to be the basis of neuron hyper excitability. Calcium channels have also an important role in cell function. Intra-cellular calcium increase contributes to depolarization processes, through kinase and determines the phosphorylation of membrane proteins that can make powerful the efficacy of the channels them-selves.

Following an acute injury, AMPA receptors are stimulated, which cause sharp pain. Receptors (areas in the body where biochemicals or drugs attach) are present in the spinal cord are called NMDA (N-methyl-D-aspartate) receptors and cause chronic pain. When these NMDA receptors are stimulated, pain becomes more severe and this extreme pain is maintained, which implies that the pain does not decrease. The brain is responsible for the suffering associated with pain. Pain results in bodily responses, especially with respect to the cardiovascular system (heart rate increases, blood pressure increases, renal arteries constrict, etc.).

When pain is severe, the brain can cause the body to increase both the heart rate and blood pressure. Extreme pain can also result in profuse sweating as well as nausea and vomiting. There are different types of nerve endings throughout the body. The pain nerve endings become hyper excitable when stimulated by injury, inflammation or a tumor. Occasionally, the nerve endings remain irritable even after the painful stimulus has been removed. Pain signals from areas in the body reach the brain by four processes (transduction, transmission, modulation and perception).

Axons carry pain fibers away from a neuron and direct them to the dendrites of the next neuron until they terminate in the brain or spinal cord. Remember that the axons and dendrites do not touch. They form synapses or clefts between the axon and dendrite. The synapse has chemicals in the axon nerve ending. These chemicals allow communication between the neurons. Drugs are chemicals that can interrupt the communication between the neurons. Hypnosis and biofeedback can disrupt pain signal transmission. Injections can also inhibit transmission of pain signals from the arms or legs to the brain.

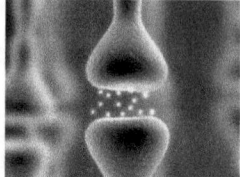

Figure 2. Chemicals are transferred between nerve endings (synapses) which cause transmission of pain signals. Pain signals may be blocked if the chemicals are inhibited from passing from one nerve to another.

Pain signals cross to the opposite side from the location of the injury and therefore, travel to the opposite side of the brain. The pain impulses will then proceed upwards to go to the brain. It is important to know that pain signals can be dampened by structures and chemicals that exist in the spinal cord.

Pain signals as mentioned previously are transmitted from the site of the injury as action potentials (Electrical impulses). Electrical and/or chemical activity between the neuron dendrites and axons propagate the axon potentials. Pain signals enter the spinal cord, then cross to the other side of the spinal cord and proceed upward to the brain. Pain on the right side goes to the left side of the brain.

It is important to understand the following processes in order to understand how your pain can be treated effectively. Transduction is a process where electrical signals originate in the nerve endings throughout the body. These impulses are chemically, mechanically and/or thermally mediated and transmitted to the spinal cord where they can be modulated and then sent to the brain.

Tissue injury or disease (including arthritis) causes the body to release biochemicals called prostaglandins. Prostaglandins themselves do not cause pain. Prostaglandins do, however, sensitize pain receptors to other chemicals in the body, which facilitate the transmission of pain impulses. Nonsteroidal drugs like ibuprofen decrease the number of prostaglandins produced in the body and may result in a decrease in pain perception.

Topical creams such as Ben Gay can decrease the process of transduction at the nerve endings.

Transmission is a process where pain signals are transported to the spinal cord. Nerves in body tissues transmit impulses to the spinal cord. Nerve blocks with anesthetics like Novocain can interrupt the transmission of pain impulses to the spinal cord. Once pain impulses reach the spinal cord, they are modulated or changed by chemicals and nerves that inhibit or lessen the number of pain impulses from going up the spinal cord to your brain. Fibers called internuncial fibers are present within the spinal cord that can decrease pain transmission.

The brain can send impulses back to these pain control fibers within the spinal cord to decrease the number of impulses that reach the pain perception center of the brain. This is the basis of hypnosis. Severe pain, however, over-whelms the nerve fibers and hypnosis essentially becomes ineffective. The spinal cord acts like a transformer to intensify or decrease the intensity of pain impulses. Narcotics and anticonvulsants can modulate pain impulses within the spinal cord. Finally, pain impulses reach the brain.

In general, the greater the tissue trauma, the more pain transmitting chemicals are produced and the worse the pain. In medical terminology, a stimulus (pin prick) produces a response (pain perception). When a stimulus such as heat produces, tissue injury chemicals are released at the site of nerve injury, which cause pain fibers to become hyperactive. These chemicals include bradykinin, histamine, substance p, acetylcholine, serotonin and histamine. These chemicals act at the nerve endings and ultimately travel to the spinal cord and brain.

GABA (gamma-amino butyric acid) in the spinal cord decreases the number of pain impulses that reach the brain. GABA inhibits pain impulse transmission. Norepinephrine and serotonin are two more chemicals in the spinal cord which attenuate the number of pain impulses, which reach the brain. The brain and spinal cord regulate pain by the production of naturally occurring narcotic-like substances that decrease pain transmission in specific areas of the brain. These narcotic-like drugs are called enkephalins, dynorphins and beta-endorphins. Some of these substances also decrease pain transmission in the spinal cord.

Enkephalins inhibit pain at the spinal cord. Enkephalins bind to narcotic receptors. When the analgesic receptors are activated, they inhibit pain signals. Dynorphins exist in both the brain and spinal cord but are more prevalent in the brain. Like enkephalins, these substances bind to narcotic receptors in the brain and spinal cord. The natural beta-endorphins in a body exhibit morphine-like activity. Following injury or stress these endorphins are released into the blood stream.

Prostaglandins sensitize pain nerve endings to pain producing tissue chemicals. Antidepressant drugs like Elavil or Prozac decrease pain by increasing norepinephrine and serotonin in the spinal cord. As previously mentioned, this two substances decrease the number of pain impulses that reach the pain perception areas of the brain. Anti-convulsant drugs like Gabitril (tiagabine) in some instances affect GABA levels in a spinal cord act by enhancing GABA blood levels decreases the number of pain signals in your spinal cord that can go to the brain. Narcotic drugs also decrease pain impulse conduction in both the spinal cord and brain. Injections of numbing medicine (local anesthetics with steroids) can decrease pain in muscle and nerves in the arms, legs and the trunk of the body.

Patients may report combinations of spontaneous pain evoked by stimuli that normally induce no/little sensation of pain. Modern neuroimaging methods (positron emission tomography (PET) and functional MRI (fMRI)) have been used to determine, whether different neuropathic pain symptoms involve similar brain structures.

PET studies have suggested that spontaneous neuropathic pain is associated principally with changes in thalamic activity and the medial pain system, which is preferentially involved in the emotional dimension of pain. Fear, suffering and pain are in different areas of the brain, but these areas are connected to each other. These interconnections ultimately can communicate with areas of the brain such as the midbrain that control heart rate and the respiratory rate as well.

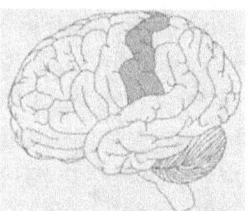

Figure 3. The brain areas (shaded) where pain signals are processed.

Aging of the nervous system is characterized by a general loss of neuronal substance. The most obvious sign is a reduced average brain weight in the elderly; brain weight was reported to be 1375 g at age 20 and 1200 g at age 80. The number of peripheral neurons also decreases, and muscles become innervated, overall, by fewer axons, possibly leading to denervation atrophy. A particular neuromuscular junction is not functionally changed with aging. Nerve conduction velocity is slightly affected by aging and tends to become slower in elderly individuals.

The overall loss of neuronal substance and decreased synaptic activity may be one explanation for the higher susceptibility of the elderly to drugs that interact with the peripheral or central nervous system. Mental capacity does show a decrease in middle age (45) and a steeper drop after 65, but individual variation is great and appears somewhat dependent on how much mental stimulation one receives. The same applies to memory. Memory losses more often affect short-term memory rather than long-term memory.

Usual aging is accompanied by a lower production of neurotransmitters, but only when the drop approaches 50% will dementia ensue. About 15% of the elderly have severe dementia. If the dementia is the result of acute electrolyte imbalances of sodium or potassium, thyroid dysfunction, drug toxicity or illness, it can be reversed upon treatment of the causal factor. It is extremely to assess pain in patients with dementia.

Pain sensation is also decreased in elderly individuals. Several studies have demonstrated that elderly patients have an increased sensitivity to opioid analgesics. It was determined by electroencephalography (EEG) that the most important difference is an increase in the sensitivity in the elderly subject compared to the younger person. In other words, compared to young patients, elderly patients will need lower opioid concentrations for an equal analgesic effect and lower loading doses for equal plasma levels. Elderly individuals will eliminate opioids from their bodies more slowly than young subjects.

Pain tolerance is the ability of the individual to handle pain. Pain threshold is the maximum level of pain that a person can tolerate. The pain threshold in the elderly is higher than in younger patients.[2] This observation may be due to degenerative nerve disease in elderly patients. Elderly women, experience more pain than aging men. Pain tolerance may, nevertheless, be decreased in both male and female elderly patients.

At high levels of pain intensity, interference decreased with age, although the age by pain intensity interaction effect was small. This evidence converges with aging theories, including socioemotional selectivity theory, which posits that as people age, they become more motivated to maximize positive emotions and minimize negative ones. The results highlight the importance of studying the mechanisms older adults use to successfully cope with pain.

Psychosocial factors associated with shortened telomeres are also common in chronic pain.[3] There is a link between premature cellular aging and chronic pain. Chronic pain is a more serious condition than has typically been recognized in terms of bodily aging. Stressful events in childhood are associated with shorter telomere length in middle-aged men and that part of this relation is explained by depressive mood and low grade inflammation.[4]

Chronic pain conditions are characterized by significant individual variability complicating the identification of pathophysiological markers. Leukocyte telomere length, a measure of cellular aging, is associated with age-related disease onset, psychosocial stress, and health-related functional decline.[5] Psychosocial stress has been associated with the onset of chronic pain and chronic pain is experienced as a physical and psychosocial stressor. Although cognitive ability, walking speed, lung function and grip strength all decline with age, they do so independently of telomere length shortening.[6]

References

1. Petrini L, Matthiesen ST, Arendt-Nielsen L. The effect of age and gender on pressure pain thresholds and suprathreshold stimuli. Perception. 2015;44(5):587-596.

2. Boggero IA, Geiger PJ, Segerstrom SC, Carlson CR. Pain Intensity Moderates the Relationship Between Age and Pain Interference in Chronic Orofacial Pain Patients. Exp Aging Res. 2015;41(4):463-474.

3. Hassett AL, Epel E, Clauw DJ, et al. Pain is associated with short leukocyte telomere length in women with fibromyalgia. J Pain. 2012;13(10):959-969.

4. Osler M, Bendix L, Rask L, Rod NH. Stressful life events and leucocyte telomere length: Do lifestyle factors, somatic and mental health, or low grade inflammation mediate this relationship? Results from a cohort of Danish men born in 1953. Brain Behav Immun. 2016.

5. Sibille KT, Langaee T, Burkley B, et al. Chronic pain, perceived stress, and cellular aging: an exploratory study. Mol Pain. 2012;8:12.

6. Harris SE, Marioni RE, Martin-Ruiz C, et al. Longitudinal telomere length shortening and cognitive and physical decline in later life: The Lothian Birth Cohorts 1936 and 1921. Mech Ageing Dev. 2016;154:43-48.

4. Pain is common in the elderly

Even though senior citizens are older patients, they should not be denied adequate pain care. Pain is a common complaint of the elderly. The elderly are often untreated or undertreated for pain. By 2030 the population of Americans 65 or older will surpass 70 million, according to a 2008 report from the Institute of Medicine. Many of them will have chronic conditions like hypertension, diabetes or osteoporosis. Unless action is taken immediately, the health care workforce will lack the capacity to meet the needs of older patients in the future. Chronic pain is associated with increased interference in older patient's daily functioning that becomes more pronounced as pain intensity increases.

Up to 40% of patients with chronic pain in cohorts aged 75, 80 and 85 years suffer from neuropathic pain. However, only a few elderly people with chronic pain used medications specifically for chronic pain, which may be due to side effects or non-willingness to experiment with these drugs. Elderly people with chronic pain rated their health and mobility to be worse and felt sadder, lonelier and more tired but were not less satisfied with their lives than those without chronic pain.[1]

Due to barriers in the health care system, the patient, and society, elders are at great risk for under treatment of pain. Barriers to effective management include challenges to proper assessment of pain; underreporting on the part of patients; atypical manifestations of pain in the elderly; a need for increased appreciation of the pharmacokinetic and pharmacodynamic changes of aging; and misconceptions about tolerance and addiction to opioids. A risk of medication-related readmissions in elderly men with adult children as caregivers however, is consistent with research showing problems in medication adherence when seniors are supported by informal caregivers.[2] Management of chronic pain in elderly adult patients is often complicated by analgesic medication related side effects.

Pain can lead to sleep deprivation, which can decrease pain thresholds, limit the amount of daytime energy and increase the incidence and severity of depression and mood disturbances. Barriers to adequate pain management in the older adult arise from three major sources: the patient, the health care community, and society at large. Patients, families and health care professionals hold strong personal beliefs and fears about the meaning of pain and pain treatment options. The prevalence of pain varies with age, living arrangements, and the general health of the population. For instance, the incidence of pain more than doubles once individuals surpass the age of 60 with pain frequency increasing with each decade.

Older patients handle pain medication differently than younger patients. For example, because kidneys become smaller with age, there is decreased blood flow and less effective removal of a drug. In addition, the liver undergoes a decrease in mass and blood flow with aging, making it harder for the liver to break down and metabolize some medications. There is a group of intractable pain patients who do not effectively metabolize oral opioids. Although gastrointestinal disease and cytochrome P450 enzymatic defects appeared to be dominant causes of oral opioid ineffectiveness, there were other possible contributing factors such as abdominal, pelvic and spine surgeries, head and neck trauma, and autoimmune disease.[3]

Opioids have become more widely accepted for treating older adults who have persistent pain, but their use requires physicians have an understanding of prevention and management of side effects. The elderly are more likely to have arthritis, bone and joint disorders, cancer, and other chronic disorders associated with pain. Between 25% and 50% of community-dwelling elderly have important pain problems.2 Nursing home–dwelling elderly have an even higher prevalence of pain, which is estimated to be between 45% and 80%.[3] Under treatment for pain can have a negative impact on the health and quality of life of the elderly, resulting in depression, anxiety, social isolation, cognitive impairment, immobility, and sleep disturbances.

As with other age groups, the elderly have pain that can be classified pathophysiologically as either nociceptive or neuropathic in origin. Alternatively, pain may be mixed, that is, having origins that are both nociceptive and neuropathic. Nociceptive pain may be either visceral or somatic and is due to stimulation of pain receptors. In the elderly, this stimulation may be the result of inflammation or musculoskeletal or ischemic disorders. Patients with nociceptive pain are treated pharmacologically with both opioid and nonopioid agents, as well as nonpharmacologic interventions.

Neuropathic pain results from a pathophysiologic disturbance of either the peripheral or the central nervous system. In the elderly, common examples include postherpetic neuralgia and diabetic neuropathy. Patients with neuropathic pain are less likely to respond to agents used to treat patients with nociceptive pain and more likely to respond to adjuvant agents such as anticonvulsants and antidepressants. Pain of mixed origins may respond to administration of agents that treat for both nociceptive and neuropathic pain.

Older adults are likely to have an increased risk of adverse reactions to the use of pharmacologic agents to manage pain. This propensity is likely due to pharmacokinetic changes such as reduced renal excretion and hepatic metabolism, as well as pharmacodynamic changes that occur with age, such as an increased sensitivity to certain analgesics, particularly the opioids. In addition, polypharmacy is a contributing factor for the increased incidence of adverse drug reactions. It has been shown that microvascular decompression for elderly patients with trigeminal neuralgia can be achieved safely with careful perioperative management which demonstrates that surgical procedures can be done on some patients with good outcomes.[4]

A comprehensive assessment should include a careful history and physical examination and diagnostic studies aimed at identifying the precise etiology of pain. Characteristics such as intensity, frequency, and location should be described. Standardized geriatric assessment tools to assess function, gait, affect, and cognition should be used.[8] Intensity should be assessed by using one of several pain scales that have been accepted for use in the elderly. A verbally administered 0-through-10 scale is an effective measurement of pain intensity in older adults. When using this scale, physicians can ask patients, "on a scale of zero to 10, with zero meaning no pain and 10 meaning the worst pain possible, how much pain do you have now?" Some older adults, particularly those with dementia, may have difficulty using this scale. Other tools such as a visual analog scale, numerical scale, pain thermometer scale, and pain faces scale can be helpful.

Even though adverse drug reactions in the elderly are a significant risk, pharmacologic intervention for pain management is the principal treatment modality for pain. Along with considering age-associated changes of pharmacokinetics and pharmacodynamics, physicians must consider the likelihood of drug-drug and drug-disease interactions. If pain is due primarily to inflammation, an anti-inflammatory agent should be given. However, if pain is predominantly neuropathic, an anticonvulsant should be used.

Most mild or moderate pain in the elderly is of musculoskeletal origin and responds well to acetaminophen given around-the-clock. This agent is well tolerated in older patients provided that both renal and hepatic functions are normal. Long-term use of nonsteroidal anti-inflammatory drugs (NSAIDs), because of their association with gastrointestinal bleeding and renal dysfunction, places the elderly at significant risk. Ginger extract nanoparticles reportedly relieves joint pain and improves problematic symptoms and improves the quality of life in elderly osteoarthritis knees.[5] In elderly adult patients with moderate to severe, chronic osteoarthritis knee or low back pain, tapentadol ER (100-250 mg bid) provided significant pain relief compared with placebo and had a better overall gastrointestinal tolerability profile than oxycodone.[6]

Administration of opioid analgesics to manage chronic noncancerous pain in the elderly has become acceptable. Short-acting opioids can be used in treatment of patients with intermittent pain, whereas sustained-release opioids should be given for continuous pain. Physicians should anticipate, prevent, and manage side effects. They should initiate prevention of constipation through the use of stool softeners and other prophylactic bowel regimens whenever opioid therapy is used in the elderly. Transdermal fentanyl should also be used with extreme caution in the elderly. It has a variable absorption rate in older adults and a long half-life even when the patch is removed. The American Geriatrics Society suggests the use of opioids to treat pain in older people not responsive to acetaminophen or nonsteroidal anti-inflammatory drugs.[7]

Clinical trial safety data following chronic administration of extended-release opioids within an older population is limited. However, safety outcomes following daily administration of extended release morphine were similar between patients aged greater or equal to age 65 years when compared to patients less than 65 years.[8] Delirium remains a major complication of hospitalized elderly patients. Chronic pain may contribute to decline in cognitive function and investigators need to determine strategies that may help in preventing or managing these potential consequences of pain on cognitive function in older adults.[9]

Tramadol hydrochloride, an analgesic that has some opioid properties and is used for mild to moderate pain, should be used with caution in the elderly because it may cause dizziness and reduce the seizure threshold. When tramadol is combined with other drugs that depress the central nervous system, such as anti-anxiety medications, narcotic pain relievers, or alcohol, the sedative effects of tramadol can be enhanced. This may be especially crucial for older adults, especially females, for whom acute or chronic pain is a common complaint and who often take other prescription medications that may interact with tramadol.[10]

In elderly adult patients with moderate to severe, chronic osteoarthritis knee or low back pain, tapentadol ER (100-250 mg bid) provided significant pain relief with less side effects compared with placebo and had a better overall gastrointestinal tolerability profile than oxycodone CR.[6]

Anticonvulsants such as gabapentin and carbamazepine are thought to be effective in neuropathic pain. Although most elderly patients require pharmacologic intervention to manage pain, nonpharmacologic approaches may have an added benefit and should be routinely considered. Although most elderly patients require pharmacologic intervention to manage pain, nonpharmacologic approaches may have an added benefit and should be routinely considered. Evidence exists that participation in regular physical activity can reduce pain and enhance functional capacity of older adults with persistent pain.

Additionally, an assessment by a physiatrist, physical therapist, or occupational therapist may be helpful, not only for recommending ways to improve muscle strength and avoid dysfunction. Analgesic use and pain in people with and without dementia in Australian residential aged are facilities have been studied. The prevalence of analgesic use was similar among residents with and without dementia.[11] Opioid-induced constipation (OIC), a common side effect of opioid treatment for chronic pain, affects patient health-related quality of life (HRQL) and may prompt some patients to lower the dose or alter adherence to their opioid medication, compromising pain relief. The importance and severity of OIC are perceived differently by patients and their physicians which results in a discordance that complicates pain management and demonstrates a need for greater communication.[12]

Anxiety disorder in the elderly is twice as common as dementia and four to six times more common than major depression and must be recognized when present.[13] Anxiety is associated with poorer quality of life, significant distress and contributes to the onset of disability. Mortality risks are also increased, through physical causes, especially cardiovascular disease, and suicide. For nursing home residents with advanced dementia and challenging behavior, providing staff with comprehensive training in behavioral management, resulted in improved behavior and less psychotropic medication use.[14] Cellular aging may be more pronounced in older adults experiencing high levels of perceived stress and chronic pain.[15]

In cases involving nursing home residents with advanced dementia and challenging behavior, it has been shown that providing staff with comprehensive training in behavioral management, resulted in improved behavior and less psychotropic medication use.[14] Although greater medical burden is associated with increased incidence of physical disability in U.S. veterans, studies suggest that initiatives designed to foster greater purpose in life may help protect against the development of physical disability in this rapidly growing segment of the population.[16]

Manifestations of pain behavior include agitation, confusion, social withdrawal, or apathy. Other indicators of pain include the following: facial expressions (grimacing, frowning); vocalization (shouting, moaning); body movements (pacing, rocking); changes in interpersonal interactions (eating alone, easily annoyed); changes in activity (no longer exercising, protecting a body part); mental status changes (increased confusion, new agitation). Meperidine is metabolized in the liver to normeperidine, which is then excreted through the urinary system. Excretion is altered in those individuals with renal dysfunction, leading to accumulation of normeperidine, and resulting in effects of central nervous system toxicity such as seizures

Intrathecal or epidural opioids, alone or in combination with local anesthetics, produce effective analgesia with minimal side effects. Neuroablative techniques such as chemical or surgical rhizotomy likewise can be effective in resistant pain. However, because of the plasticity of the nervous system, alternate pathways can transmit pain over time. Thus, ablative procedures are generally reserved for patients with a life expectancy of less than 12 months.

Postthoracotomy pain is quite intense. Epidural analgesia has long been the gold standard but is often associated with hypotension and urinary retention. It appears that intraoperative intercostal injections with bupivacaine liposome at 6 levels during thoracotomy provided significantly better pain control in postoperative days 1 and 3, compared to epidural anesthesia.[17]

It has been shown that patients with dementia are at risk of receiving insufficient treatment for pain after a hip fracture. lower doses of opioids may reflect uncertainty about how to treat pain patients with dementia.[18] Pain after total joint arthroplasty can be severe and difficult to control in elderly patients. A large series of elderly patients who had total joint arthroplasty procedures experienced pain relief after the introduction of liposomal bupivacaine as part of an established multimodal protocol.[19]

In patients with knee osteoarthritis who were eligible for unilateral total knee replacement, treatment with total knee replacement followed by nonsurgical treatment resulted in greater pain relief and functional improvement after 12 months than did nonsurgical treatment alone.[20] However, total knee replacement was associated with a higher number of serious adverse events than was nonsurgical treatment, and most patients who were assigned to receive nonsurgical treatment alone did not undergo total knee replacement before the 12-month follow-up.

Physical NPTs include the use of physical movement, heat, cold, massage, acupuncture or acupressure, and transcutaneous electrical nerve stimulation (TENS). Physical movement such as sports, dance, or Tai Chi decreases pain from chronic pain syndromes such as osteoarthritis, fibromyalgia, or peripheral vascular disease. Activity improves joint function and flexibility, increases muscle strength for improved alignment and reduced muscle spasms, and promotes collateral circulation, minimizing symptoms of claudication.

The application of heat or cold can be helpful as well. Massage offers many therapeutic effects that reduce pain, including release of muscle tension, improved circulation, increased joint mobility, and decreased anxiety. Chiropractic manipulative treatment (CMT) can reduce low back pain in elderly patients as well.[21] The costs of care for the episode and per episode day were lower for patients who used a combination of CMT and conventional medical care than for patients who did not use any CMT. These findings support initial CMT use in the treatment of, and possibly broader chiropractic management of, older multiply-comorbid chronic low back pain patients.

References

1. Rapo-Pylkko S, Haanpaa M, Liira H. Chronic pain among community-dwelling elderly: a population-based clinical study. Scand J Prim Health Care. 2016;34(2):159-164.

2. Olson CH, Dey S, Kumar V, Monsen KA, Westra BL. Clustering of elderly patient subgroups to identify medication-related readmission risks. Int J Med Inform. 2016;85(1):43-52.

3. Tennant F. Why oral opioids may not be effective in a subset of chronic pain patients. Postgrad Med. 2016;128(1):18-22.

4. Amagasaki K, Watanabe S, Naemura K, Shono N, Nakaguchi H. Safety of microvascular decompression for elderly patients with trigeminal neuralgia. Clin Neurol Neurosurg. 2016;141:77-81.

5. Amorndoljai P, Taneepanichskul S, Niempoog S, Nimmannit U. Improving of Knee Osteoarthritic Symptom by the Local Application of Ginger Extract Nanoparticles: A Preliminary Report with Short Term Follow-Up. J Med Assoc Thai. 2015;98(9):871-877.

6. Biondi DM, Xiang J, Etropolski M, Moskovitz B. Tolerability and efficacy of tapentadol extended release in elderly patients >/= 75 years of age with chronic osteoarthritis knee or low back pain. J Opioid Manag. 2015;11(5):393-403.

7. Guerriero F, Roberto A, Greco MT, Sgarlata C, Rollone M, Corli O. Long-term efficacy and safety of oxycodone-naloxone prolonged release in geriatric patients with moderate-to-severe chronic noncancer pain: a 52-week open-label extension phase study. Drug Des Devel Ther. 2016;10:1515-1523.

8. Setnik B, Pixton GC, Webster LR. Safety profile of extended-release morphine sulfate with sequestered naltrexone hydrochloride in older

patients: pooled analysis of three clinical trials. Curr Med Res Opin. 2016;32(3):563-572.

9. van der Leeuw G, Eggermont LH, Shi L, et al. Pain and Cognitive Function Among Older Adults Living in the Community. J Gerontol A Biol Sci Med Sci. 2016;71(3):398-405.

10. Bush DM. Emergency Department Visits for Adverse Reactions Involving the Pain Medication Tramadol. The CBHSQ Report. Rockville (MD)2013.

11. Tan EC, Visvanathan R, Hilmer SN, et al. Analgesic use and pain in residents with and without dementia in aged care facilities: A cross-sectional study. Australas J Ageing. 2016.

12. LoCasale RJ, Datto C, Wilson H, Yeomans K, Coyne KS. The Burden of Opioid-Induced Constipation: Discordance Between Patient and Health Care Provider Reports. J Manag Care Spec Pharm. 2016;22(3):236-245.

13. Koychev I, Ebmeier KP. Anxiety in older adults often goes undiagnosed. Practitioner. 2016;260(1789):17-20, 12-13.

14. Pieper MJ, Francke AL, van der Steen JT, et al. Effects of a Stepwise Multidisciplinary Intervention for Challenging Behavior in Advanced Dementia: A Cluster Randomized Controlled Trial. J Am Geriatr Soc. 2016;64(2):261-269.

15. Sibille KT, Langaee T, Burkley B, et al. Chronic pain, perceived stress, and cellular aging: an exploratory study. Mol Pain. 2012;8:12.

16. Mota NP, Tsai J, Kirwin PD, Sareen J, Southwick SM, Pietrzak RH. Purpose in Life is Associated with a Reduced Risk of Incident Physical Disability in Aging U.S. Military Veterans. Am J Geriatr Psychiatry. 2016.

17. Khalil KG, Boutrous ML, Irani AD, et al. Operative Intercostal Nerve Blocks With Long-Acting Bupivacaine Liposome for Pain Control After Thoracotomy. Ann Thorac Surg. 2015;100(6):2013-2018.

18. Jensen-Dahm C, Palm H, Gasse C, Dahl JB, Waldemar G. Postoperative Treatment of Pain after Hip Fracture in Elderly Patients with Dementia. Dement Geriatr Cogn Disord. 2016;41(3-4):181-191.

19. Barrington JW, Olugbode O, Lovald S, Ong K, Watson H, Emerson RH, Jr. Liposomal Bupivacaine: A Comparative Study of More Than 1000 Total Joint Arthroplasty Cases. Orthop Clin North Am. 2015;46(4):469-477.

20. Skou ST, Roos EM, Laursen MB, et al. A Randomized, Controlled Trial of Total Knee Replacement. N Engl J Med. 2015;373(17):1597-1606.

21. Weeks WB, Leininger B, Whedon JM, et al. The Association Between Use of Chiropractic Care and Costs of Care Among Older Medicare Patients W(2):63-75 e62.ith Chronic Low Back Pain and Multiple Comorbidities. J Manipulative Physiol Ther. 2016;39

5. Pain Assessment

The move to offering patients senior patient pain clinics are much more likely to accurately assess and treat pain in the aging population than general population pain clinics. Stressful events in childhood are associated with shorter telomere length in older patients and part of this relation is explained by depressive mood and low grade inflammation.[2] Cellular aging may be more pronounced in older adults experiencing high levels of perceived stress and chronic pain.

The only way to manage pain is to assess the effectiveness of the treatment. If the pain was at a 7 prior to a medication, and an hour after the medication it was a 2, the treatment has been pretty effective. If the pain remained the same the treatment was not effective. Behaviors that may indicate the presence of pain in a patient unable to communicate verbally include: facial expressions, vocalizations, body movements, changes in interpersonal interactions, changes in routines, and mental status changes.

Several different techniques are available for the doctor to use in determining the level of pain. Commonly used techniques include verbal, visual, and psychological tests. Both a patient and the doctor are responsible for documenting and recording trends in the intensity and frequency of the pain. This information tells each of a patient whether the pain has really improved or whether it has worsened. Charting the pain levels will help the doctor see the long-range pain trends, which are ultimately more important than the day-to-day pain trends.

A patient may wonder why a patient needs to measure his/her pain. A pain experience measurement is extremely valuable to both a patient and the doctor. It provides a baseline for the doctor to assess any therapy or medications a patient are currently taking, and it also helps the doctor to prescribe future therapy methods. The doctor also needs to be able to determine how much disability a patient have in order to prescribe the appropriate types of therapy for a patient.

Many of the test instruments that mentioned in this chapter enable doctors to diagnose a specific pain condition. They also help doctors determine whether the patient is truly in pain or just making it up. A patient should be able to easily understand the test a patient are being given so that it is as accurate as possible at measuring the level of pain. A patient and the doctor can use several different pain assessment forms to monitor the pain-medicine therapy.

Which assessment form is best for a patient? There is no definite answer to this question. The assessment form that a patient feels most comfortable with is the best pain assessment for both a patient and the doctor. These assessment scales help a patient and the doctor plan an individualized pain-management program. Look over the pain-assessment evaluations carefully. If a patient is not decreasing the pain, or if the pain is becoming worse, a patient and the physician must evaluate other treatments for the pain. A patient and the doctor must develop a partnership in the control of the pain. A large number of pain assessment tools exist, and their content varies. No generally accepted pain classification yet exists on which to base such tools.

The doctor will depend on a patient for accurate and reliable answers to questions about the pain a patient feel. Because pain involves many aspects such as sensory, emotional, and behavioral factors, it is difficult to measure the amount of pain a patient feel based on one thing. The doctor will carefully instruct a patient as to how to report the pain when going through a pain-assessment test. The choice of a pain-assessment test depends on the needs of both a patient and the doctor. A functional evaluation, such as reports of the daily activities, must be included in the assessment. If the doctor does not ask about the daily activities, voluntarily tell him the further limitations with respect to work, recreation, dressing, fixing meals, and any other daily activities.

The five most important aspects of the pain experience which should be addressed by a pain assessment tool are: pain intensity, temporal pattern, treatment and exacerbating / relieving factors, pain location and pain interference. Inadequate pain assessment prevents optimal treatment in palliative care. The content of pain assessment tools might limit their usefulness for proper pain assessment, but data on the content validity of the tools are scarce.[2]

Positive effects of therapy are best assessed when the doctor keeps a database of the pain progression. This type of data is easily stored on a computer. This type of database is even more because the doctor can graph important data from each of the visits. The assessment and measurement of pain has received considerable attention in the past two decades. Progress continues to be made in developing pain-assessment tools. A patient or the doctor should not oversimplify the pain assessment. The objective reports a patient are able to give, as well the observations the doctor is able to make about the behavior, are important to accurate pain management decisions.

Because pain is subjective and can be observed only by a patient, it is important that the reports of the pain levels come from a patient. This will give the doctor a more accurate measurement of the type of pain a patient is experiencing. For example, if a patient just complains of a toothache, the doctor will have almost no way of knowing how severe the pain is. On occasion, the doctor will need to rate the level of pain if a patient are not able for some reason to identify the level of pain. In general, a patient should be able to accurately describe the level of pain. If a patient is not able to rate the pain, it should be done by a relative or other type of health-care provider.

Each doctor's approach to managing pain may differ. Therefore, it is important that a patient and the doctor have a healthy doctor-patient relationship and that the doctor understands the situation. The causes of each person's pain differ, and therefore the doctor may suggest different combinations of methods to help relieve the pain. The current methods doctors have available to measure pain are imperfect. The perception of pain is based on many things that affect a patient, and can range from memories of a previous painful event to psycho-logical influences. Pain is not necessarily just a sensory experience, but it is also a result of processes that occur at a higher level in the brain, making pain a psychological experience.

There is no general consensus among pain medicine doctors as to the best test for the measurement of pain. An ideal test for the assessment of pain must bring together experimental as well as clinical knowledge. Right now, there are no adequate tests that can differentiate gender with respect to the assessment of pain. In order to provide adequate pain management, a doctor must combine all of the data given by a patient concerning the pain complaints.

Hopefully a universally accepted pain assessment test will become available in the near future. In the meantime, a patient and the doctor must talk not only about pain complaints, but also about the feelings of depression and anxiety during each office visit. A patient and the doctor must develop a healthy relationship so that the appropriate pain modalities can be rationally prescribed specifically for a patient.

Pain is subjective and does not allow itself to be measured accurately. In other words, it is impossible to visualize "pain." When the doctor interviews a patient about the pain complaints, he or she will begin by asking the following questions: the time of the onset of the pain, the location of the pain on the body, how long it lasts, and how often it occurs during the day.

The doctor also will ask a patient whether the pain is sharp, dull, or cramping. A patient should tell the doctor whether the pain is mild, moderate, or severe. Women in general are more able to express their pain experiences than men. A patient must provide the doctor with enough information so that he or she can come up with a reasonable and accurate diagnosis for a patient.

What follows is an initial pain-assessment form. This assessment addresses the pain and psychosocial issues and leaves room for the doctor's evaluation of the condition. The doctor will give a patient a copy of this assessment form. A patient will be asked questions such as when the pain began, how long it lasts, what makes it worse, what makes it better, what medications a patient are taking, what effects medications are having on the pain, and what the emotional status is during episodes of pain. One way of assessing the pain is to use a verbal numeric scale. This is the simplest method for attempting to measure the pain. During this test, a patient is asked to rate the pain on a scale of 0 to 5 or to use words such as "none," "slight," "moderate," or "severe."

This assessment is also a quick, simple, and reliable way to evaluate the effectiveness of any medications a patient are taking to manage the pain. On the numeric scale, 0 equals no pain, 1 equals mild pain, 2 equals moderate pain, 3 equals distressing pain, 4 equals horrible pain, and 5 equals excruciating pain confining a patient to bed rest. This method is easily understood and may be helpful in guiding the treatment plans the doctor creates for a patient. Another type of verbal scale asks a patient to rate the pain on a scale of 1 to 10, with 1 being equivalent to pain that is barely noticeable and 10 relating to excruciating pain. A verbal numeric scale is easily understood. All a patient has to do is choose a number to represent the level of pain.

The following numeric pain-intensity scale is the most popular test used by pain-medicine specialists. A patient circle a number on the scale that corresponds to how much pain a patient feel. It only uses numbers from 0 through 10 along the length of the horizontal scale. A score of 0 indicates no pain, whereas a score of 10 means that a patient feel the worst pain ever imagined.

Numeric Pain Intensity Score

0 1 2	3 4 5	6 7	8 9 10
No Pain	Moderate Pain	Severe Pain	Worst Pain

Another method used by some doctors is a pain diary. This is a descriptive report a patient keep to assess the pain. The pain diary shows a written account of the day-to-day experiences. It can be used to help diagnose the cause of the pain. The value of the pain diary is that a patient and the doctor can monitor the day-to-day variation of painful states and the response to therapy. A patient needs to keep a diary of the pain patterns when a patient are sitting, standing, and lying down. A patient also must note the amount of pain medication a patient are taking and whether it lessens the pain. Because pain can interfere with eating patterns, keep a diary of the amount of food a patient eat and at what time a patient ate. One needs to include any types of recreational activities and whether the pain felt better or worse afterward.

The following is a sample of a pain diary that a patient may find useful. A patient has to be diligent in the record keeping. This form enables a patient to record an entire month of pain-intensity scores, the activities, the location of the pain, and a medication log. The physician will find this diary extremely helpful in working with a patient to plan the pain therapy.

Date_____   Daily Pain Assessment

Time	Where is the pain? Rate the pain (0-10), or list the word from the scale that describes your pain	What were you doing when the pain started or increased?	Did you take medicine? What did you take? How much?	What other treatments did you use?	After an hour, what is your pain rating?	Other problems or side effects? Comments.
morning						
noon						
evening						

Pain drawings offer a visual way to evaluate pain. A patient will be asked to shade in areas on a human figure outline that correspond to the areas of the pain. The drawing will help the doctor determine where the pain is coming from and how widespread it is on the body. Over time, the pain drawings can be compared to show the changes of the pain and how a patient is responding to therapy.

The following is a sample pain-assessment tool that includes diagrams for a patient to shade to tell the doctor whether the pain is confined to one area of the body or whether the pain is widespread throughout the body. This form allows a patient to shade the areas of the body where a patient is feeling the pain. It is a simple way of evaluating where a patient is experiencing pain. It is helpful when patients have trouble communicating where he or she is hurting and is especially helpful in patients who have had a stroke injury.

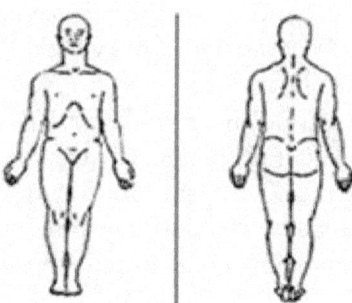

A common method of determining the behavioral component of the pain is for a patient to be directly observed by the doctor. A patient must be observed while sitting, walking to and from the office, and getting in and out of vehicles. The doctor will focus his or her attention on the area of the major pain complaint. Behavioral influences affecting the perception of pain include the amount of medications a patient use and the number of doctor visits required. Limping and facial grimacing also are appropriate behavioral evaluations of pain. Depression and anxiety are emotional factors that can be measured by tests.

Because the experience of pain is impossible to measure directly, the doctor must observe the displays of appropriate or inappropriate physical behavior. After observing the behavior, the doctor may classify a patient using the following four-class system: Class 1 consists of patients with low physical injury but high levels of abnormal behavior patterns related to their pain. Class 2 consists of patients with lower physical injury and low behavior pattern abnormalities. Class 3 consists of patients with significant tissue injury in addition to high behavioral pattern abnormalities. Class 4 consists of patients with a high tissue injury and normal behavioral patterns.

A visual analog scale is another method of assessment that attempts to measure the level of pain. Instead of choosing a number, a patient are asked to mark a point on a horizontal line that is labeled with "no pain" at one end and "the worst possible pain" at the opposite end. It is slightly more difficult to administer than the numeric method, but some doctors and researchers think that the visual analog scale is more accurate than the numeric scale for pain measurements.

+_____+

Visual Analog Scale

Patients with dementia can be difficult to assess. One solution is the clinician or nursing care observations of facial expressions and vocalizations which are accurate means for assessing the presence of pain, but does not measure its true intensity.

References

1. Persons AGSPoPPiO. The management of persistent pain in older persons. J Am Geriatr Soc. 2002;50(6 Suppl):S205-224.
2. Holen JC, Hjermstad MJ, Loge JH, et al. Pain assessment tools: is the content appropriate for use in palliative care? J Pain Symptom Manage. 2006;32(6):567-580.

6. Psychological assessment

Various psychological approaches to the treatment of elderly patients including activity and stimulation programs, reality orientation, environmental approaches and behavior modification can be used in elderly pain patients. Psychological treatment can be considered for any intense and recurrent pain problem that has not responded to initial medical and/or surgical treatment. Chronic pain is one of the most common complaints in the elderly, associated with much impairment of quality of life.[1] Up to now clinical research has focused little attention on pain in old age.

Pain is often classified as an inevitable phenomenon in the elderly. But present studies show that differences between older and younger patients appear less important than similarities. The studies also make evident that proved psychological pain management is transferable to elderly patients. The knowledge of effective psychological treatment in case of chronic pain in the elderly has been seldom realized in clinical practice.

Psychological strategies for the treatment of chronic pain are an important component of the necessary multidimensional treatment for patients in chronic pain. These techniques including relaxation training, biofeedback, hypnosis and cognitive-behavioral therapy have demonstrated efficacy. The impact of these techniques is on the sensory aspect of pain and the psychological distress and on the maladaptive coping mechanism people develop in response to pain.

Pain is perceived differently by men and women. Anxiety, pain thresholds, and pain tolerance influence pain intensity. The International Association for the Study of Pain (IASP) defines pain as an unpleasant sensory and emotion experience associated with tissue injury as a result of trauma (for instance, bone fracture) or disease (for instance, cancer or shingles).

Pain is psychological in that it is a mental processing of sensation impulses that reach the pain center in the brain, whereas pain "intensity" depends on how an individual reacts to pain. Injury or illness experienced when young may influence the way an individual relates to pain. When pain becomes chronic, it becomes a personal problem. However, pain can also become a social problem, perhaps disrupting the family and resulting in loss of self-esteem.

The following findings relate to how an individual's psychological state influences his or her perception of and response to pain: Patients who have strongly negative emotions about a situation experience more pain. Women have more negative emotions about situations in general than men and, therefore, have a higher incidence of pain. However, women cope better with pain than men. Family members' and friends' pain may influence an individual's own pain.

For example, women whose immediate family members were experiencing significant pain experienced more clinical pain and complained of more severe pain themselves. In general, men do not demonstrate this effect.

In general, women have a lower tolerance to pain than men. A higher level of anxiety in women may be somewhat responsible for their increased pain sensitivity. In 1998, a Washington Post article reported that although women are more sensitive to pain than men, they appear better able to handle it. In 1998, the Wall Street Journal reported that women and men report different responses to pain. An article in the Journal of the American Medical Association in 1998 reported that girls and boys have different responses to pain and that these pain responses begin early in their lives.

As already stated, pain is an unpleasant sensory as well as an emotional response to tissue trauma. "Nociception" is the avoidance of a painful stimulus. For example, if a match is placed against your skin, you will quickly move away from the heat of the match. This is a nociceptive response to prevent tissue damage. Following the initial tissue response, the psychological aspects of suffering then become manifest. However, we do observe this in children following a fall. Some children cry loudly and seek attention, whereas others pick themselves up and continue what they were doing without a whimper. Even though the tissue trauma can be the same for multiple individuals, the response to pain is individualized based on education, psychological makeup, gender, and cultural influences.

"Pain medicine" as a specialty has evolved in a short time to realize that pain is a multidimensional entity influenced by psychological, neurological, social, ethnic, and cultural factors. Before the advent of this specialty, many doctors looked only at tissue injury and not at the patient as a whole.

Pain cannot be observed or objectively measured. Instead, a pain "diagnosis" is based on verbal and nonverbal communication from the individual suffering pain. People communicate their pain through their behavior. These behaviors, such as limping or grimacing, can be seen by others and result in attention being given to the suffering individual.

Doctors should diagnose pain based on both physical and psychological data. Physical data may include a physical examination and interpretation of x-rays, CT scans, and multi resonance imaging (MRI) images. Doctors use this information to tailor therapies (successful, one hopes) to the individual patient. Features unique to pain assessment in older adults include the likelihood of multiple diagnoses contributing to chronic pain, the ability of older adults to self-report, including those with mild to moderate cognitive impairment, and recognition that some older adults with cognitive impairment may demonstrate various behaviors to communicate pain.[2]

Pain management is best accomplished through a multimodal approach, including pharmacologic and nonpharmacologic treatments, physical rehabilitation, and psychological therapies. Interventional pain therapies may be appropriate in select older adults, which may reduce the need for pharmacologic treatments. To promote early engagement in skill-focused treatments, providers can routinely evaluate pain coping strategies in older adults using a treatment algorithm.[3]

For reasons not entirely understood, women suffer from more disability than men in general. Further research is needed to unlock the mystery of human behavior and its relationship to disabling painful states so that chronic pain will cease to become a major cause of both physical and psychological disability. Because emotional factors can affect pain perception and intensity, a pain specialist's complete assessment of pain should include not only a physical examination but also analysis of the psychological, emotional, and behavioral aspects of pain. Such analysis may prove challenging because many patients are reluctant to discuss painful psychological issues with their pain-management doctor (and it is more socially acceptable to seek medical rather than psychiatric care).

The purpose of "behavioral medicine" is to relieve anxiety and depression and to decrease pain intensity. Techniques used include biofeedback, relaxation training, and hypnosis. Because anxiety and depression can make people less able to cope with persistent pain, consultation with a behavioral medicine specialist can prove extremely beneficial. Sadness, hopelessness, insomnia, and feelings of worthlessness are all associated with depression. Anxiety is characterized by apprehension and fear or a sense of doom. Doctors need to recognize the stressors that are causing anxiety and address them with their patients. Signs and symptoms of anxiety include loss of appetite, diarrhea, fainting, increased heart rate, and sexual dysfunction.

Personality greatly influences an individual's response to pain and his or her chosen coping strategies. In general, people who have underlying anxiety are more likely to seek higher doses of pain medications. Understanding how people cope with stress is helpful; this is a task aided by discussion with the patient's family. A psychological history should include questions about depression, sleep disruption, preoccupation with body pain, reduced "everyday activities," fatigue, and loss of sexual interest. People with "psychogenic" pain make illness and hospitalization a primary goal. Psychological stresses such as anxiety and depression make pain more intense and less tolerable.

Psychologists have analyzed pre-injury personalities to identify types of people who may be more likely to develop pain syndromes. These studies conclude that there does not appear to be an unstable personality that predisposes to reflex sympathetic dystrophy or other chronic pain syndromes. Reflex sympathetic dystrophy, an extremely painful nervous system condition, was once thought to be caused by psychological disorders.

According to psychological studies made after reflex sympathetic dystrophy and similar types of neuropathic (nerve injury) pain syndromes have resolved, a predisposing psychological factor is rarely associated with the pain syndrome. In some instances, however, a person's psychological makeup may control his or her sympathetic nervous system.

In 1964, the behavioral aspects of seven patients' chronic reflex sympathetic dystrophy involving an extremity were reported. In each of these seven cases, financial compensation was the main motivating factor, for which these seven individuals maintained signs and symptoms of reflex sympathetic dystrophy, including each individual's chronic disability. Anxiety over potential long-term disability can actually lead to a disability in some patients.

Pain is a subjective complaint and is affected by a patient's emotions. Unfortunately, persistent pain can change a patient's behavior. Persistent pain can increase patient anxiety and depression. As a result, it is difficult for a doctor to ascertain whether the pain came first or the psychological dysfunction. Most pain patients can benefit from behavioral treatments designed to improve their ability to cope with pain.

Psychotherapy may help patients realize what is actually causing pain to be chronic. In some instances, a psychiatrist or a neuropsychologist can significantly decrease a patient's pain. Psychologists and psychiatrists often operate multidisciplinary pain centers. Psychologists not only diagnose and treat behavioral disorders; they may also suggest pain-treatment alternatives. "Pain" is difficult to define because it relates to people's subjective complaints and behaviors.

As previously stated, pain varies in duration and intensity. Most people with pain, whether acute or chronic, are able to adapt in a normal manner. Other people have an extreme disruption of their lives and develop chronic pain syndromes in which the pain itself becomes a disease, serving no useful biological purpose. At the time of injury, pain serves a useful purpose: warning the body to cease activity and allow healing. When pain persists after the tissue has healed, it serves no known biological purpose.

In 1976, Fordyce suggested that pain behavior is a learned response that can be modified. If a patient receives extra attention from a spouse or family members, the pain behavior is "reinforced." This is an example of pain causing a benefit or a "positive reinforcement." On the other hand, if an individual loses work and income because of pain, pain intensity usually decreases, allowing the individual to return to work. This is an example of "negative reinforcement."

Both the patient and the doctor need to identify situations that reinforce pain behavior. Patients can use a pain diary to help identify what behavior signals pain, and a family conference may help to identify the positive reinforcements (rewards) of pain, such as a doting spouse, being excused from household chores, and so on. Some people appreciate extra attention given them by family members, attention that perhaps was not available before the painful condition. Others use pain to avoid psychologically painful situations, such as workplace problems with co-workers or a supervisor, and use it to avoid going to work and dealing with colleagues. People may also use pain to avoid social or family gatherings.

When doctors fail to relieve pain, patients may find that a consultation with a behavioral medicine specialist such as a psychologist or psychiatrist may prove helpful. If pain provides a way to escape difficult psychological situations, this should be addressed. Most people with pain respond to routine treatments, such as oral medication and nerve injections of anti-inflammatory drugs (corticosteroids, for instance) as well as physical or manipulative therapy. When an individual fails to respond to these methods, psychological intervention is necessary

Pain patient behaviors that should be closely watched include frequently talking about pain, moaning, and frequently going to doctors and refusing to work. Doctors should observe and note blatant pain manifestations. Pain behavior is influenced by environmental consequences. Suffering is the conceptual component of pain that denotes a persistent negative affect. Suffering is composed of depression, fear, and isolation. The concept of pain is complex. Philosophers have argued for years whether pain is an emotion or a sensation.

Some theologians in the Middle Ages thought that pain was a penalty. It has been described as a punishment for sin. Pain is essentially a behavioral subjective phenomenon. Patients with chronic pain share many of the following characteristics: preoccupation with pain, strong dependency needs, feelings of isolation, an inability to attend to self needs, and an inability to appropriately deal with repressed anger and hostility.

Many patients with chronic pain exhibit masochistic behavior patterns. Pain can gratify an individual's need to suffer and receive constant attention from a family member or health-care professional. Pain and disability can cause dependency upon others to assist in activities of daily living, such a cooking, cleaning, laundry, and so on.

Many chronic pain patients have suffered emotionally traumatic childhoods; a history of this trauma should be sought by the doctors caring for these patients. Pain may significantly increase when there is low self-esteem. When an individual attempts to suppress emotions, muscle tension may occur. Muscle tension can contribute to both body pain and tension-type headaches

Emotional disorders can also be associated with chronic pain, including somatoform disorders, somatization disorder, conversion disorder, psychogenic pain disorder, and hypochondriasis. These emotional disorders will affect a patient's response to a chronic pain syndrome. In a somatoform disorder, physical symptoms are compatible with a physical disorder, but there is no evidence of any clear psychiatric or physical problem. These patients overanalyze their bodies and have a tendency to look for abnormal symptoms.

Somatization disorders usually persist throughout the patient's life. It also tends to run in families. Some psychiatrists think that the high female-to-male ratio in this disorder reflects the cultural pressures on women in North American society and the social "permission" given to women to be physically weak or sickly.

A somatization disorder is a chronic disorder that usually begins before age 30 and primarily affects women. With it, an individual complains of many symptoms but has few physical findings to confirm their complaints. These individuals consult many doctors to validate their symptoms and may even consent to multiple injections by a pain-management doctor or even a surgical procedure for the treatment of pain. The diagnosis of somatoform disorders in elderly patients is frequently difficult due to the presence of a mixture of symptoms related to organic pathological changes, medication side effects and mental processes.

A conversion disorder results from an emotional conflict unrelated to bodily disease but resulting in loss of function of a part of the body. An example is losing the use of a hand without an obvious physical problem or injury. These individuals exaggerate the magnitude of their complaints. The expression of the psychic apparatus into the body, and its various clinical manifestations, has no direct specificity in the elderly. Psychogenic pain disorders are complaints of pain without adequate physical findings. These individuals exhibit neurotic behavior. Neurotic behavior is a behavior that you realize is abnormal such as anxiety. Individuals seeking financial compensation may exhibit psycho-genic pain disorders.

Hypochondriasis is a disturbance that involves an unrealistic interpretation of physical disease. These individuals have a preoccupation with the belief that they have a serious disease and are preoccupied with their physical symptoms. The persistence of less intense hypochondriacal concerns after remission of depression suggests that these features may represent a mixture of trait phenomena in elderly depressives. Malingering is uncommon but implies a conscious fabrication of an illness for personal gain. These individuals are often seeking financial compensation or may be seeking narcotic analgesic drugs.

However, before diagnosing an individual of faking an illness, a doctor must thoroughly investigate a patient's complaint and exclude any possible real illness. The pain-prone patient is often an individual who had a traumatic childhood, perhaps with a history of physical and/or emotional abuse or a history of chronic pain or disability. Individuals who feel unloved are prone to use pain to meet ungratified needs. These individuals frequently try to manipulate others and have a tendency to burden their families.

Various psychological tests are available to evaluate pain patients. A common test is the Minnesota Multiphase Personality Inventory Test (MMPI), which evaluates multiple dimensions of a pain patient. The Beck Depression Scale can be used to assess depression. The MMPI, consisting of 566 questions, is widely used by psychologists working with pain patients, but cannot consistently distinguish between psychogenic and tissue damage pain. However, people with high hypochondriasis and hysteria scores and lower depression scores may have a physical basis for their pain, rather than a conversion reaction. The MMPI test also proves useful in assessing emotional disorders that occur secondary to a pain experience and personality factors that could affect an individual's response to pain treatment.

A problem with labeling pain as psychogenic is the assumption that the actual cause of the affected patient's pain is unknown. Elderly patients may have many age related ailments that can cause chronic pain. The assumption that an elderly patient's pain is psychogenic may be false, because the physical reason for many pain syndromes may be unclear or unknown. This is a problem in workman's compensation or bodily injury cases. If, following an examination, a doctor paid by an insurance company cannot find a reason for a claimant's pain, the patient is often labeled as a malingerer, which unfortunately ruins the patient's credibility with a judge or jury. Remember, however, that the diagnosis of psychogenic pain is a diagnosis only of exclusion. That is, a diagnosis made by excluding the diseases to which only some of your symptoms may belong, leaving one disease as the most likely diagnosis, although no conclusive tests or findings establish that diagnosis for certain.

Most chronic pain patients are not malingers. Acute and chronic pain is disabling. Most patients do not want to suffer. A desire to avoid pain is a strong desire. Most pain doctors want to minimize the use of drugs and medicines. No medicine is without potential dangerous side effects. This is why most pain-management doctors use injection therapy and prescribe physical and/or occupational therapy and make referrals to chiropractors or other nonconventional health-care providers.

In the past, the failure of injections or drugs to relieve pain resulted in referral to a psychologist or a psychiatrist for treatment of psychiatric or behavioral problems. Today these specialists are essential to pain management. In fact, a psychiatrist is a medical doctor, and a psychologist has a Ph.D. Not only can psychiatrists prescribe medications for pain, they also attend to mental and emotional conditions that may be contributing to pain. (A psychologist cannot prescribe medications.)

Psychological assessments and treatment are now part of the total approach to managing those experiencing chronic pain. Psychologists can teach relaxation techniques and biofeedback and use hypnosis to decrease pain, complementing physical therapy, pharmacological therapy, and injections.

Placebo medicine studies help us to further understand the role of psychology in chronic pain. Pain may be considered a result of a tissue injury signaling the brain to experience pain. However, placebo medications, defined as inactive drugs such as sugar pills, can significantly decrease pain. When doing any type of study evaluating the analgesic effects of a particular new medicine, a placebo group must be included.

For example, chronic migraine headache sufferers asked to participate in a study evaluating a new headache medication will be divided into two groups. One group will be prescribed the active, or "study," drug, whereas the other will be given either an inactive drug or no drug. If a participant experiences significant pain relief from the inactive drug or the sugar pill, he or she has experienced a placebo effect: essentially, pain relief from no medication.

The placebo effect demonstrates that a psychological component affects the perception of painful stimuli. People with high expectations that the drugs they are receiving are powerful pain relievers will likely experience a decrease in pain after taking placebo drugs. The expectation of significant pain relief psychologically causes relief.

People's expectations when seeing a pain doctor or receiving medications, nerve injections, and psychological therapy will also affect their pain response. Those who do not expect relief, on the other hand, will probably not experience pain relief. For this reason, each individual has control of his or her painful situation.

A dog or cat can be struck by an automobile and sustain significant trauma. In most instances, however, the animal is back functioning within a short time. An animal has no secondary gain issues and does not anticipate having significant monetary compensation for an injury caused by a careless driver. However, humans can have prolonged pain following an accident only to have the pain relieved following a large jury settlement. This observation is referred to as the "green poultice department" treatment.

The effect of prayer also has been documented as a powerful analgesic. An orthopedic surgery textbook tells of an individual with two lumbar disk ruptures. This individual had weakness in a leg. The orthopedic surgeon used MRI images and clinical evaluation of the patient to determine surgery was necessary. The patient also had significant pain. However, when the patient's church congregation prayed for his relief, his pain dissipated in a day. A repeat MRI revealed no disk rupture. The numbness in the extremity also disappeared. This is one of many documented cases of the power of prayer.

Another study looked at post surgery cancer patients who were given saltwater (saline) injections and had a significant decrease in post-surgery pain. Individuals may even have side effects associated with placebos. If you are a participant in a study, the side effects of the actual drug studied are noted and written down for you. A placebo response can be as high as 35 percent with side effects experienced in as many as 19 percent of cases. For instance, individuals responded to flavored water with demonstrated signs of drunkenness when they were compared to a group that had flavored alcohol drinks.

Some researchers report that the placebo effect is related to the body's release of endorphins, naturally occurring chemicals that we have in our bodies to control pain. A placebo, furthermore, may reduce anxiety. Anxiety can increase the perception of pain. People with positive expectations prior to taking medications generally have more positive results. This finding may be related to endorphin release from the brain and spinal cord. Expectation is a learned trait. This is one reason why a placebo response is not evident in children. Expectation depended on an individual's life experience and personality. Hostility with a treating doctor will decrease expectation. On the other hand, respect for a doctor's abilities will increase positive expectations for successful pain relief.

Other methods used by psychologists for the management of pain include relaxation and biofeedback training. These methods are used to treat both acute and chronic pain syndromes. Relaxation is also frequently used to control pain associated with labor contractions. Used properly, relaxation can also decrease the body's metabolic activity and preserve energy. Learning to manage pain through relaxation methods enables people to consciously control pain and become proactive in their own pain management.

Biofeedback is another method frequently used by psychologists to manage pain. An electromyogram, which measures muscle contractions in different parts of the body, can be used for biofeedback training and pain evaluations. Other measurements include skin temperature and brainwave forms. When muscles are tense, skin temperature is less than in surrounding tissues because of a decrease in blood flow.

Biofeedback techniques can increase blood flow to muscles and skin and increase a patient's temperature. This can be used in combination with relaxation training to manage pain; both techniques are more commonly used by women than by men. Biofeedback has been used to treat many chronic pain syndromes, including muscle-tension headaches. People with migraine headaches, phantom limb pain, and reflex sympathetic dystrophy can also respond to biofeedback training.

Migraine headaches have been successfully treated with biofeedback. On average, females have a higher incidence of migraine headaches than males. Biofeedback training can result in a 50 percent reduction in severe migraine headache pain. Some studies advocate combining biofeedback and relaxation training for the treatment of migraine headaches.

Relaxation treatment has also been shown to be effective for the management of lower back pain. Most back pain is caused by sustained muscle tension. Relaxation training relaxes muscles and increases blood flow and oxygen delivery while removing excessive buildup in muscles of lactic acid.

Hypnosis can decrease or inhibit pain impulses to the brain's pain center as well as pain impulses in the spinal cord. Hypnosis can create the expectation of pain reduction. People with headaches can find relief with hypnosis. Imagery is an important component of hypnosis. Hypnosis causes a deeply relaxed state, diverting attention from pain. Although hypnosis is used to reduce pain, it is difficult to completely eliminate it. However, it can decrease pain to a tolerable state.

Understanding the destructive and preventable nature of arthritis may facilitate early detection and increased uptake of appropriate treatment options for osteoarthritis that have the ability to modify disease trajectories.4 A psychologist will teach a patient that pain is a set of multiple problems rather than one single entity.

Psychosocial factors in telomere degradation.[5] Social isolation affects telomere length, which supports the hypothesis that telomeres provide a biomarker indicating exposure to chronic stress.[6] Results from a racially/ethnically diverse community sample of men and women provide initial evidence that low social support is associated with shorter telomere length in adults aged 65 years and older and is consistent with the hypothesis that social environment may contribute to rates of cellular aging, particularly in late life.[7]

There is evidence that a major depressive disorder is associated with shortened telomeres.[8] Strong evidence supports that living in disadvantaged neighborhoods has direct unfavorable impact on mental and physical health. An association between perceived neighborhood quality and cellular aging exists over and above a range of individual attributes. Biological aging processes may be impacted by socioeconomic milieu.[9] Childhood maltreatment could influence cellular aging as well.[10]

References

1. Persons AGSPoPPiO. The management of persistent pain in older persons. J Am Geriatr Soc. 2002;50(6 Suppl):S205-224.

2. Bicket MC, Mao J. Chronic Pain in Older Adults. Anesthesiol Clin. 2015;33(3):577-590.

3. DiNapoli EA, Craine M, Dougherty P, et al. Deconstructing Chronic Low Back Pain in the Older Adult - Step by Step Evidence and Expert-Based Recommendations for Evaluation and Treatment. Part V: Maladaptive Coping. Pain Med. 2016;17(1):64-73.

4. Harris ML, Byles JE, Sibbritt D, Loxton D. "Just get on with it": qualitative insights of coming to terms with a deteriorating body for older women with osteoarthritis. PLoS One. 2015;10(3):e0120507.

5. Mathur MB, Epel E, Kind S, et al. Toward a mechanistic understanding of psychosocial factors in telomere degradation. Brain Behav Immun. 2016;56:413.

6. Aydinonat D, Penn DJ, Smith S, et al. Social isolation shortens telomeres in African Grey parrots (Psittacus erithacus erithacus). PLoS One. 2014;9(4):e93839.

7. Carroll JE, Diez Roux AV, Fitzpatrick AL, Seeman T. Low social support is associated with shorter leukocyte telomere length in late life: multi-ethnic study of atherosclerosis. Psychosom Med. 2013;75(2):171-177.

8. Hartmann N, Boehner M, Groenen F, Kalb R. Telomere length of patients with major depression is shortened but independent from therapy and severity of the disease. Depress Anxiety. 2010;27(12):1111-1116.

9. Park M, Verhoeven JE, Cuijpers P, Reynolds Iii CF, Penninx BW. Where You Live May Make You Old: The Association between Perceived Poor Neighborhood Quality and Leukocyte Telomere Length. PLoS One. 2015;10(6):e0128460.

10. Tyrka AR, Price LH, Kao HT, Porton B, Marsella SA, Carpenter LL. Childhood maltreatment and telomere shortening: preliminary support for an effect of early stress on cellular aging. Biol Psychiatry. 2010;67(6):531-534.

7. Physical therapy

Pains belong to the most frequent reasons for a doctor's visit. In elderly people, it is the result of progressive degenerative processes (e. g. , arthrosis, osteoarthritis, degenerative spinal changes) and a higher prevalence of cancer disease to a further increase of the patients who suffer unnecessarily from pain.1 It is not exceptional longevity but one's function and health that may be associated with telomere length.2

Physical therapy is an important modality that can be used to help manage pain. Physical therapy and rehabilitation are used to treat elderly patients suffering from illness, disease or injury. Physical therapists work with patients who have impairments, limitations, disabilities, or changes in physical function and health status resulting from injury, disease or other causes. Their role includes examination, evaluation, diagnosis, prognosis and interventions toward achieving the highest functional outcomes for each patient or client.

Physical therapy includes aspects of pathophysiology, impairment, functional limitation and disability. Physical therapy can help restore function, improve mobility, relieve pain, and prevent or limit permanent physical disabilities. Physical therapists also use electrical stimulation, hot packs or cold compresses, and ultrasound to relieve pain and reduce swelling. Therapists also teach patients to use assistive and adaptive devices such as crutches, prostheses and wheelchairs. They also may show patients exercises to do at home to expedite their recovery.

Geriatric physical therapy is a proven way for elderly parents of all levels of physical ability to build confidence, improve balance and strength, and stay active. The interpersonal relationship that develops between physical therapist and patient is an important aspect of the treatment program. According to the National Institutes of Health, physical therapy is good for improving strength, balance, mobility and overall fitness. Those are factors that all aging parents could benefit from, as each contributes to the physical ability of maintaining independence for a longer period of time.

The main goal of physical therapy is to help boost overall functionality, minimize pain and increase mobility resulting in an improvement in balance and strength. Therapy can improve their mobility, strength, flexibility, coordination, endurance, and even reduce pain. The goal of physical therapy is therefore, to restore, maintain, or promote optimal physical function.

Individuals suffering from arthritis can benefit greatly from physical therapy. The exercises used in physical therapy will help preserve joint mobility and increase strength. Previous studies have demonstrated the trainability of stroke survivors and documented beneficial physiological, psychological, sensorimotor, strength, endurance, and functional effects of various types of exercise.

By the age of 65, most people suffer from arthritis in the spine. Physical therapy can help improve strength, balance and motion with the use of aquatic therapy, hot packs, electrical stimulation, and ice to reduce swelling.

Osteoporosis can be treated with balance exercises and extension exercises to help improve posture and prevent dangerous falls. One of the most common reasons an older person requires physical therapy is that they suffer from a fall. Physical therapy can help ease pain from injuries and improve balance. Many conditions that often plague older adults are well-suited for physical therapy treatment, including: arthritis, osteoporosis, pain associated with cancer, strokes, dementia, Alzheimer's, and incontinence. One of the best improvements gained by physical therapy is improved independence.

Vertebral compression fractures are the most common type of fracture secondary to osteoporosis. These fractures are associated with significant rates of morbidity and mortality and annual direct medical expenditures of more than $1 billion in the United States.

Although many patients will respond favorably to nonsurgical care contemporary natural history data suggest that more than 40% of patients may fail to achieve significant pain relief within 12 months of symptom onset. As a result, percutaneous vertebral vertebral augmentation kyphoplasty and vertebroplasty is often used to hasten symptom resolution and return of function.[3]

Physical and pharmacologic modalities of pain control and exercises or physiotherapy to maintain spinal movement and strength are important components in the care of vertebral fracture patients.[4] Conservative treatment is a reasonable option for the primary initial treatment for isolated, symptomatic, nontraumatic, supraspinatus tears in older patients.[5]

Osteoarthritis and osteoporosis are known to occur in an older population. A patient must tell the therapist when the pain gets worse during the day or if increased pain occurs with certain activities. A therapist will examine the range of motion of a patient's joints, including the range of motion of the neck and lower back. Movements of a patient's joints, neck, and lower back will be done to assess flexibility.

Any atrophy of the extremities will be addressed. A therapist will target this area to increase strength and muscle mass. The goal of physical therapy is to identify the cause of a patient's pain with an attempt to treat the cause of the pain syndrome.

A physical therapist will attempt to correct any mechanical flaws in a patient's body that could lead to further injury, such as posture. A therapist may do a muscle and joint stabilization program to increase strength and flexibility. Physical therapists can help you decrease your muscle tension. Your therapist also can educate you on how to decrease muscle tension yourself. Most muscle tension is related to the stress of everyday life.

When one experiences stress, the body has a protective mechanism that increases muscle tightness. This is an early part of the fight-or-flight response to stressful situations. Physical therapy helps older adults stay strong and maintain their independence and productivity. Geriatric physical therapy is a proven way for elderly parents of all levels of physical ability to build confidence, improve balance and strength, and stay active.

The high efficacy of inpatient physical rehabilitation is a means of improving functional independence. Hospital rehabilitation should be recommended for elderly people, not only in cases of absolute indications for hospital admission, but also periodically for patients at risk of physical disability. It is not exceptional longevity but one's function and health that may be associated with increased telomere length which may be affected by physical therapy.[3]

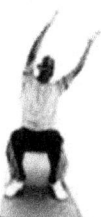

Figure 1. A physical therapist will demonstrate proper exercises to do.

Occupational therapy is a treatment that incorporates meaningful activity to promote participation in everyday life. Many people do not understand how occupational therapy differs from physical therapy. The primary difference is that the occupational therapist assesses the patient's ability to perform his daily "occupations" or activities and the physical therapist focuses on improving mobility.

When a physical therapist treats a person with a hip fracture his goal may be for the patient to walk and use the stairs. An occupational therapist, on the other hand, may recommend bathtub grab bars and a raised toilet seat to increase safety and independence during self-care "occupations".

The first step in occupational therapy for the elderly is an assessment of the individual's capabilities and the surrounding environment. Safety is an important consideration for elderly patients, who may not have good balance or can be hampered by visual problems. The occupational therapist will identify potential risks such as stairs without handrails or throw rugs that can cause falls, and make recommendations to make the home or living quarters safer. A physical examination will identify the patient's strengths, weaknesses, capabilities and cognitive function, which affects the ability to follow instructions and learn new ways of doing things.

Occupational therapy focuses on self-care activities and improvement of fine motor coordination of muscles and joints, particularly in the upper extremities. Unlike physical therapy, this focuses on muscle strength and joint range of motion. Occupational therapy focuses on activities of daily living and includes eating, dressing, bathing, grooming, toileting, and transferring.

The effects of occupational therapy on patients with Alzheimer's disease or related conditions have been evaluated. The results show a real improvement in the quality of their daily life.[6]

Occupational therapy includes preparing meals; communicating by telephone, writing, or computer; managing finances and daily drug regimens; cleaning; doing laundry, food shopping, and other errands; managing finances; traveling as a pedestrian or by public transportation; and driving. Driving is particularly complex, requiring integration of visual, physical, and cognitive tasks.

References

1. Eiche J, Schache F. [Pain Management in geriatric patients]. Dtsch Med Wochenschr. 2016;141(9):635-641.
2. Terry DF, Nolan VG, Andersen SL, Perls TT, Cawthon R. Association of longer telomeres with better health in centenarians. J Gerontol A Biol Sci Med Sci. 2008;63(8):809-812.
3. Goldstein CL, Chutkan NB, Choma TJ, Orr RD. Management of the Elderly With Vertebral Compression Fractures. Neurosurgery. 2015;77 Suppl 4:S33-45.
4. Kendler DL, Bauer DC, Davison KS, et al. Vertebral Fractures: Clinical Importance and Management. Am J Med. 2016;129(2):221 e221-210.

5. Kukkonen J, Joukainen A, Lehtinen J, et al. Treatment of Nontraumatic Rotator Cuff Tears: A Randomized Controlled Trial with Two Years of Clinical and Imaging Follow-up. J Bone Joint Surg Am. 2015;97(21):1729-1737.

6. Labbaci S, Gonthier R, Auguste N, Achour E. [Impact of occupational therapy on the experience of carers]. Soins. 2016(803):42-44.

8. Alternative medicine

Large-scale surveys in the United States and abroad suggest that 35-60% of adults have used some form of complementary and/or alternative medicine (CAM). Because conventional medications can have adverse effects in aged patients, CAM may be of benefit for pain management. However, no studies to date have focused on predictors and patterns of CAM use among elderly persons. Findings suggest that there is significant interest in and use of complementary or alternative medicine among elderly persons. These results suggest the importance of further research into the use and potential efficacy of these therapies within the senior population.

"Conventional medicine" is considered to be practiced by individuals who have a medical doctor degree (M.D.) or a doctor of osteopathy degree (D.O.). Traditional medicine also includes methods practiced by allied health-care professionals such as physical therapists, occupational therapists, psychologists, and registered nurses. Other terms for conventional medicine include allopathy, mainstream medicine, and orthodox medicine. In contrast, complementary and alternative medicine is referred to as unconventional or nonconventional medicine as well as unproven health care.

Practitioners of alternative medicine hold to the theory that germs can cause illness only if there is an imbalance in various body systems allowing the germs to thrive. They believe that the body's internal environment is healthy and must be kept fit, and that everyday exposure to germs does not result in illness.

The following is a definition for alternative medicine specialties by the National Center for Complementary and Alternative Medicine. "Complementary and alternative medicines are practices and products that are not currently considered to be part of conventional medicine." Complementary and alternative medicine practices change and update continually.

Those therapies that have been thoroughly investigated and that are proven to be safe and effective eventually do become adopted into the traditional health-care system. Complementary and alternative medicines, unlike many conventional medicine therapies, are designed to help one develop control over their overall health. Medical professionals are beginning to recognize the benefits of alternative medicine. As an example, the National Institute of Health Office of Alternative Medicine was established in 1992. In addition, there has been a significant increase in professional interest in the area of alternative medicine. Right now, about 30 medical schools are currently offering at least one elective course on alternative medical therapies. The attitudes of medical school faculty toward the use of complementary medicine practices are important to alternatives gaining acceptance.

A study was done to evaluate the efficacy of massage therapy in breast disease. All participants felt that massage therapy was effective in helping them relax, and 34 felt that it was very or somewhat effective in reducing muscle tension. More than 75% reported that massage therapy was effective in reducing fatigue, creating a general feeling of wellness, and improving sleep quality and their ability to think clearly.[1] Other investigators evaluated massage therapy in breast cancer patients an concluded that this modality was also effective in breast cancer patients.[2,3]

Here are some other ways that alternative medicine is gaining acceptance: Some health plans have announced their intention to incorporate payment for some alternative medicine practices into their insurance coverage. Some managed care corporations have revealed their intentions to include alternative medicine practices for payment. Some state governments are considering legislation pertaining to the practice of alternative medicine by health-care professionals. A vitamin is a supplement and is not used to treat a disease per se. Not all CAM treatments are safe. For example, cyanide intoxication by apricot kernel ingestion as complimentary cancer therapy could be fatal.[4]

Seventy percent of older Americans turn to alternative medicines to treat their health problems. This is surprising because so-called alternative treatments are seen more as cutting edge and out of the realm of common medical practice with fewer studies to back them. It should be advised that an elderly person be selective; however, in adopting naturopathic recommendations.

Seniors are more likely to use chiropractors than any other practitioners of alternative treatments and there are least likely to use acupuncturists. Seniors may be taking herbs or other over-the-counter products that could interfere with commonly prescribed drugs. If a senior is going to use alternative treatments, they, or someone in charge, should talk with their doctor and go over the medications.

In addition, the alternative medications a patient takes could react with the prescription medications a doctor has given a patient and cause even more problems. If in doubt, consult the Physician's Drug Reference for herbal medicines. This will advise a patient about safe doses, and any precautions and drug interactions that one may need to be aware of.

In 1994, Congress passed the Dietary Supplement Health and Education Act. In passing this act, Congress recognized that many individuals believed that dietary supplements offered health benefits. The bill gave dietary supplement manufacturers freedom to produce more products and to provide information about their products' health benefits.

The Food and Drug Administration (FDA), on the other hand, is responsible for overseeing any claims by the dietary supplement manufacturers to the truthfulness of these claims. The Federal Trade Commission regulates the advertising of all the dietary supplements. A patient should be aware that the quality control standards for natural substances are a problem within this industry. Some of the manufacturers of these products will not have the amount of substance in the natural medication as stated on the container label.

Obesity is a rapidly growing epidemic that now affects approximately 30% of the adult population in the United States. The prevalence of obesity in the geriatric population makes it one of the fastest growing groups due to aging baby boomers. Because of the limited number of available treatments for obese adults, they often turn to supplements and alternative medicine sources to help them lose weight. One such group of supplements contains plant metabolites flavonoids, which includes catechins from tea, quercetin from fruits and vegetables, and isoflavones from soy products.[5] Some flavonoids such as catechins and soy isoflavones can modestly reduce weight.

Despite widespread public use of complementary and alternative medicine (CAM) therapies, no standardized CAM curriculum is available to medical educators, and evaluation of such curricula is limited. A course that provides students with the opportunity to delve into the vast area of CAM though site visits, small group discussions, lectures, and independent research projects may be an effective means of providing a CAM curriculum.[6] Education at medical school does influence attitudes to CAM.

As their orthodox medical training proceeds, medical students seem to increase their skepticism about CAM. Complementary medicine should be evaluated as rigorously as conventional medicine to protect the public from charlatans and unsafe practices. However, many practitioners of complementary medicine are reticent about evaluation of their practice. Sceptics maintain that this is because of fear that investigations will find treatments ineffective and threaten livelihoods.[7] In defense, many practitioners argue that research methods dissect their practice in a reductionist manner and fail to take into account complementary medicine's holistic nature leading to invalid evaluation.

Vitamin D for example, prevents falls among elderly patients and has been found that it reduces the risk by one quarter. This is an important finding for a couple of reasons. First, falls are a major problem affecting one-third of American elderly people each year, sending nearly 10% of them to the emergency room. Broken hips, wrists, ankles, shoulders and serious head injuries are the result of falls.

The NIH does however award grants for the study of research in complementary as well as alternative medicines. Clinical trials are being done throughout the United States with respect to complementary and alternative medicines. You may want to participate in one of these trials. Trials with respect to herbal medicines are an important part of the medical research process. The results from clinical trials can define better ways to treat your painful conditions.

Always remember that clinical trials have risks. Before participating in a clinical trial, discuss this trial with a primary-care physician. To find out about ongoing clinical trials for example, studies on arthritis and neurological disorders go to www.nccam.nih.gov. One also may want to access the National Library of Medicine online (www.pubmed.com). Pub Med contains a database from which you can search for "complementary medicine" to find citations to recently published scientific articles on this subject.

In Scotland, men and women use complementary medicines at about the same rate. In the Netherlands, however, women use complementary or alternative "medicines" more than men. In the United States and Canada, elderly women use complementary and alternative "medical care" more than men. These women generally tended to have higher incomes and were more educated than the general population.

Homeopathic medical therapy may also play a beneficial role in the long-term care of older adults with chronic diseases. Very little is known about the range of diagnoses, course of treatment and long-term outcome in elderly patients who choose to receive homeopathic medical treatment. Homeopathic specialists prescribe dilutions of natural substances from plants, minerals, and animals.

Homeopathy has been around for more than 200 years. About 500 million people around the world receive homeopathic treatment each year. The World Health Organization has recommended that homeopathy is a system of traditional medicine that should be integrated with conventional medicine, which is considered the traditional approach to medicine.

It is important to know that the U.S. Food and Drug Administration recognizes homeopathic remedies as official drugs and regulates their manufacture. This is unlike the herbs used for medicinal use. Homeopathy qualities of medicine are used frequently by conventional physicians in Europe. In Britain, homeopathy is a part of the national health system.

The basic principles of homeopathy are that a disease can be destroyed and removed by a type of medicine that can produce the disease in humans. In other words, a substance that in large doses would produce symptoms of a disease can be used in very minute doses to cure it. In conventional medicine, this is called the theory of antibiotics. Homeopathic practitioners adhere to the fact that the more a substance is diluted, the more potent it is. In conventional medicine, it is believed that a higher dose of the medicine will lead to a greater effect.

The purpose of diluting out substances in homeopathic medicine is to avoid side effects. Homeopathic practitioners adhere to the fact that illness is different for every person. Homeopathic treatments are unique for each patient. Homeopathic medicine emphasizes that patients are individuals and have individual signs and symptoms of an illness and should be treated only on an individual basis. The entire individual is treated, which includes the physical, psychological and spiritual portions of each person.

Naturopathic medical care involves the diagnostic evaluation of the whole person in finding the root cause, prevention and treatment of disease through non-invasive natural therapies, stimulating the body's innate power to heal itself. Galen, the successor of Hippocrates, established diet and nutrition as the main form of medicine for healing the majority of illnesses.

Naturopathic medicine, therefore, treats disease by using the body's natural ability to heal itself. Naturopathic practitioners invoke healing processes by using a variety of treatment options based on your particular needs. In naturopathic medicine, disease symptoms are a sign of the body's attempt to heal itself naturally. Naturopathic medicine gets its data from Chinese, Native American, and ancient Greek cultures. Naturopaths recommend healing of the person and not the disease. Naturopathic medicinal treatments will include doses of natural substances that are much higher than those used by practitioners of homeopathic medicine.

Tai chi, a traditional Chinese exercise, combines meditation with gentle movement sequences that involve the whole body but do not strain joints or muscles. Tai chi practice is believed to promote good health, and studies have found that it can reduce blood pressure, improve heart health, increase muscle strength, improve balance, and reduce the risk of falling. It has also been shown to reduce both anxiety and depression, and to promote an overall sense of well-being. Recently, it has been reported to help manage fibromyalgia.

A patient should not be afraid to approach a doctor with the fact that he or she is taking herbal medications. This is important not only because of possible drug interactions, but because some substances such as garlic and gingko can decrease the blood's ability to form a blood clot normally. This could result in excessive bleeding. It is extremely important if a patient is about to have a surgical procedure that one let the surgeon know the patient is are taking an herb that can thin the blood. The surgery may need to be delayed until the blood's ability to form a normal clot has been restored.

Be aware that when a patient is using alternative medicines that these medicines are not strictly controlled with respect to dosage and the amount of drug in a pill, capsule, or tea. All plants have different amounts of substances in them. A true dose of a medication is unknown in many instances. You should look carefully at the label before taking one of these substances and not take more than the label recommends. The overall drug interactions of herbal substances have not been established because they are not required to be strictly studied by the FDA.

To best choose a natural product to decrease pain, one should know which chemicals in the body produce pain. With this knowledge, an individual can pick the analgesic best suited to relieve the pain. For joint pain, for instance, one will want to use an alternative medicine that has anti-inflammatory properties. If a patient is injured or has inflammation, the body makes a variety of chemicals that transmit pain impulses to a pain-processing center in the brain. These chemicals include the prostaglandins, cytokines, substance P, glutamic acid, and nitric oxide. Nitric oxide is a gas that is also a pain chemical transmitter in your nervous system.

The following remedies are anti-inflammatory substances that one may want to use as a prostaglandin inhibitor to relieve your pain in some situations: Turmeric has anti-inflammatory and antioxidant effects and has been shown to inhibit prostaglandin formation. This drug should not be used if a patient has gallbladder disease. No significant health risks or side effects with use of this drug have been reported to date. The average dose is 3 grams of turmeric per day. This dose can be divided up into 1-gram doses and be taken 3 times per day with meals. For example, a patient may take 1 milligram with each meal for a total dose of 3 grams.

Ginseng has anti-inflammatory effects and is used in homeopathic medicine for the treatment of rheumatoid arthritis. A patient should not use this medicine if he or she has hypertension. A patient should not use ginseng with caffeine. Exercise caution if a patient uses ginseng along with any diabetic medicine or insulin.

A patient should not use ginseng with MAOI inhibitors, which are used to decrease blood pressure. One should not use ginseng in combination with diuretics. Side effects include sleep deprivation, nosebleeds, headaches, nervousness, and vomiting. The average daily dose of this root is 1 to 2 grams. Do not take more than 2 grams per day. The 2 grams can be divided up and taken 3 times a day.

Resveratrol is an antioxidant and a COX-2 inhibitor that some believe prevents heart disease and cancer. It is largely found in the skin of red grapes. Therefore, many people obtain resveratrol by drinking red wine. This substance can prevent clot formation, whereas the conventional COX-2 inhibitors do not prevent clot formation. The usual dose is no more than 600 mg per day. There are no known side effects or drug interactions for resveratrol itself.

Fish oils contain the omega-3 fatty acids and can decrease prostaglandins. Fish oils are used for the treatment of rheumatoid arthritis. One also may use fish oils for the control of joint pain. The most common side effect that a patient may experience with fish oil supplementation is mild stomach upset. The fish oils can decrease ones blood's ability to clot. If a patient is taking blood-thinning drugs, the patient should not take fish oils, because it will give the individual an increased risk of bleeding.

N-acetyl cysteine is an amino acid produced by the body that will decrease prostaglandin formation. It can help prevent some diseases and boost the immune system. A patient should not take this drug if he/she is taking carbamazepine (Tegretol). Side effects include headaches, nausea, vomiting, and stomach upset. The recommended dose is 200 milligrams three times a day.

Cayenne is an anti-inflammatory medication that is beneficial for the treatment of muscle pain and arthritis. This drug may be helpful for inhibiting the release of substance P as well. Cayenne side effects include diarrhea and intestinal colic. It can decrease the body's ability to form a normal blood clot. It also can reduce the effects of aspirin, so a patient should be aware of this fact if he/she is taking aspirin as a blood thinner. High doses of cayenne over a prolonged time can cause kidney and liver damage. A patient should not use this drug for more than two days in a row. After two weeks, one may use it again for two days. The daily dose of cayenne should not exceed 10 grams.

Ipriflavone can be used as a prostaglandin inhibitor. Women also use it to decrease the incidence of osteoporosis. This medicine can actually stop bone loss. It can decrease the risk of bone fractures in females. This drug, like the other drugs that are prostaglandin inhibitors, can increase the blood-thinning activity of other drugs that you may be taking, such as Coumadin. It also can increase the effects of some asthma drugs such as theophylline, so a patient should avoid taking ipriflavone if he/she is using such medications.

Side effects are mostly stomach upset. The average dose is 200 milligrams three times a day.

Procyanidolic oligomers are natural substances extracted from grape seeds. They are useful for their antioxidant effects. They can decrease arthritis pain. However, another important effect of this medicine is that it can decrease the effects of nitric oxide. Nitric oxide is released from cells in your bloodstream. Nitric acid essentially exists in a gas form to transmit pain impulses. There are no significant side effects associated with this drug. The daily dose of this drug ranges from 150 to 300 milligrams per day.

Cytokine inhibitors include the fish oils, as previously mentioned. Cytokines are chemicals produced in your bloodstream that enhance pain impulses. They contribute to the formation of substances that can destroy joint linings if a patient has rheumatoid arthritis.

Substance P inhibitors include cayenne and ginseng. Substance P is a neurotransmitter chemical that can be associated with nerve pain, such as shingles. Histamine also can provide pain relief. Histamine released from certain cells in the body can cause a patient to develop a rash, a headache, and itching all over the body. However, in extremely small doses, histamine may relieve pain. There have not been any placebo-controlled studies to date that compare a histamine cream to a placebo cream. In contrast, one animal study did conclude that morphine may exert its pain-relieving effect in the brain and spinal cord by releasing histamine into the central nervous system.

Hydroxy tryptophan is an amino acid that naturally occurs in the body. It has been found to significantly decrease substance P formation. Because substance P may be involved in fibromyalgia, this medicine can improve your fibromyalgia pain. It also may be helpful for the treatment of headaches, shingles, and neuropathic pain entities such as carpal tunnel syndrome. Nausea is a common side effect of this drug. A patient also may experience drowsiness, dry mouth, and stomach pain. In 1989, some people taking this drug developed joint pain, high fever, weakness in their arms and legs, and had shortness of breath.

The Center for Disease Control concluded that the drug came from a Japanese manufacturer and was contaminated. Drug interactions reveal severe effects if a person is taking an antidepressant medicine from their doctor. A patient should not take this drug if he/she has Parkinson's disease and are not taking the drug Sinemet. A patient should not use this drug if he/she has scleroderma. This drug also may interfere with the effects of drugs that a patient may be taking for migraine headaches. Adults should take no more than 50 milligrams 3 times a day.

Cannabinoids are another natural substance for the control of pain. State legislation throughout the United States will eventually decide on the use of cannabinoids for medical purposes. Marijuana has been used since antiquity. In 1942, marijuana was reported to be a dangerous, harmful, and habit-forming drug. In 1970, marijuana was classified as causing addiction drug with no accepted medical use.

However, in 1996, voters in Arizona and California passed referenda to legalize marijuana for medicinal use. Other states have legalized marijuana as well. There has been a recent discovery of two cannabinoid receptors in your body, CB-1 and CB-2. Now the scientific medical community is interested in this substance. Cannabinoids are now reported to have therapeutic value as pain relievers. There have not been any controlled clinical trials for the use of this drug to date.

Cannabinoids do exhibit some anti-inflammatory properties. However, they are no more effective than the current anti-inflammatory medications available. If a patient suffers from pain involving nerves, such as shingles or reflex sympathetic dystrophy, one may be able to note some pain relief with the use of marijuana. To date, the safety and efficacy of marijuana have not been found. In 1997, the American Medical Association House of Delegates recommended to allow adequately designed controlled studies of cannabinoids with respect to their effect on pain as well as other illnesses. This recommendation was adopted by the AMA House of Delegates as a policy during the 2001 AMA Annual Meeting.

References
1. Pruthi S, Degnim AC, Bauer BA, DePompolo RW, Nayar V. Value of massage therapy for patients in a breast clinic. Clin J Oncol Nurs. 2009;13(4):422-425.
2. Ashikaga T, Bosompra K, O'Brien P, Nelson L. Use of complimentary and alternative medicine by breast cancer patients: prevalence, patterns and communication with physicians. Support Care Cancer. 2002;10(7):542-548.
3. Knight A, Hwa YS, Hashim H. Complementary alternative medicine use amongst breast cancer patients in the Northern region of peninsular Malaysia. Asian Pac J Cancer Prev. 2015;16(8):3125-3130.
4. Seghers L, Walenbergh-van Veen M, Salome J, Hamberg P. Cyanide intoxication by apricot kernel ingestion as complimentary cancer therapy. Neth J Med. 2013;71(9):496-498.

5. Hurt RT, Wilson T. Geriatric obesity: evaluating the evidence for the use of flavonoids to promote weight loss. J Nutr Gerontol Geriatr. 2012;31(3):269-289.

6. Torkelson C, Harris I, Kreitzer MJ. Evaluation of a complementary and alternative medicine rotation in medical school. Altern Ther Health Med. 2006;12(4):30-34.

7. Mason S, Tovey P, Long AF. Evaluating complementary medicine: methodological challenges of randomised controlled trials. BMJ. 2002;325(7368):832-834.

9. Chiropractic

Complementary and alternative medicine (CAM) is the term for medical products and practices that are not part of standard medical care. Chiropractic is a health care profession dedicated to the non-surgical treatment of disorders of the nervous system and/or musculoskeletal system. Generally, chiropractors maintain a unique focus on spinal manipulation and treatment of surrounding structures. Manual therapies commonly used by chiropractors are generally effective for the treatment of lower back pain as well as for treatment of lumbar herniated disc for radiculopathy and neck pain.

At one time conventional medicine practitioners viewed chiropractic care as quackery. Now chiropractic therapy enjoys wide acceptance by conventional medicine practitioners. Some chiropractors have been appointed to workmen's compensation boards. Some are even on staff at hospitals. Some chiropractors work closely with pain-medicine doctors. Following injections into the small joints in the back, a chiropractor may come to a hospital to adjust the back and realign the spine.

Chiropractors are involved in sports medicine Spinal manipulative therapy (SMT) and exercise may be used to treat neck pain. SMT resulted in greater pain reduction after 12 weeks of treatment.[1] Chiropractors provide medical expert testimony with respect to whiplash injuries and other injuries of the spine in courtrooms. Be aware that the relationship between chiropractors and medical doctors has improved over the past decade.

The definition of chiropractic therapy is the correction of problems that exist in the spinal column. This enables the body to function at its peak level without medications, surgical procedures, or steroid injections. In 1999, more than 25 million Americans were treated by chiropractors. Not only do chiropractors take care of back injuries, they also can help with the neck, hip, leg, ankle, foot, arm, and hand pain. Most back and neck pains are the result of mechanical disorders in one's spine.

People treated with chiropractic medicine recover faster than non-chiropractic treated patients. The problem with chiropractic medicine is that it has been maligned for a long time in the United States. However, it is now widely accepted. In Canada, which is under a national health-care system, chiropractic care is included among treatment methods that are reimbursed by the national system.

Chiropractic medicine focuses its attention on the relationship between the structure of the spine and how it affects the nervous system. A patient has 24 back bones and 31 nerves that come off of the spinal cord. The nerves come out of a hole in the bones called foramina. If the spine is not in alignment due to slouching or poor posture, this can cause some of the nerves to be compressed.

The bones in one's back form protection for the spinal cord. Be aware that the nerves coming off of the spinal cord can go to your organs and glands as well as to your muscles, bones, and nerves in your arms and legs. Your brain, which functions as a computer, sends electrical impulses that essentially regulate all of your bodily functions. When the spine is not aligned correctly, it can cause tension in muscles that will in turn affect the nervous system.

If the neck and back are not in alignment there will be a decrease in the range of motion. It can cause muscle spasms, pain, and even headaches. Be aware that blood vessels also run next to nerves that go to the arms, legs, and organs. If the spine is not aligned, there could be compression some of the blood vessels, which will make the arms and legs, feel cold. Therefore, the goal of chiropractic therapy is to correct the misalignment throughout the spine to allow the body to restore itself.

In older adults with a neuromusculoskeletal complaint, a study was done to evaluate risk of injury to the head, neck, or trunk after an office visit for chiropractic spinal manipulation compared with office visit for evaluation by primary care physician. Among Medicare beneficiaries aged 66 to 99 years with an office visit risk for a neuromusculoskeletal problem, risk of injury to the head, neck, or trunk within 7 days was 76% lower among subjects with a chiropractic office visit than among those who saw a primary care physician.2

Chiropractors complete six to seven years of college, including postgraduate study. There are 17 accredited chiropractic colleges in the United States. Chiropractors complete two years of undergraduate courses before going to chiropractic school. Chiropractors must pass a national exam and obtain a state license just like your regular medical doctor before they can practice.

The early Egyptians practiced spinal manipulation. However, in 1895, the founder of chiropractic medicine, Daniel Palmer, was a student of both physiology as well as anatomy and studied the effect of spinal manipulation on neck and back pain. The overall goal of chiropractic medicine is to treat the cause of one's pain as opposed to just treating symptoms. Periodic chiropractic adjustments can prevent everyday wear and tear on joints and ligaments throughout the spine. A chiropractor will emphasize increases in motion around the neck and back. If one receives regular chiropractic care, he or she may have better long-term relief with this method as opposed to conventional medicine methods.

Be aware that chiropractic medicine is safer than conventional medicine in the fact that no narcotics, muscle relaxants, and other potentially addicting drugs are prescribed by chiropractors. All drugs can have some side effects as well as cause some allergies. It has been shown that only sixty percent of people with back pain actually receive relief with surgery.

Among Medicare B beneficiaries aged 66 to 99 years with neck pain, incidence of vertebrobasilar stroke was extremely low. Small differences in risk between patients who saw a chiropractor and those who saw a primary care physician are probably not clinically significant.[3] Compared with routine method for cervicogenic sudden hearing loss, additional chiropractic can improve hearing and relieve neck pain effectively.[4]

Chiropractic medicine results in high patient satisfaction. This is due to the hands-on application of a chiropractor as opposed to a conventional medical specialist. A patient may be afraid that if a chiropractic physician manipulates the neck or back that one may become paralyzed. The chance of these occurrences is extremely rare. Remember, if a patient has a steroid injection in the neck or back, there is a small chance that he or she could become paralyzed as well. Studies also have shown that chiropractic medicine is cost-effective. Whether availability of chiropractic care affects use of primary care physician (PCP) services is unknown. Greater availability of chiropractic care in some areas may be offsetting PCP services for back and/or neck pain among older adults.[5]

Some chiropractors limit their practice to the spine. Other chiropractors emphasize not only spinal manipulation but treat arm and leg pain and provide nutritional counseling as well. Often chiropractors will use traction, cold packs, electrical stimulation, ultrasound, and cryotherapy to help control pain. These methods are similar to those used by physical therapists. Cryotherapy, it is the application of cold packs to tissue. The cold decreases tissue swelling and decrease pain fiber nerve ending sensitivity. Some chiropractors can even perform acupuncture and recommend herbal medicines. A large percentage of acute and importantly chronic lumbar disc herniation patients treated with chiropractic spinal manipulation reported clinically relevant improvement.[6]

A chiropractor may do a manipulation of the spine on the first visit. It is difficult to estimate how many treatments a patient will need before the pain has been significantly decreased. After the spine has been misaligned for any length of time, a body may have a tendency to resume that misalignment again. Therefore, periodic visits with a chiropractor are recommended. A chiropractor can treat neck and back injuries. Some chiropractors also treat carpal tunnel syndrome and sports injuries that limit range of motion.

A chiropractor will address a patient's posture. Steroid injections are not permanent and the effects only last from weeks to months. Chiropractic manipulation can be utilized for the rest of a patient's life. There is a limit to the amount of steroids that a patient can receive in a year and there also is a limit to the amount of medications that one can take. Remember that all of these methods can have potential side effects.

There are three degrees of ligament or muscle injuries that a patient should be aware of. An injury to a muscle is called a strain, whereas an injury to a ligament is called a sprain. If one sustains a grade I soft-tissue injury, this means that the fibers of the muscle and ligaments remain intact. A grade II injury is more serious and the fibers of the muscle or ligaments are partly torn. A grade III injury, implies that muscles or ligaments are completely ruptured or torn. At this time, the arm, leg, shoulder, hip, or knee has essentially no functional use. Grades II and III injuries need to be addressed by an orthopedic surgeon.

A chiropractor may treat a patient with the following methods: cryotherapy, paraffin baths, hydrocolator packs, and whirlpool baths. Infrared lamps and ultraviolet light also can be used to treat your pain with these methods that release heat. Ice and cold water are used to treat swelling in arms and legs after an injury. Heat is used to increase blood flow to the painful tissue. The heat can relax muscles as well. If pain is immediately under the skin, an infrared heat lamp can be used to treat pain or to relax the upper muscles in the neck and back. The heat can increase the blood flow in the skin and superficial muscles. The superficial heat also can relax some of the muscles immediately under the skin.

Another superficial method of treating pain is cryotherapy, which uses ice packs, cold sprays, cold whirlpools, or even ice massage to the body. The cold will decrease the blood flow to muscles and skin. The purpose of the reduction in the blood flow to these tissues is to decrease the swelling that follows an acute injury to tissues. Cold can decrease pain transmission to nerves. Cold spray has been used to treat the pain associated with muscle pain syndromes. Be aware that cold can decrease the speed of nerve conductions. Therefore, cold will decrease the amount of pain impulses that reach the spinal cord and ultimately the pain impulses that go to the brain.

Deep heat is another form of heat therapy that can be used to manage pain. The use of ultrasound heat is common in both chiropractic medicine as well as in physical therapy. This deep heat can provide significant pain relief and is used to treat a wide range of disorders, including bursitis and deep muscle spasms. Ultrasound consists of sound energy.

The sound waves will get the molecules of your tissue to vibrate. The vibration creates friction between the molecules of tissue and the friction is converted into heat. This type of heat goes deep into the body. Overall, ultrasound will increase circulation in many situations and provide pain relief. Deep-heat therapy as well as superficial heat therapy should not be used if a patient has had a recent injury within the past 72 hours.

Another procedure used along with the deep-heat therapy is phonophoresis. During this procedure, medications are driven under the skin to a depth of about 2 millimeters. Phonophoresis is ultrasound mixed with steroids or numbing medicine such as lidocaine. The purpose of the phonophoresis is to apply the medication at the area of your pain. All the ultrasound treatments can be used in muscle pain as well as tendonitis and bursitis.

Diathermia also is another deep-heat method. This type of heat can use microwave energy waves. This device can provide heat to the deeper muscles which can relax muscles as well as increase the blood flow to deeper muscles.

Electricity can be used to treat pain as well. Over the years, many claims have been made for the therapeutic application of electrical current for the treatment of some pain syndromes. Electrical current is applied to the body by placement of electrodes, which are patches with adhesive that stick to the body. The current is directed over the painful areas of the body.

Electrical current can vibrate the molecules of tissues similar to ultrasound therapy. The vibration produced by friction between the molecules of r tissues will increase tissue temperature. As a result, heat is produced. As electrical current passes through your tissue, some nerves are excited while others are not.

It has been shown that electricity can stimulate tissue growth and repair and is sometimes used by orthopedic surgeons to stimulate bone growth following bone surgery. Sometimes stimulators can be placed following orthopedic surgery to enhance bone growth. Theoretically, the electrical current should speed up the healing time.

A popular electrical current emitting device that is used frequently in pain medicine by conventional physicians, chiropractic physicians, and physical therapists is the transcutaneous electrical nerve stimulator (TENS). A TENS unit applies electrical current to the body through electrodes that are adhered to the body. The TENS unit is used for pain control. The power source is battery operated. TENS unit therapy became popular in the late

1960s and early 1970s. The use of a TENS unit for the treatment of chronic pain is well documented.

A TENS unit has an amplitude knob that lets one control pain relief. These TENS units are about the size of a pager. The TENS unit patches can be placed over muscles or nerves for the management of pain both in muscles as well as the nerves in the arms and legs. a TENS may be used pain control without any significant side effects. Some people however, have allergic reactions to the adhesive in the patches.

There are nonallergen TENS patches that can be purchased. A TENS unit can reduce pain as well as stress. Iontophoresis is the use of an electrical current to drive medications through the skin. Different medications can be applied through the skin to decrease pain. Not only is electrical current used for pain relief, it can also hasten tissue healing.

Traction is another method that is frequently used by chiropractors and physical therapists. Traction involves mechanical forces that separate adjacent body parts away from each other. If a patient has problems with a disc in the neck or back, traction can separate the bones in the back and increase blood flow to injured tissue, which can expedite healing.

Therapeutic massage can significantly help control pain, especially if the pain is caused by muscle spasms. Massage can decrease stress as well as decrease headaches and pain associated with whiplash injuries.

Massage therapy promotes generalized body relaxation. Massage is the application of touch to muscles or ligaments that does not cause tissue to move or change position of a joint. Massage therapy can decrease lower back pain as well as neck pain. It also has been effective to reduce pain associated with sciatica. Massage therapy can decrease the pain associated with headaches and can relieve muscle spasms as well.

There are different types of massage therapy. The Swedish massage is the most common form of massage therapy in the United States. Swedish massage works on the superficial layers of the skin as well as the superficial muscles of the body. Swedish massage promotes relaxation and improves circulation in the superficial muscles. Another type of massage is deep-tissue massage. This is more direct pressure on the deeper muscle layers of the body. Deep-tissue massage is highly effective for the treatment of lower back pain.

Sports massage combines Swedish massage with deep-tissue massage. This type of massage therapy can decrease your pain following a vigorous athletic workout. It may not be a good idea to use therapeutic massage if you have certain forms of cancer, heart disease, or some infectious diseases. If you have these conditions, massage therapy could cause some spread of your tumor if done over your tumor. Talk with your doctor before beginning massage therapy if you have any of these conditions. Women are more willing to use massage therapy. This finding should suggest that men may benefit from massage therapy if they were encouraged to use it and if they were educated in this method. Menstrual status can affect the effectiveness of massage when it is used for pain relief.

Aromatherapy is rarely practiced by conventional medical doctors in the United States but is practiced by many chiropractors. However, in France, aromatherapy is practiced by medical doctors. Studies are still being conducted on this method. To date there are no state licensing boards for practitioners of aromatherapy.

Acupuncture is another popular method that can be used for the treatment of pain. Acupuncture can decrease both pain as well as stress. Acupuncture originated in China more than 5,000 years ago. Acupuncture is based on the belief that health is determined by a balanced flow of vital life energy referred to as chi. There are 12 major energy pathways in the body called meridians. Each meridian is linked to a specific internal organ. There are more than 1,000 acupoints within the meridians of the body.

Stimulation of these meridians enhances the flow of vital life energy. Needles are inserted just under the skin to stimulate these meridians and provide pain relief. It is believed that acupuncture releases the body's own chemicals that relieve pain, called endorphins and enkephlins. These two chemicals are the body's natural pain-killing chemicals. Acupuncture can decrease the production as well as the distribution of substances that cause pain nerve impulses to go to the brain. Acupuncture, therefore, can decrease the need for conventional pain pills. Acupuncture has been demonstrated to decrease muscle-tension headaches as well.

After an examination, an acupuncturist will place 10 to 12 needles in any of the 1,000 acupoints throughout the body depending on the location of the pain complaints. The needles are small. Acupuncture is essentially painless. A patient must tell the acupuncturist if he or she is experiencing any pain during the procedure. Some treatments performed by the acupuncturist may only last several minutes, whereas other procedures can last up to 45 minutes. Instead of needles, some practitioners apply pressure to the acupoints for pain control.

In 1997, the U.S. Food and Drug Administration classified acupuncture as an actual medical device. It also has been classified as a safe method. In 1997, the National Institutes of Health endorsed acupuncture for postoperative pain, dental pain, tennis elbow, and carpal tunnel syndrome. In the

United States, people make approximately 10 million visits per year to acupuncturists.

The World Health Organization has reported that acupuncture can treat migraine headaches, trigeminal neuralgia, sciatica, and arthritis. Acupuncture also can be used to treat fibromyalgia, neck pain, and back pain. A CAM study has been shown to be effective in the control of pain in some cancer patients.[7] This study could be used to develop holistic nursing interventions and CAM use by patients undergoing cancer treatment.

Acupuncture is now being accepted by conventional medical practitioners. More than 30 percent of all conventional medical schools include reference to acupuncture as an accepted scientific method that can be used in the health-care system. Acupuncture predates Western civilization. Acupuncture, which is used more often in women, is continuing to be studied by the scientific community.

In some states there is no licensing required to be an acupuncturist, whereas other states limit the practice to medical doctors and chiropractors. In some states acupuncturists are considered primary health-care professionals and may see you without your doctor's referral. Some states require that an acupuncturist graduate from an approved school and pass a state licensing examination.

To find physicians that practice acupuncture, go to the website www.medicalacupuncture.org. Furthermore, the American Association of Oriental Medicine has a website, www.aaom.org, which is a national trade organization of acupuncturists who have met acceptable standards of competency. This organization can provide individuals with the names and locations of competent members of this organization in one's community.

The diagnosis and treatment of interstitial cystitis/bladder pain syndrome (IC/BPS) in female patients has shifted from organ-specific to a multifactorial, multidisciplinary and individualized approach. Patients with refractory and debilitating symptoms may respond to complementary and alternative medical treatments.[8] Furthermore, in females, acupuncture point injection of vitamin K3 has been shown to relieve menstrual pain rapidly.[9]

References

1. Maiers M, Bronfort G, Evans R, et al. Spinal manipulative therapy and exercise for seniors with chronic neck pain. Spine J. 2014;14(9):1879-1889.

2. Whedon JM, Mackenzie TA, Phillips RB, Lurie JD. Risk of traumatic injury associated with chiropractic spinal manipulation in Medicare Part B beneficiaries aged 66 to 99 years. Spine (Phila Pa 1976). 2015;40(4):264-270.

3. Whedon JM, Song Y, Mackenzie TA, Phillips RB, Lukovits TG, Lurie JD. Risk of stroke after chiropractic spinal manipulation in medicare B beneficiaries aged 66 to 99 years with neck pain. J Manipulative Physiol Ther. 2015;38(2):93-101.

4. Zhou X, Luo HS, He JY, Wang R, Zhuang Y, Zhan Q. [A randomized controlled trials on treatment of cervicogenic sudden hearing loss with chiropractic]. Zhongguo Gu Shang. 2015;28(1):62-65.

5. Davis MA, Yakusheva O, Gottlieb DJ, Bynum JP. Regional Supply of Chiropractic Care and Visits to Primary Care Physicians for Back and Neck Pain. J Am Board Fam Med. 2015;28(4):481-490.

6. Leemann S, Peterson CK, Schmid C, Anklin B, Humphreys BK. Outcomes of acute and chronic patients with magnetic resonance imaging-confirmed symptomatic lumbar disc herniations receiving high-velocity, low-amplitude, spinal manipulative therapy: a prospective observational cohort study with one-year follow-up. J Manipulative Physiol Ther. 2014;37(3):155-163.

7. Korkmaz M, Tavsanli NG, Ozcelik H. Use of Complementary and Alternative Medicine and Quality of Life of Cancer Patients: Turkish Samples. Holist Nurs Pract. 2016.

8. Atchley MD, Shah NM, Whitmore KE. Complementary and alternative medical therapies for interstitial cystitis: an update from the United States. Transl Androl Urol. 2015;4(6):662-667.

9. Wade C, Wang L, Zhao WJ, et al. Acupuncture point injection treatment of primary dysmenorrhoea: a randomised, double blind, controlled study. BMJ Open. 2016;6(1):e008166.

10. Nutrition

Nutrition and lifestyle, known to modulate aging process and age-related diseases, might also affect telomerase activity.[1] Short and dysfunctional telomeres rather than average telomere length are associated with longevity in animal models, and their rescue by telomerase maybe sufficient to restore cell and organismal viability. Improving telomerase activation in stem cells and potentially in other cells by diet and lifestyle interventions may represent an intriguing way to promote health-span in humans.

The fundamental principles of optimal health and optimal ageing are abstaining from smoking, modest alcohol consumption, regular physical exercise and a diet rich in fish and plants and low in condensed calories, sugar and dairy products. Pain management can pose special challenges for the elderly, as many geriatric patients take various medications to alleviate elevated blood pressure, high cholesterol, to prevent blood clots, etc.[2]

Supplementation with vitamins has little effect on ageing/prevention of chronic diseases, but anti-inflammatory molecules like polyphenols are more effective, especially when combined with reduced intake of calorie-condensed foods.[2] Drugs prescribed for pain relief may interact with existing medications, causing further health complications. The goal of geriatric pain management is to retain physical independence and well-being. Treating pain with a combination of medications, nutrition, injections, physical therapy and exercise can decrease elderly patients' pain and subsequently provide greater independence for these patients. To minimize the risk of drug interactions, doctors and patients should explore options for treating pain that do not involve pain medications.

One solution is proper nutrition to control a patient's pain. Comprehensive lifestyle changes significantly increase telomerase activity and consequently telomere maintenance capacity in human immune-system cells.[3] Anti-inflammatory molecules like polyphenols are more effective, especially when combined with reduced intake of calorie-condensed foods.

Proper nutrition, however, can be a challenge because increasing age has effects on gastrointestinal function that can ultimately affect nutrition. Secretion of gastric acid, intrinsic factor and pepsin is decreased, which then reduces the absorption of vitamins B6, B12, folate, iron and calcium. Many medications alter nutritional status in numerous ways (e.g. altered taste, dry mouth, nausea, vomiting, diarrhea or constipation). Dietary omega 3 can help to slow the aging process for example.[4]

It is recommended that a patient consult a dietician before beginning any nutritional program and discuss the program with his/her primary care physician. Increases in relative telomere length were found after bariatric surgery in the long term, presumably due to amelioration of metabolic traits. This may overrule the influence of age and baseline telomere length and facilitate telomere protection in patients experiencing pronounced weight loss.[5]

Telomerase deficiency and hence short telomeres impair replicative capacity of pancreatic beta-cells to cause impaired insulin secretion and glucose intolerance, mechanistically defining diabetes mellitus as an aging-associated disorder.[6] Regular consumption of sugar-sweetened sodas might influence metabolic disease development through accelerated cell aging.[7]

The principles of integrative nursing advocate that food be considered as a primary intervention for health promotion, risk reduction, and generally improved well-being.[8] Food provides information to the body, signaling basic biological functions and normalizing physiological processes. Health care professionals should query patients about their nutritional intake, recognizing that adjustments in the types of foods consumed can often address long-standing symptoms that create distress, including pain, fatigue, anxiety, and gastrointestinal dysfunction.

In another study, mean pain scores were significantly reduced following meals compared with the no food. The maximum reduction in pain occurred 1.5 hours after ingestion, and a significantly greater effect was exerted by the high-fat low-carbohydrate meal compared with a high-carbohydrate low-fat meal. These results demonstrate that food, significantly reduced pain in healthy human subjects.[9]

The main difference between a Nutritionist and a Dietitian is the specific credentials achieved by the individual. The definition of a Nutritionist would be any professional with an education in nutritional science of any kind, working in a capacity where they are trusted to instruct, recommend and or assist with the nutrition, diet and wellness of their clients or patients.

A Dietitian, on the other hand, under current regulations, must earn a four-year degree in dietetics or nutritional sciences from an accredited college or university, complete a regulation internship in the nutrition science field as well as pass the Registered Dietitian (RD) or Dietetic Technicians, Registered (DTR) examination authorized by the Commission on Dietetic Registration. Since the title 'nutritionist' has been used by many unqualified people to describe their involvement in food and nutrition related practice, one should be careful when choosing a qualified nutritional professional.

A previous study was done to assess the dietary quality of older women with and without rheumatoid arthritis (RA). Living with RA was associated with significantly lower dietary quality. Since even small changes in dietary quality can translate into better nutritional status, future interventions should focus on increasing dietary quality in this high-risk group.[10]

Emerging data suggest that vitamin D has a significant role in inflammatory bowel disease (IBD). Low vitamin D levels are common in IBD patients and are associated with higher morbidity and disease severity, signifying the potential importance of vitamin D monitoring and treatment.[11]

An improper diet can cause one's body to form free radicals which are chemicals, which can cause inflammation in one's body. An incorrect diet can furthermore, cause one's body to form prostaglandins. These chemicals are like hot water, which can cause pain conduction nerves to become active. These chemicals also cause inflammation in one's joints and cause muscle irritation. A pain reduction diet can reduce the stress caused by foods on one's bodily systems. A pain reduction diet can decrease effects on one's tissues by decreasing free radicals in the body which in turn can decrease inflammation. An improper diet can cause a body to form free radicals which are chemicals, which can cause inflammation in a body.

An incorrect diet can furthermore, cause a body to form prostaglandins. These chemicals are like hot water, which can cause pain conduction nerves to become active. These chemicals also cause inflammation in joints and cause muscle irritation. A pain reduction diet can reduce the stress caused by foods on bodily systems. A pain reduction diet can decrease effects on tissues by decreasing free radicals in a body which in turn decrease inflammation in a body.

Vitamin D is a potent inhibitor of the pro inflammatory response and thereby diminishes turnover of leukocytes. Leukocyte telomere length is a predictor of aging-related disease and decreases with each cell cycle and increased inflammation.[12] Higher vitamin D concentrations, which are easily modifiable through nutritional supplementation, are associated with longer telomere length, which underscores the potentially beneficial effects of this hormone on aging and age-related diseases.

In order to know something about inflammation and nutrition, a person needs to understand the concept of free radicals. Free radicals are molecules responsible for aging, tissue damage, and some diseases like arthritis. These free-radical molecules are very unstable; therefore, they look to bond with other molecules. Antioxidants, present in many foods, are molecules that prevent free radicals from harming healthy tissue. Free radicals do not have an even number of electrons, and search for an extra electron to become stable. In other words, an atom will try to fill its outer shell by gaining or losing electrons to either fill or empty its outer shell.

Free radicals can cause the disruption of a living cell. Environmental factors such as pollution, radiation, cigarette smoke and herbicides can also spawn free radicals. Normally, the body can handle free radicals, but if antioxidants are unavailable, or if the free-radical production becomes excessive, cell and tissue damage can occur. The vitamins C and E are thought to protect the body against the destructive effects of free radicals. Antioxidants neutralize free radicals by donating one of their own electrons to the free radical. Inflammation is a protective attempt by one's body to remove the injurious stimuli and to initiate the healing process. Chronic inflammation however, can lead to rheumatoid arthritis, osteoarthritis etc.

Consistent with well-known evidence of benefit or harm for chronic age-related diseases, dietary antioxidants and consumption of antioxidant-rich, plant-derived foods help maintain telomere length.13 In contrast, total and saturated fat intake and consumption of refined flour cereals, meat and meat products, and sugar-sweetened beverages relate to shorter telomeres. In one large study, greater adherence to the Mediterranean diet was associated with longer telomeres. These results further support the benefits of adherence to the Mediterranean diet for promoting health and longevity.14

Chronic inflammation is characterized by simultaneous destruction and healing of one's tissue from the inflammatory process. Inflammation is often a significant factor in causing pain. It is best to eat a low-carbohydrate diet rich in fruits and vegetables and high in Omega-3 fatty acids as found in fish and grass-fed-meats (Pasture raised beef is lower in total fat than regular beef and is rich in Omega-3 fatty acids). Most grass fed beef is organic beef.

Omega-3 fatty acids help to decrease inflammation in one's body. It appears that when one's body is inflamed, increased pain occurs. The amino acid, tryptophan (found in avocados, bananas, grapefruit, nuts, seeds, papayas, peaches, and tomatoes) encourages production of the calming neurotransmitter, serotonin. Serotonin can decrease the intensity of pain signals to one's brain.

Beneficial foods for pain reduction include broccoli, cauliflower, winter squashes, sesame seeds and flax seeds. Strawberries contain natural salicylates (aspirin like substances), and are anti-inflammatory. Inflammation as mentioned at the beginning of this chapter is often a factor in pain causation. Enzymes, present in unheated vegetables, reduce inflammation, which is usually a factor in one's pain.

Apples contain boron, a mineral that may reduce the risk of developing osteoarthritis and help decrease joint pain, swelling and stiffness in people who have arthritis. Some people report arthritis pain relief with apple cider vinegar. Apples are a great food to relieve irritable bowel pain. However, one's should peel the apple before eating it.

Chile peppers contain capsaicin. It has been demonstrated that after ingesting capsaicin containing foods the reduction in pain is directly proportional to the concentration of capsaicin present. When capsaicin is applied to inflamed oral mucosa, the pain diminishes as the burning sensation caused by capsaicin subsides. Green tea is an effective anti-oxidant as well, and has various other properties, which will help in treating arthritis pain.

Black bean broth has been proven to be very effective in relieving one's body's inflammatory response and acts as an analgesic on pain nerves and works within the brain to reduce pain sensitivity. An extract made from avocado and soybean oils placed in a tea can improve the pain and stiffness of knee and hip osteoarthritis and reduce the need for non-steroidal anti-inflammatory drugs. It appears to decrease inflammation and stimulate cartilage repair in joints.

Patients who suffer from gallbladder pain may want to eat beets because they may relieve gallbladder pain in some individuals. In addition, they benefit the liver and the betaine they contain has also been shown to improve the function of liver cells. Cherries contain anthocyanins 1 and 2 that researchers believe can have a significant impact on relieving muscle and joint soreness more quickly. Cherries' powerful bundle of antioxidants and carbohydrates offer added nutrition active people need.

Vitamin B1, B2, B5, B6, B12 rich foods, such as fish, peas, broccoli, prunes, raisins, oatmeal, avocados, asparagus, bananas, spinach, walnuts, sunflower seeds, broccoli, Brussels sprouts, mushrooms, brown rice, cabbage, cantaloupe, salmon, seafood, yogurt, whole grains and nuts may help alleviate some types of headache pain. For pulsating, stabbing headaches eat Vitamin A rich foods, such as apricots, asparagus, beet greens, broccoli, carrots, cantaloupe, collards, dandelion greens, fish oil, garlic, papaya, peaches, red peppers, sweet potatoes, and yellow squash.

The specific arthritis fighting nutrients like folate and vitamin B6 is in the right proportion in a banana. In general for full chronic pain eat a wide range of deep-sea food. Raw cabbage juice has been shown to help relieve ulcer pain. Bananas also can help lower stomach acids and coats the stomach with a special compound that gives a protective lining, allowing the ulcer to heal.

Garlic taken orally strengthens one's immune system and facilitates back pain healing. Garlic may relieve tooth pain as well. Daily doses of raw or heat-treated ginger are effective for relieving muscle pain following strenuous exercise. Ginger can relieve pain for those patients with rheumatoid arthritis and osteoarthritis. Its uses for pain relief cover many different kinds of pain. One may want to cook one's food in extra-virgin olive oil.

Extra-virgin olive oil contains a compound called oleocanthal that acts in the same way ibuprofen does to relieve pain. Oleocanthal acts as a natural anti-inflammatory by inhibiting COX-2 enzymes in the same way Celebrex does. COX-2 enzymes take part in the process of joint inflammation that can lead to arthritic pain.

The olive oil may relieve some of the pain associated with fibromyalgia. Olive oil which includes genomic instability, telomere attrition, epigenetic alterations, loss of proteostasis, deregulated nutrient sensing, mitochondrial dysfunction, cellular senescence, stem cell exhaustion and altered intracellular communication.

Virtually all these hallmarks are targeted by dietary olive oil, particularly by virgin olive oil, since many of its beneficial effects can be accounted not only for the monounsaturated nature of its predominant fatty acid (oleic acid), but also for the bioactivity of its minor compounds, which can act on cells though both direct and indirect mechanisms due to their ability to modulate gene expression.[15] Greater vegetable consumption might modify telomere-related hypertension risk[16]

One's diet should include foods that contain the antioxidants Vitamin A, Vitamin C, Vitamin D, and Vitamin E. Vitamin A is in yellow-orange fruits and vegetables, such as apricots, sweet potatoes, pumpkin, carrots, peaches, and winter squash. It is also in dark green leafy vegetables such as broccoli, spinach, collard greens and parsley. Vitamin C is in cantaloupe, grapefruit, papaya, kiwi, oranges, mangoes, raspberries, pineapples, strawberries, Brussels sprouts, collard greens, cabbage and asparagus. Concentrated food sources of vitamin D include salmon, sardines, shrimp, milk, cod, and eggs. Vitamin E is found in cold-pressed olive oil, sunflower seeds, wheat germ, nuts, avocados, whole-grain breads and cereals, dried prunes, and peanut butter.

Apples and grapes contain minerals called boron, which is known to reduce the risk of developing osteoarthritis. And by itself, boron has been shown to help build strong bones and reduce the pain of those who already have the disease. Garlic contains sulfur, which is used to treat arthritis. Curry contains quite a few powerful antioxidants that fight pain and inflammation. Mushrooms may be effective for treating fibromyalgia, and chronic fatigue.

Beverages can help one's decrease one's pain as well. Drinking eight glasses of water a day is the recommended amount, which in the case of arthritis, flushes uric acid from one's body, thereby reducing pain. Juicing is one of the most efficient ways to get a large amount of nutrients and vitamins into one's diet as well.

In chronic hepatitis C, coffee consumption induces a reduction in oxidative damage, correlated with increased telomere length, with lower collagen synthesis which are factors that mediate the protection exerted by coffee with respect to disease progression.[17] Coffee is an important source of antioxidants, and consumption of this beverage is associated with many health conditions and a lower mortality risk. Higher coffee consumption is associated with longer telomeres in individuals. Future studies are needed to better understand the influence of coffee consumption on telomeres, which may uncover new knowledge of how coffee consumption affects personal health and longevity.[18]

There are some foods and beverages that one should avoid. Avoid all fried foods. These foods may increase one's free radicals which can cause inflammation in the body. Alcohol, cola drinks, sugar and chocolate should also be avoided. Some elderly persons drink alcohol for pain relief. Wine can be heart protective in moderation, but it does not decrease one's pain. Alcohol has no direct pain relieving properties. Alcohol abuse advances osteoporosis and some forms of arthritis, especially gouty arthritis which may cause severe pain. Alcohol consumption can also lead to muscle atrophy, which can increase muscle pain and weakness as well. Chronic excessive intake of alcohol can cause destruction of one's pancreas resulting in severe chronic pain, and may cause pancreatic cancer.

Some foods and drinks can make irritable bowel (IBS) pain worse. Foods and drinks that may cause or worsen symptoms include; fatty foods like French fries, milk products, cheese or ice cream, chocolate, alcohol, caffeinated and carbonated drinks. One should avoid sugar and sugar products. In the body, sugar that isn't used immediately to create energy is stored in the body. Sugar causes the body to release insulin from the pancreas. The insulin takes the glucose to one's cells that have insulin receptors and utilizes it in one of three places: about 50% is used for immediate energy, 2) about 10% is stored in one's muscle and liver as glycogen and 3) approximately 40% is stored as fats. Many people will notice an increase in joint, muscle or headaches soon after sugar intake.

One needs to be aware that cancer cells have many times more insulin receptors compared to normal cells and require more glucose for growth. Therefore, high sugar intake may associate with an increased cancer risk. A patient also needs to know that when carbohydrates are broken down for energy formation in the body, certain vitamins and minerals that are antioxidants are needed for proper carbohydrate processing. As a result, vitamin and mineral depletion may take place. This action could increase one's pain by increasing inflammation throughout the body.

References

1. Boccardi V, Paolisso G, Mecocci P. Nutrition and lifestyle in healthy aging: the telomerase challenge. Aging (Albany NY). 2016;8(1):12-15.
2. Bengmark S. Impact of nutrition on ageing and disease. Curr Opin Clin Nutr Metab Care. 2006;9(1):2-7.
3. Ornish D, Lin J, Daubenmier J, et al. Increased telomerase activity and comprehensive lifestyle changes: a pilot study. Lancet Oncol. 2008;9(11):1048-1057.
4. Laye S. What do you eat? Dietary omega 3 can help to slow the aging process. Brain Behav Immun. 2013;28:14-15.
5. Laimer M, Melmer A, Lamina C, et al. Telomere length increase after weight loss induced by bariatric surgery: results from a 10 year prospective study. Int J Obes (Lond). 2016;40(5):773-778.
6. Kuhlow D, Florian S, von Figura G, et al. Telomerase deficiency impairs glucose metabolism and insulin secretion. Aging (Albany NY). 2010;2(10):650-658.
7. Leung CW, Laraia BA, Needham BL, et al. Soda and cell aging: associations between sugar-sweetened beverage consumption and leukocyte telomere length in healthy adults from the National Health and Nutrition Examination Surveys. Am J Public Health. 2014;104(12):2425-2431.
8. Sandquist L. Food First: Nutrition as the Foundation for Health. Creat Nurs. 2015;21(4):213-221.
9. Zmarzty SA, Wells AS, Read NW. The influence of food on pain perception in healthy human volunteers. Physiol Behav. 1997;62(1):185-191.
10. Grimstvedt ME, Woolf K, Milliron BJ, Manore MM. Lower Healthy Eating Index-2005 dietary quality scores in older women with rheumatoid arthritis v. healthy controls. Public Health Nutr. 2010;13(8):1170-1177.
11. Kabbani TA, Koutroubakis IE, Schoen RE, et al. Association of Vitamin D Level With Clinical Status in Inflammatory Bowel Disease: A 5-Year Longitudinal Study. Am J Gastroenterol. 2016;111(5):712-719.
12. Richards JB, Valdes AM, Gardner JP, et al. Higher serum vitamin D concentrations are associated with longer leukocyte telomere length in women. Am J Clin Nutr. 2007;86(5):1420-1425.

13. Freitas-Simoes TM, Ros E, Sala-Vila A. Nutrients, foods, dietary patterns and telomere length: Update of epidemiological studies and randomized trials. Metabolism. 2016;65(4):406-415.

14. Crous-Bou M, Fung TT, Prescott J, et al. Mediterranean diet and telomere length in Nurses' Health Study: population based cohort study. BMJ. 2014;349:g6674.

15. Fernandez del Rio L, Gutierrez-Casado E, Varela-Lopez A, Villalba JM. Olive Oil and the Hallmarks of Aging. Molecules. 2016;21(2):163.

16. Lian F, Wang J, Huang X, et al. Effect of vegetable consumption on the association between peripheral leucocyte telomere length and hypertension: a case-control study. BMJ Open. 2015;5(11):e009305.

17. Cardin R, Piciocchi M, Martines D, Scribano L, Petracco M, Farinati F. Effects of coffee consumption in chronic hepatitis C: a randomized controlled trial. Dig Liver Dis. 2013;45(6):499-504.

18. Liu JJ, Crous-Bou M, Giovannucci E, De Vivo I. Coffee Consumption Is Positively Associated with Longer Leukocyte Telomere Length in the Nurses' Health Study. J Nutr. 2016;146(7):1373-1378.

11. Opioids

Pain management is an ongoing issue in the elderly, and remains underestimated and under-treated in this fragile population. Pain management in the elderly has increasingly become problematic in the USA as the aged population grows. The proportion of the population over 65 continues to climb and may eclipse 20 % in the next decade.[1]

The use of opioid drugs is sometimes necessary for the management of pain in elderly patients. Opioids are a type of medication used to relieve pain. Guidelines from the American Geriatrics Society (AGS) say elderly people with chronic pain may be better off taking opioid painkillers such as codeine rather than over-the-counter products such as ibuprofen. Analyses of Medicare Part D data demonstrated a substantial growth in opioid prescriptions from 2007 to 2011 and large variation in opioid prescriptions across states.[2]

Opioids are a class of drugs, which depress the central nervous system to relieve pain. An opioid is a drug that acts similarly to morphine. Some opioids are found naturally in the environment, whereas others are made in a lab. Opioids as a class, applies to drugs like morphine as well as to any type of substance that could cause one to become dependent on it. Chronic pain has a high prevalence in the aging population. Strong opioids also should be considered in older people for the treatment of moderate to severe pain or for pain that impairs functioning and the quality of life.[3]

Compared with younger patients, elderly patients show measurable pharmacokinetic differences that result in higher, more prolonged plasma drug concentrations, which may cause more adverse effects, toxicity, and unfavorable drug interactions. In addition, drug effects can be different for aged patients, even when their plasma drug concentrations are similar to those of younger patients. A retrospective analysis of patients who used fentanyl-based intravenous patient-controlled analgesia (IV-PCA) after surgery, evaluated the difference between young and elderly patients on their characteristic of adverse effects.[4] When fentanyl-based IV-PCA is used for postoperative pain control, a larger proportion of young patients required rescue analgesics while elderly patients required more rescue antiemetics.

The elderly patient's clinician should start analgesics at low doses. In general, one should begin with half of the usual adult dose and slowly titrate upward. Medications with a short half-life decrease the risk of over accumulation while they are being titrated to steady state. Prescribing one drug at a time avoids unnecessary additive effects.

Pain is a widespread symptom in clinical practice. Older adults and chronically ill patients are particularly affected. In multi morbid geriatric patients, pharmacological pain treatment is an extension of previously existing multi medications. Besides the efficacy of pain treatment, drug side effects and drug-drug interactions have to be taken into account to minimize the health risk for these patients.[5] Apart from the number of prescriptions, the age-related pharmacokinetic and pharmacodynamic changes significantly increase the risk among older adults.

The risk of sedation in combination with other drugs, tramadol and other opioids can induce the serotonin syndrome. Among older adults, especially in the case of polypharmacy, an individualized approach should be considered instead of sticking to the pain management recommended by the World Health Organization in order to minimize drug-drug interactions and adverse drug reactions.

Over a third of patients with rheumatoid arthritis use opioids in some form, and in more than a tenth use is chronic. Use has increased in recent years. Patients aged 50-64 with rheumatoid arthritis use substantially more opioids than their non-rheumatoid arthritis RA counterparts.[6]

Morphine is the drug that has been studied the most with respect to the treatment of pain. Morphine was named after Morpheus, the Greek god of dreams. It is prepared from the liquid of the opium poppy plant. Morphine was the first opioid ever used for pain relief. Morphine is primarily metabolized in the liver, and its metabolites are excreted by the kidneys. Thus, elderly patients with liver or kidney disease need lower dosages or longer dosing intervals. Morphine is metabolized in the body primarily to morphine-3-glucuronide (M3G) and morphine-6-glucuronide (M6G). M6G has high pain relieving properties.

Naturally occurring types of opioid drugs include morphine and codeine. Man-made types of opioids include fentanyl, meperidine (Demerol), and methadone. Altering naturally occurring opioids will produce a semisynthetic drug, such as heroin. It is not uncommon for a doctor to prescribe opioids for treating severe pain. However, doctors are sometimes afraid of prescribing these drugs because of the potential for abuse. If prescribed correctly, nevertheless, opioid drugs are safe and effective for treating both cancer and noncancerous types of pain. It is important that the patient and their physician understand how opioids work and how the patient should use them appropriately if they are prescribed for the treatment of their pain.

Opioids bind themselves to receptors on nerves in the body that are located in the central nervous system and in the peripheral nerves in the arms and legs. When the opioid attaches to one of the receptors, it turns on the receptor. When the receptor is turned on, the numbers of pain sensations that reach the brain are lessened. Opioid drugs can either be classified as weak or strong, depending on how they interact with the opioid receptors in the body. Codeine and propoxyphene (Darvon) are considered weak opioids. Darvon has been taken off the market because of heart problems associated with this drug. All others are considered strong opioids.

All opioid drugs provide pain relief by decreasing the amount of chemicals that transmit pain in the nervous system. With this decrease in the chemicals that transmit pain, the overall numbers of pain impulses are dampened or may not even reach the brain at all. Some opioid medications can alter the mood or occasionally cause the patient to experience euphoria or excitement.

Changes in the chemicals that exist in the brain cause these types of mood changes. When a patient takes opioids over a large time span of weeks or months, the patient can build up a tolerance to the effect of the opioids. When the patient becomes tolerant to the opioid, its ability to relieve the pain is lessened, and more of the drug is needed to relieve it.

Opioid drugs can be further classified into three categories: agonist, antagonist, and mixed agonist/antagonist. The agonist drugs such as morphine attach to two of the three opioid receptors in the brain and spinal cord to provide pain relief by switching the receptors on. Antagonist drugs bind to all three types of receptors throughout the body. When they bind to the receptor, they do not switch the receptor on. The mixed agonist/antagonist drugs stimulate activities at the opioid receptors, but do not allow them to be switched on.

Morphine is classified as a naturally occurring agonist drug. It has been made into a slow-release formula. The slow-release morphine (MS Contin) needs to be taken only every 12 hours. It allows a gradual release of morphine as the pill passes through the stomach and intestine. Codeine is considered a weak agonist drug and is not commonly used for severe pain management. It is often used for mild pain, whereas morphine is used for more extreme types of pain. Codeine also is less likely to cause addiction than other opioids. When codeine enters the body, it is converted into morphine, which produces its pain-relieving effects.

An example of a synthetic opioid is methadone. Methadone lasts a long time in the body. This drug offers an advantage to patients because less-frequent dosing is required. Methadone is an excellent medication for use in patients who have some component of their pain that is related to nerve inflammation such as shingles or reflex sympathetic dystrophy.

Propoxyphene (Darvon) is a drug that is not sold by pharmacies nor is it prescribed anymore. It is related in its chemical structure with methadone. Its pain-relieving effects have been claimed to be less than that of aspirin. The advantage of this drug is that it has Novocain like activity. It has been shown in animals to be a potent local anesthetic. This drug may be effective in patients suffering from mild cases of shingles or mild cases of nerve inflammation as seen in the later stages of reflex sympathetic dystrophy where the patient is getting progressively better.

Darvon has been removed from the pharmaceutical market because it caused heart problems. The opioid analgesic propoxyphene was withdrawn from the US market in 2010, motivated by concerns regarding fatality in overdose and adverse cardiac effects.[7] Multiple studies have found propoxyphene to be no more effective than acetaminophen, yet propoxyphene causes opioid side effects and has been involved in many drug-related deaths.[8]

Meperidine (Demerol) can cause seizures if it is administered for a long time in patients. The medication fentanyl was originally used for anesthesia during surgery. However, fentanyl can now be administered by a patch or by a lozenge. It also is available in a sucker form for administering to children. Fentanyl is one of the most powerful drugs that have been previously mentioned.

The fentanyl (Duragesic) patch was introduced in the late 1980s. It became popular for the treatment of chronic cancer pain. In patients who are unable to swallow or have persistent diarrhea, the patch will provide continuous pain relief. The effects of fentanyl are 70 times more powerful than morphine. It is readily absorbed through the skin. The patch holds the fentanyl in a small amount of alcohol in a gel. The gel is deposited in a drug reservoir within the patch.

Between the reservoir and the skin is a membrane that is regulated by various-size holes. An adhesive layer keeps the patch attached to the skin. When the patch is applied to the skin, the drug spreads through the holes in the membrane to the skin. The fentanyl is then concentrated in the outermost layer of the skin. As the drug is deposited in the skin, it is gradually taken from the skin into the bloodstream. It takes at least 60 minutes before any fentanyl actually is detected in a patient's blood.

It takes approximately six hours before pain relief is noted after applying the patch. After the initial patch, placement of subsequent patches does not have a delay in the onset of pain relief. It should be noted that an increase in temperature will increase the absorption of the drug from the patch. This can cause side effects or even an overdose of the fentanyl. The patients using the fentanyl patch should not use a heating blanket, sun lamp, or a warm bathing tub. In cancer patients, patient acceptance is high. Occasionally, patients using the patch will have an episode of temporary pain called breakthrough pain. This pain is seen if a patient becomes overly active.

Fentanyl patches may cause significant mental and cognitive side effects in elderly patients. Thus, a patient and his spouse or caregiver should be aware of the possible side effects of a fentanyl patch and know what to do if experienced. The effects of the patch can be altered in elderly patients because of minimal fat stores, muscle wasting, altered clearance rates, improper administration, and non-adherent patches.

In addition, absorption of fentanyl might be increased in a hot environment. It is also important to remember that when titrating the dose, the shortest titration period is three days because of the extended time required for the plasma concentrations of the drug to stabilize. A fentanyl lozenge (Actiq) has been introduced, which has a relatively fast onset. The fentanyl lozenge can be used to enhance the effects of the fentanyl patch.

Tramadol (Ultram) is a synthetic chemical similar to codeine. Tramadol is indicated for the management of moderate to moderately severe pain in adults. It also increases serotonin and norepinephrine in their brain and spinal cord. These are two chemicals within the central nervous system that decrease feelings of depression. Serotonin and norepinephrine also decrease the number of pain impulses that ultimately reach their brain. Tramadol also can be combined with acetaminophen (Ultracet) to provide mild pain-relieving effects.

In general, dose selection for an aging patient over 65 years old should be cautious, usually starting at the low end of the dosing range, reflecting the greater frequency of decreased hepatic, renal or cardiac function and of concomitant disease or other drug therapy. For elderly patients over 75 years old, the total dose should not exceed 300 mg/day.

Tramadol would appear to be particularly useful in the elderly population affected by osteoarthritis because, unlike nonsteroidal anti-inflammatory drugs, it does not aggravate hypertension or congestive heart failure, nor does it have the potential to cause peptic ulcer disease. Compared with narcotics, tramadol does not induce consequential respiratory depression, constipation, or have consequential abuse potential. Serotonin is a chemical a body produces that's needed for nerve cells and brain to function. But too much serotonin causes symptoms that can range from mild (shivering and diarrhea) to severe (muscle rigidity, fever and seizures). A severe serotonin syndrome can be fatal if not treated.

Butorphanol (Stadol nasal spray) and nalbuphine (Nubain) are agonist/antagonist drugs. Butorphanol is available as a nasal spray and is now in a generic form. Nalbuphine is another agonist/antagonist drug that is available only intravenously. Elderly patients may be sensitive to butorphanol. In clinical studies of nasal Stadol, elderly patients had an increased frequency of headache, dizziness, drowsiness, vertigo, constipation, nausea and/or vomiting, and nasal congestion compared with younger patients.

Side effects of opioids can include drowsiness, alteration in mood, and mental clouding. If the dosage is too high, ther ability to concentrate can be affected. Opioid drugs can decrease their breathing rate. If the dosage of the opioid is high enough, it is possible for the patient to completely quit breathing. Nausea and vomiting are common with all the opioids. The opioid drugs can decrease pupil size. This is a result of stimulation of part of a nerve of the eye that controls the opening and closing of the pupil.

The morphine like drugs decrease the cough reflex and can be useful in this matter. If the dose of the opioids is too high, it can decrease ther blood pressure. Opioids can cause constipation. They cause constipation by decreasing the ability of the stomach and bowel to push food through to the rectum. Some of the agonist drugs also can cause hives.

Oxymorphone is an opioid that is not broken down in the liver to another substance. Oxycodone is broken down in ther liver to oxymorphone. This is why some physicians prescribe Opana, which is available in an immediate release form and an extended release form. This drug may be useful if the patients are taking many different medications.

Nucynta (tapentadol) is a medicine used in adults to treat moderate to severe pain. Be aware that this medication may cause a serious side effect if a patient is taking antidepressant medications. A serotonin syndrome is a rare, life-threatening problem that could happen if the take Nucynta with certain antidepressant/psychiatric medications and with migraine treatments known as triptans.

Animal studies have demonstrated the differences between males and females with respect to responses to opioids. Male rats have demonstrated greater pain relief with morphine than female rats following painful stimuli. In another laboratory study, there were no sex differences reported with fentanyl and buprenorphine. The same types of effects have been found in people. There is no information on the effects of opioids in older animals and the younger animals.

Gender-specific issues exist with respect to opioids. Elderly men respond better to some opioids than women. For example, women have more side effects than men do while taking Oxycontin. It is interesting to note that when a placebo (sugar pill) is given to men and women in clinical drug studies, their response to the placebo is equal.

The difference between the effects of opioids on men and women may be related to the different sex hormones that are located on their receptors. Receptors on cells differ between men and women. One study has shown that when the female hormone estrogen is given to males, and the male hormone androgen is given to women; the effects are different from when female hormones are given to women, and male hormones are given to men. This observation implies that ther receptors are affected by their sex hormones. Kappa opioid analgesia is greater in females than in males, even in elderly patients when compared to males.

The amount of drugs and the frequency of dosing also should differ between men and women. Examinations of pharmacological textbooks as well as the Physician's Desk Reference do not specify gender differences in the dosing and frequency of dosing. These factors need to be addressed with future studies. More women are addicted to cocaine than men. The reason for this observation may be due to the effects of female hormones on the addictive pathway in the female central nervous system.

Older women may need less morphine analgesia postoperatively, while pain sensitivity tends to increase particularly in elderly men. However, the net effects of changes in opioid pharmacology with age on clinical opioid analgesia remain unclear, probably due to the significantly greater variability in body function with increasing age.

Testosterone can affect the response to opioids in both men and women. Testosterone is usually decreased in both elderly men and women. Their doctor may evaluate their testosterone levels when treating the elderly patient with opioids.

Older Americans are becoming addicted to prescription drugs. Barriers to effective pain management are, however, well documented. Elderly women represent one of the fast-growing age groups impacted by the increased abuse of prescription drugs throughout our society. A significant barrier between doctors and patients' families is a fear that the use of opioid analgesics to manage pain will contribute to the development of drug addiction. If they are suffering from both acute and chronic pain, one should share a concern about these issues.

Lack of doctor as well as patient knowledge about addiction and the proper use of opioids can lead to a phobia of opioids and result in an under use of these medications based on the fear of drug addiction. Drug abusers exhibit significantly shorter telomere lengths.9 The time before relapse also presented an inverse correlation with telomere length. Drug abusers who had used heroin and diazepam displayed shorter telomere lengths than those taking other drugs.

It is imperative that the patient's pain be controlled, and that the must be treated with both dignity as well as compassion by the treating doctor even if they have a history of substance abuse. The problem exists in that many drug-seeking individuals will seek out a pain-medicine doctor to receive opioid drugs. This type of behavior eventually leads to state regulations that eventually make it more difficult for legitimate patients to get prescriptions for their medications.

Most pain-medicine specialists require that a patient sign a pain contract when the patient is admitted into the doctor's practice. The contract states that the patient will obtain pain-relieving medications from only one doctor and will use just one pharmacy. These contracts are usually mandated by state medical boards. Urine drug screens are randomly done to ensure compliance with respect to taking the prescribed medications.

A doctor treating a patient with significant pain must provide comfort to the patient. Each year, more than a million patients are prescribed opioid analgesics but do not develop addiction. A study published in 1996 reported that there was no significant difference in the rate of substance abuse among patients with severe chronic back pain versus a controlled group without back pain. An important conclusion was derived. These investigators concluded that severe pain is not associated with an increased risk for substance abuse. If the patients are taking medications for pain relief, their chances of becoming addicted are extremely low.

It is important in the management of any severe chronic pain condition that the patient and their family overcome the fear that the pain patient will become an addict. The patient and other patients must have the opportunity to use proper opioid medications to control extreme pain. It is imperative that the patient and other patients do not endure unnecessary pain and suffering.

Over the past 10 years, pain treatment has been given much more attention by the media. The lay press has provided news coverage of new medications as well as new technologies for pain management. However, the majority of the news articles fail to mention that opioids as a class remain the safest and most effective way to manage significant painful conditions.

Opioid medications are readily used in the cancer patients. In contrast, opioids have been underused in noncancerous patients suffering from severe chronic pain. For the majority of the past century, the prevailing medical opinion was that the use of opioids for the treatment of noncancerous pain was inappropriate. This thinking was at the state medical board level. However, following the neurobiological studies that began in the 1970s, the medical community has, for the most part, changed their attitudes toward opioid prescribing. Opioid drugs are now being used more aggressively in both cancer pain management as well as noncancerous pain management.

The demand for an increased use of opioids exists. However, this demand comes at a time when the United States is confronted with widespread drug abuse and drug trafficking. An examination of the history of opioid use over the centuries demonstrated that there have been periods of liberal opioid use for the treatment of pain which were followed by periods that prohibited the prescribing of opioids. It is felt that this is a result of the adverse patient consequences associated with opioid prescribing.

In today's medical environment, doctors must use opioids for their pain relieving qualities but at the same time minimize adverse effects of the drugs that may result from their chronic use. The prescribing doctor may require the patient to have a urine drug screen on occasion. The patient will urinate in a cup. The cup will be sent to a laboratory. Using mass spectrometry, the laboratory can identify which drug patients are taking as well as which prescribed drug the patients are not taking.

References

1. Jones MR, Ehrhardt KP, Ripoll JG, et al. Pain in the Elderly. Curr Pain Headache Rep. 2016;20(4):23.

2. Kuo YF, Raji MA, Chen NW, Hasan H, Goodwin JS. Trends in Opioid Prescriptions Among Part D Medicare Recipients From 2007 to 2012. Am J Med. 2016;129(2):221 e221-230.

3. Lazzari M, Marcassa C, Natoli S, et al. Switching to low-dose oral prolonged-release oxycodone/naloxone from WHO-Step I drugs in elderly patients with chronic pain at high risk of early opioid discontinuation. Clin Interv Aging. 2016;11:641-649.

4. Koh JC, Lee J, Kim SY, Choi S, Han DW. Postoperative Pain and Intravenous Patient-Controlled Analgesia-Related Adverse Effects in Young and Elderly Patients: A Retrospective Analysis of 10,575 Patients. Medicine (Baltimore). 2015;94(45):e2008.

5. Gosch M. [Analgesics in geriatric patients. Adverse side effects and interactions]. Z Gerontol Geriatr. 2015;48(5):483-492; quiz 493.

6. Zamora-Legoff JA, Achenbach SJ, Crowson CS, Krause ML, Davis JM, 3rd, Matteson EL. Opioid use in patients with rheumatoid arthritis

2005-2014: a population-based comparative study. Clin Rheumatol. 2016;35(5):1137-1144.

7. Ray WA, Murray KT, Kawai V, et al. Propoxyphene and the risk of out-of-hospital death. Pharmacoepidemiol Drug Saf. 2013;22(4):403-412.

8. Mort JR, Schroeder SD. Propoxyphene and pain management in the elderly. S D Med. 2009;62(11):433-435.

9. Yang Z, Ye J, Li C, et al. Drug addiction is associated with leukocyte telomere length. Sci Rep. 2013;3:1542.

12. Addiction

In 2000, people aged 65 and older made up 12.4 percent of the U.S. population. It has been estimated that pain occurs in from 45 percent to 85 percent of the geriatric population. Much of it is undertreated. Undertreated pain leads to other problems, including reduced quality of life, decreased socialization, depression, sleep disturbances, cognitive impairment, and malnutrition.[1]

Alcohol and drug abuse affect people at all ages, including the elderly population. An individual may have been abusing drugs or alcohol for years, or may start as a way of dealing with feelings of grief, financial difficulties, loneliness, or medical problems. Some senior citizens may begin abusing medications that were prescribed to them for legitimate medical issues. Nearly 25 percent of all prescription drugs dispensed in the United States are consumed by the elderly. Results of one study suggest that smoking dependence may predict more frequent use of opioids.[2]

Prescription drug abuse is present in 12% to 15% of aging individuals. Elderly patient substance abuse is often linked to medical problems and the emotional trauma that can accompany old age. There is now an increase in heroin and cocaine addiction at the front end of the baby-boom wave. Many times, seniors will hide their abuse by visiting several different doctors and not fully informing their doctors of their current prescription intake.

Drugs are chemicals that have a profound impact on the neurochemical balance in the brain. This action affects how one feels and acts. People, who are suffering emotionally, sometimes use drugs to escape from their problems. This can lead to drug abuse and addiction.

Some physicians are afraid to prescribe scheduled drugs because of the possibility of causing addiction. Addiction is a chronic relapsing brain disease. Brain imaging shows that addiction severely alters your brain areas critical to decision-making, learning and memory, and behavior control, which may help to explain the compulsive and destructive behaviors of addiction.

Frail older adults have a high prevalence of chronic pain with major effects on function and quality of life. Many analgesics, including opioids, have adverse effects on older adults with multiple co-morbidities. It has been reported that methadone is an excellent choice for pain management in frail older adults.[3]

The impact of poorly managed chronic pain on the quality of life of elderly patients and the problems related to its management are widely acknowledged. Underutilization of opioids is a major component of poor pain management in this group of patients, despite good evidence for the effectiveness of opioids and published guidelines directing their usage.[4]

Reasons for this underutilization are, among others, poor assessment of pain in this age group; fear of polypharmacy and opioid phobia; and avoidance of opioids because of concerns about tolerance, physical dependence, addiction and adverse effects. With appropriate dosing, vigilant management, and careful tapering, opioids are a safe and effective choice for pain management in older adults.[5]

An addiction is a recurring problem by an individual to engage in some specific activity, despite harmful consequences to the individual's health, mental state or social life. An addiction can occur with drugs, gambling, overeating, etc. Narcotic drugs can make one euphoric. As a result, a patient may request more and more drugs to maintain this euphoria.

Drug abuse or substance abuse, involves the repeated and excessive use of prescription or street drugs. In one way or another, almost all narcotic drugs over stimulate the pleasure center within the brain, flooding it with the neurotransmitter dopamine which produces euphoria. That heightened sense of pleasure can be so compelling that the brain wants that feeling back, again and again.

Addiction is frequently found in people with a wide variety of mental illnesses, including anxiety disorders, unipolar and bipolar depression, schizophrenia, and borderline and other personality disorders. Methadone can be used for the treatment of pain in addicted patients. Methadone is also an opiate that prevents users from getting high on heroin by competing with the much more potent opiates for the body's opiate receptors. Buprenorphine is another drug that is effective in the treatment of addiction and is in addition an analgesic.

Drug abusers exhibit significantly shorter telomere length than controls. The time before relapse also presented an inverse correlation with telomere length. Drug abusers who had used heroin and diazepam displayed a shorter telomere length than those taking other drugs. Drug abusers who had ingested drugs via snuff exhibited longer telomere lengths than those using other methods. These observations may offer a partial explanation for the effects of drug addiction on health.[6]

Addiction and drug dependence occur when drugs become so important that a patient is willing to sacrifice work, home and even one's family. Once the brain and body get used to the substances a patient is taking, a patient begins to require increasingly larger and more frequent doses, in order to achieve the same effect. Narcotics such as Heroin may over-stimulate the pleasure centers within the brain producing euphoric effects that cause compulsive drug-seeking behaviors. The severities of withdrawal symptoms associated with narcotics include chills, shakes, muscle pain, nausea, vomiting, and headaches and cravings.

A clinician must be able to distinguish between legitimate patients with chronic pain, and individuals engaged in non-therapeutic drug seeking behavior. Physicians have for years recognized the value of opioid analgesics in relieving lasting pain. Unfortunately, drug seekers may also request opioid analgesics. They do this by feigning illnesses, and seek controlled substances from multiple doctors and by forge prescriptions. Drug seekers may be difficult to distinguish from true chronic pain sufferers.

In general, drug seekers prefer illicit drugs such as heroin and cocaine in contrast to prescription drugs. Prescription drugs, however, have advantages over illicit drugs. Third-party insurers or welfare-entitlement programs may pay for prescribed narcotic drugs. Prescription pharmaceuticals are obtained in the safety of the physician's office. Drug abuse and addiction have a devastating impact on society. Heroin use alone is accountable for the epidemic number of new cases of HIV/AIDS and hepatitis. Drug abuse is responsible for increased healthcare costs, and an escalation of domestic violence and violent crimes.

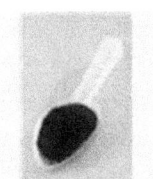

Figure 1. Drug addiction is a serious public health problem in the United States.

An estimated 20 percent of people in the United States have used prescription drugs for nonmedical reasons. Central nervous stimulants, depressants and opioids are prescription drugs that are frequently abused. Central nervous system depressants (e.g. Valium) are used to treat anxiety, panic attacks, and sleep disorders. Examples are Nembutal (pentobarbital sodium), Valium (diazepam), and Xanax (alprazolam). Long-term use can lead to physical dependence and addiction. Central nervous system stimulants are used to treat narcolepsy and the attention-deficit/hyperactivity disorder. Examples include Ritalin (methylphenidate) and Dexedrine (dextroamphetamine).

Opioids, also known as narcotic analgesics are used to treat pain. Opioids are the most commonly abused prescription drugs. Examples include morphine, codeine, OxyContin (oxycodone), Vicodin (hydrocodone) and Demerol (meperidine).

One may obtain drugs by the following means: prescription forgery, by telephone (faking to be a physician's office), multiple doctors, and indiscriminate prescribing by physicians. Pain clinicians who prescribe chronic opioids are aware that there is an illicit market for opioid analgesics. For example, OxyContin can be sold for $1.00 per milligram. One 80 mg pill can be sold therefore, on the street for $80.00. This may be a source of income for an elderly individual who is dependent on a fixed income.

Telephone scams occur when the drug seeker claims to be a patient of one of the other physicians in the on-call group, and asks for a prescription for an analgesic to last until they can see their regular physician. Sometimes, the drug seeker uses a telephone to impersonate a practicing physician.

Prescription forgery is a common activity among drug seekers. Drug seekers can modify a legitimate prescription to increase the dosage or quantity of an opioid. The easiest method is to increase the number of tablets on the prescription.

Numerous episodes of noncompliance raise an alert of drug seeking behavior as well as multiple episodes of prescription loss. The patient with chemical dependency loses control over drug taking. The patient cannot take medications as prescribed.

The physician will notice that the drug seeker frequently requests early renewals of prescriptions. A pain physician must, however, be aware that aggressive complaining about the need for more drugs may indicate inadequate pain management in contrast to drug seeking behavior. A patient should not be allowed to suffer. It should be understood that substance abusers can suffer from chronic pain, which should be treated in a humane manner. Unapproved use of opioids to treat another symptom such as sleep deprivation should not be tolerated. However, the pain management physician must objectively identify a patient's pain complaint with the appropriate medical test before prescribing an opioid.

Opioid analgesics are powerful tools in the armamentarium of the pain clinician. Criminal and chemically dependent drug seekers may attempt to obtain such drugs from the physician. A pain medicine physician must therefore, use safe prescribing strategies. A physician has no legal obligation to prescribe opioid analgesics on demand.

A reasonable precaution to be taken by the pain medicine physician with an unfamiliar patient is to establish a policy of not prescribing opioid analgesics pending a complete assessment, including corroboration of the patient's history. Some patients or patient's families are afraid of addiction. However, a significant number of individuals do not understand the difference between addiction and tolerance.

The American Academy of Pain Medicine, the American Pain Society, and the American Society of Addiction Medicine recognize the following definitions and recommend their use.

I. Addiction

Addiction is a primary, chronic, neurobiologic disease, with genetic, psychosocial, and environmental factors influencing its development and manifestations. It is characterized by behaviors that include one or more of the following: impaired control over drug use, compulsive use, continued use despite harm, and craving. An entity termed pseudo-addiction exists which is not true addiction. Pseudo-addiction occurs when pain is under treated. Pseudo-addiction resolves when the pain resolves. Addictive behavior, on the other hand, persists in spite of increasing the patient's pain medication.

II. Physical Dependence

Physical dependence is a state of adaptation that is manifested by a drug class specific withdrawal syndrome that can be produced by abrupt cessation, rapid dose reduction, decreasing blood level of the drug, and/or administration of an antagonist.

III. Tolerance

Tolerance is a state of adaptation in which exposure to a drug induces changes that result in a diminution of one or more of the drug's effects over time. Most specialists in pain medicine and addiction medicine agree that patients treated with prolonged opioid therapy usually do develop physical dependence and sometimes develop tolerance, but do not usually develop addictive disorders. Addiction is a primary chronic disease and exposure to opioid medications is only one of the etiologic factors for its development. Therefore, good clinical judgment must be used in determining whether the pattern of behaviors signals the presence of addiction or reflects a different issue.

Drug abusers exhibited significantly shorter telomere lengths in one study. Drug abusers who had used heroin and diazepam displayed a shorter LTL than those taking other drugs.[6] Other study results support previous findings associating telomere shortening drug addiction.[7]

The elderly substance abuser should be treated in an environment in which there are other aged persons. The behavior of older addicts is different than a younger substance abuser. Seniors usually prefer to not be in group therapy sessions with younger patients. For this reason senior specific treatment programs are more productive if one surrounds the recovering addict with other individuals that he or she can relate to. Furthermore, group therapy sessions may be more relaxed for the substance abuser and therefore, be more productive than individual treatments.

Improving pain management in nursing homes for example requires improving provider knowledge and attitudes, enhancing diagnostic precision, standardizing pain treatment, and achieving an institutional commitment.[8] Furthermore, it must be realized that patient-controlled analgesia use should not be hindered by age differences in beliefs about postoperative pain and opioids. Younger and older patients attained comparable levels of analgesia and were equally satisfied with their pain control.[9]

References
1. Robinson CL. Relieving pain in the elderly. Health Prog. 2007;88(1):48-53, 70.
2. Skurtveit S, Furu K, Selmer R, Handal M, Tverdal A. Nicotine dependence predicts repeated use of prescribed opioids. Prospective population-based cohort study. Ann Epidemiol. 2010;20(12):890-897.
3. Gallagher R. Methadone: an effective, safe drug of first choice for pain management in frail older adults. Pain Med. 2009;10(2):319-326.
4. Auret K, Schug SA. Underutilisation of opioids in elderly patients with chronic pain: approaches to correcting the problem. Drugs Aging. 2005;22(8):641-654.
5. Schneider JP. Chronic pain management in older adults: with coxibs under fire, what now? Geriatrics. 2005;60(5):26-28, 30-21.
6. Yang Z, Ye J, Li C, et al. Drug addiction is associated with leukocyte telomere length. Sci Rep. 2013;3:1542.
7. Levandowski ML, Tractenberg SG, de Azeredo LA, et al. Crack cocaine addiction, early life stress and accelerated cellular aging among women. Prog Neuropsychopharmacol Biol Psychiatry. 2016;71:83-89.
8. Tarzian AJ, Hoffmann DE. Barriers to managing pain in the nursing home: findings from a statewide survey. J Am Med Dir Assoc. 2005;6(3 Suppl):S13-19.
9. Gagliese L, Jackson M, Ritvo P, Wowk A, Katz J. Age is not an impediment to effective use of patient-controlled analgesia by surgical patients. Anesthesiology. 2000;93(3):601-610.

13. Anti-inflammatory medications

Elderly persons represent the largest single group of prescription consumers in the United States today. They only represent 13 percent of the population, yet they consume nearly 30 percent of all medications. Nonsteroidal anti-inflammatory drugs (NSAIDs) are used by more than 13 million arthritis sufferers. Since the number of arthritic conditions increase with age, most patients taking NSAIDs are elderly. For example, nonsteroidal anti-inflammatory drugs (NSAIDs) can decrease pain if one suffers from the following: rheumatoid or osteoarthritis, headaches, menstrual pain, or generalized acute and prolonged pain.

Some of the NSAIDs are used for pain and for inflammation. As a group, elderly patients are more likely to experience an adverse drug reaction (ADR) from a medication. There are many effective treatment modalities available as potential therapeutic interventions for elderly patients, including but not limited to analgesics such as NSAIDs and opioids, as well as multiple interventional pain techniques.1

The American Geriatrics Society (AGS) guideline recommends that acetaminophen be considered for initial and ongoing treatment of persistent pain. Like opioids, NSAIDs are a class of drugs that have similar chemical structures and properties and are effective for many forms of pain. Unlike opiods, NSAIDs do not cause addiction. However, NSAIDs can have serious side effects, including bleeding from the stomach and intestines, and are responsible for as many as 10,000 deaths per year when used in prescribed doses. The AGS recommends that nonselective NSAIDs and cyclo-oxygenase-2 (COX-2) selective inhibitors "be considered rarely".

Aspirin is the prototype NSAID. Approximately, 2,400 years ago, Hippocrates prescribed bark from a white willow tree to his patients for various painful ailments. The chief ingredient of aspirin is more than 1,000 years old. NSAIDs have progressed since the time of Hippocrates. Aspirin was the first NSAID. The active ingredient of willow bark is salicin. This is a bitter-tasting chemical. Chemists took salicin and converted it to salicylic acid in the nineteenth.

It was noted then that salicylic acid could decrease fever. In the late 1880s, a 29-year-old man named Felix Hoffmann changed the chemical structure of salicylic acid. His research resulted in what is now aspirin. The Bayer Company was the company that Felix Hoffmann worked for. The Bayer Company coined the term "aspirin" for an unknown reason. Bayer aspirin became available in January 1899. Aspirin is still in common use today.

Alka-Seltzer, Bufferin, and Excedrin are products that contain aspirin. Initially, aspirin could be purchased only with a prescription. The German Bayer Company eventually opened a Bayer Company in the United States as well as in Latin America. Following World War I, the Bayer Company was accused of sending profits to Germany, and the company was sold to Sterling Products, Inc.

After World War I, people became worried that aspirin could have adverse effects on the heart. The Sterling Company published an ad that stated that the aspirin did not affect the heart. It is currently known that aspirin has a beneficial effect on the heart, and that it can prevent heart attacks. It is at present, one of the first drugs of choice following a myocardial infarction.

An article was published in 1944 in the Journal of the American Medical Association (JAMA) that stated that aspirin was not safe and could adversely affect the heart as well as the stomach. However, as time progressed, physicians began telling people to take a daily aspirin to prevent a heart attack. An article published in the 1980s revealed that aspirin could decrease the risk of heart attacks by 44 percent. Research went on to discover that regular aspirin use could decrease the risk of colon cancer by nearly 50 percent. Furthermore, esophageal cancer could be decreased about 80 percent and ovarian cancer by approximately 25 percent. Unfortunately, age or gender differences were not addressed in any of these studies.

The problems associated with long-term aspirin use include bleeding ulcers, gastritis, bleeding into the brain causing a stroke, and asthmatic reactions. Original aspirin studies were done on men. Current research is now being done directed toward the risk of heart attack versus stroke in men versus women. The incidence of heart attacks in men is greater than in women. In 1982, a British pharmacologist, Sir John Vane, discovered that aspirin blocked the formation of chemical substances called prostaglandins. It was noted that the prostaglandins affected pain and can also lessen fevers. Aspirin was noted to stop the enzyme that is involved in the production of prostaglandins. Further studies have recently shown that aspirin can decrease dementia associated with Alzheimer's disease.

The NSAIDs, including aspirin, are widely used worldwide. They may be the most vastly used drug in the United States. These drugs are used not only for menstrual cramps but also for arthritis, headaches, and minor muscle strains and ligament and tendon sprains. The newer NSAIDs are used for post-operative pain and are noted to be effective for the control of pain in general. NSAIDs were not traditionally given for postoperative pain because NSAIDs can inhibit clotting mechanisms and cause one to bleed from a surgical incision.

Telomere shortening is closely associated with severity of H. pylori-induced gastritis and CDH1 methylation status. Also, telomere shortening is accelerated by NSAID usage especially in H. pylori-negative subjects.[2] On the other hand, the regeneration of human skeletal muscle are expedited by ingestion of nonsteroidal anti-inflammatory medication.[3]

The newer NSAID (Celebrex) can be given to one after surgery for pain control, and one will not have any bleeding problems associated with one of these drugs. The NSAIDs in general are classified as weak acids. This means that they are absorbed from oner stomach or small intestine at different rates into one's bloodstream at a rate that is dependent on the pH of oner stomach or small intestine. That is why aspirin is buffered.

Acetaminophen (Tylenol) does have some weak anti-inflammatory properties. Acetaminophen is a nonacid drug. Acetaminophen exerts it effects in the brain and spinal cord as well as in one's arms and legs. This drug is recommended for elderly patients.

The nonsteroidal anti-inflammatory medications are used to decrease the overall pain experience without resorting to the need for the increased use of morphine like medications. Opioid drugs act primarily in the brain and spinal cord. The nonsteroidal anti-inflammatory drugs exert their pain-relieving effects in the peripheral nervous system as well as in the brain and spinal cord. By combining these two different mechanisms, a physician can have better control of pain that originates from the peripheral nervous system.

Prostaglandins desensitize nerves that propagate painful stimuli. Prostaglandins are important in many normal physiological states as well as pathological states. Prostaglandins are ultimately synthesized as a result of trauma or normal secretion from the outer aspects of various cells. Within the cell membrane are fatty substances that contain arachidonic acid. Arachidonic acid is present in all cell membranes. In response to a cell stimulus, the arachidonic acid in the cell membrane is released and is quickly converted to different types of prostaglandins. A chemical in the body called cyclooxygenase (COX) ultimately converts the arachidonic acid to the various prostaglandins.

Arachidonic acid formation from cell membranes can be broken down in and mixed with other chemicals to form leukotrienes. These leukotrienes are formed and released from the white blood cells. These chemicals are important in the formation of inflammation (redness, swelling, warmth) in areas of the body as well as allergic reactions. Histamine production in the body are released from mast cells which are involved in allergic reactions.

There are two types of cyclooxygenase chemicals in the body called cyclooxygenase I (COX I) and cyclooxygenase II (COX II). Prostaglandins causing pain can be formed in the body as a result of tissue trauma and COX 2 activities, but the body needs "good prostaglandin" to maintain normal physiologic functions. When prostaglandins are formed, they sensitize the peripheral nerve endings to other pain-causing substances in the body, which enhances pain.

The prostaglandins do not cause pain themselves but make the nerve endings more sensitive to other pain-producing chemicals such as bradykinins in the body. Occasionally, the pain can become more pronounced than one would expect with a normal painful stimulus. The prostaglandin can make the skin more sensitive.

Prostaglandin inhibition in the brain and spinal cord produces pain relief. In the past decade, the two structures of cyclooxygenase were discovered. Enzymes in the body speed up biological reactions. COX-1 is present in most tissues under normal conditions. COX-2 is formed following tissue trauma. The older NSAIDs decrease the effects of both COX-1 and COX-2 activity. Side effects exhibited by NSAIDs are the result of inhibition of the COX-1 chemicals. Recently, NSAIDs have been developed that are specific for the COX-2 chemicals. These new drugs do not inhibit the COX-1 chemicals. This is significant because one needs a normal level of COX-1 enzymes in the body.

Patients with chronic renal failure are vulnerable to deterioration in renal function on exposure to non-steroidal anti-inflammatory drugs, as elderly patients may have renal function that is compromised by renal vascular disease and/or the effects of ageing upon the kidney. Leukocyte telomere length predicts risk of esophageal adenocarcinoma in patients with Barrett's esophagus independently of smoking, obesity, and NSAID use. These results show the ability of leukocyte telomere length to predict the risk of future cancer and suggest that it might also have predictive value in other cancers arising in a setting of chronic inflammation.[4]

Nonsteroidal anti-inflammatory drugs (NSAIDs) are divided into different classes, depending on the drug's chemical structure. There are three classes of NSAIDs. The first are the carboxylic acid and enolic acid groups. This general class includes ibuprofen, naproxen, indomethacin, and ketorolac. The second are the benzenesulfonic acid derivatives such as Celebrex. The third group is the phenol group, which includes acetaminophen. In spite of having different chemical structures, all these medicines do provide anti-inflammatory effects. One should be aware that acetaminophen has only mild anti-inflammatory properties.

Great optimism abounds since the release of the cyclooxygenase-2 inhibitors. The advent of these drugs is important because NSAIDs are the most commonly used analgesics worldwide. Prostaglandins can be formed within minutes following tissue injury. The problem with the COX-2 enzyme inhibitors is that some moderate pain requires inhibition of both COX-1 and COX-2 enzymes. In these instances, a physician may prescribe a mild analgesic such as Ultram (tramadol). A new NSAID is being developed with both COX-1 and COX-2 inhibition that has equal pain-relieving properties against each of the two COX enzymes but has minimal side effects.

Recent studies report that the COX-2 enzyme may be involved in some forms of cancer. COX-1 and COX-2 may also be involved in the formation of atherosclerotic plaque. COX inhibition may provide one with relief or even prevention of plaques and cancer. COX-2 inhibitors have been approved by the FDA for the treatment of individuals with osteoarthritis as well as rheumatoid arthritis. Celebrex has been approved by the FDA for the treatment of patients suffering from acute muscle and bone pain. If one suffer from arthritis, both COX-1 and COX-2 enzymes may be present in inflamed joints.

COX-2-inhibiting NSAIDs are now used for minor post-surgical pain management. These COX-2 drugs are useful because they do not result in postsurgical bleeding. The usual NSAIDs can increase bleeding during or after a surgical procedure. Some recent studies have advocated the pre surgical use of the new COX-2-inhibiting NSAIDs to prevent postsurgical pain associated with RSD following hand or foot surgery. The rationale for using NSAIDs postoperatively is to decrease the need for opioid medications.

Post surgically, the adverse effects of NSAIDs in elderly patients are similar to the adverse effects of NSAIDs in the general population. Gastrointestinal hemorrhage has been reported even with the new COX-2-inhibiting drugs. Delayed healing of fractures can be seen with the traditional NSAIDs. In rabbits, COX-2 inhibitors decrease healing of bone fractures. However, in humans, there is no evidence to date that indicates that a COX-2-inhibiting drug will delay fracture healing.

Celebrex and other NSAIDs can also lead to liver damage. Warning signs include nausea, vomiting, tiredness, appetite loss, itching, yellow coloring of skin or eyes, flu-like symptoms and dark urine. Patients experiencing any of these symptoms should discontinue use of Celebrex immediately and consult their physician. The COX-2 inhibitors can be used for mild to moderate pain of essentially any etiology, including some gynecological disorders. The NSAIDs and especially the COX-2-inhibiting NSAIDs are extremely useful for the management of joint pain.

Arthritic entities that can be successfully treated include osteoarthritis as well as rheumatoid arthritis and ankylosing spondylitis. NSAIDs have been shown to drastically improve the quality of life if one has arthritis. Opioid medications are indicated for pain management if the pain becomes intolerable.

In addition to joint pain, the COX-2-inhibiting NSAIDs can be used for muscle pain, including fibromyalgia. Other uses for NSAIDs that one might find useful include the treatment of migraine headaches as well as tension headaches. NSAIDs can be used for pain management in cancer patients who have mild to moderate pain. If the pain worsens, opioid medications can be used. NSAIDs are especially useful in bone pain. Some tumors can invade bone. This pain can be agonizing.

In addition to the treatment of arthritic conditions such as osteoarthritis and rheumatoid arthritis, it is possible that the COX-2 inhibitors may provide protection against some forms of cancer as well as Alzheimer's disease. A concern has been addressed in the academic community regarding an increased incidence of heart attack in individuals in a study who were taking COX-2 inhibitors. The older NSAIDs are known to decrease the clotting of blood and can decrease the risk of a heart attack.

Because the COX-2 drugs do not affect clotting, it was suspected that their use could be associated with a higher incidence of a myocardial infarction risk. The consensus now is that if a patient is prone to have a heart attack (obesity, hypertension, and angina) one should take an aspirin with the COX-2 inhibitor. It is recommended that one take the aspirin initially in the morning, and toward the afternoon, one should take the COX-2 inhibitor. A baby aspirin in addition to the COX-2 inhibitor may be given instead of a whole aspirin.

Some prostaglandins can have beneficial effects on the body. Some prostaglandins inhibit acid production in the stomach. These "good" prostaglandins can stimulate mucus production in the upper gastrointestinal tract. This effect can decrease the incidence of ulcers. The older NSAIDs would decrease these "good" prostaglandins in the body and could cause ulcers. These older NSAIDs could also cause one to have gastritis, which in turn would cause stomach pain, nausea, vomiting, and diarrhea. A small number of patients would develop gastrointestinal bleeding and would die. If one has a history of ulcers, one should not use the traditional NSAIDs.

In addition to causing ulcers, the older NSAIDs could cause a patient to bleed from the stomach or elsewhere. The older NSAIDs inhibit proper platelet function. Platelets are needed by the body to form blood clots. NSAIDs that decrease the COX-1 enzymes in the body could cause bleeding. A patient should not take NSAIDs if he or she is taking blood thinners. One should not take aspirin for 10 to 14 days prior to any surgery or major dental work.

One must not use garlic, gingko, or vitamin E when taking NSAID medications. These herbal remedies can cause one to bleed if one are taking NSAIDs. Increased bleeding following the use of NSAIDs has been reported in patients having abdominal surgery, hysterectomies, or tonsillectomies. Patients who use NSAIDs are more prone to postoperative bleeding than individuals who do not regularly use NSAIDs.

One should not use NSAIDs regularly if one has a history of any of the following: A history of a gastrointestinal bleed, a history of a peptic ulcer or gastrointestinal intolerance to these medications, a bleeding history or a history of bruising easily, if one are taking blood thinners like Plavix, or have a history of kidney disease.

"Good" prostaglandins regulate blood flow to the kidneys. These good prostaglandins contribute to normal excretion of water from the kidneys. On the other hand, other prostaglandins can cause a decrease in the blood flow to the kidneys and disrupt renal function. In kidney failure, sodium and water retention occurs, causing one to appear swollen. Potassium can be elevated in the bloodstream as well. If the potassium becomes too high, the heart rhythm can be adversely affected. Overall hypertension may occur. Ultimately, the chronic use of nonsteroidal anti-inflammatory drugs can cause significant damage to the kidneys. The development of more recent NSAIDs does not spare the effects of NSAIDs on kidney function.

Liver damage can occur following chronic nonsteroidal anti-inflammatory use, and one must be aware of this side effect. Liver damage occurs in approximately 3 percent of patients receiving NSAIDs. Therefore, liver function tests must be performed periodically if one is taking NSAIDs long term. Even though nonsteroidal anti-inflammatory drugs are used for inflammatory pain such as arthritis, the Food and Drug Administration (FDA) has approved some of the NSAIDs for mild to moderate pain. Ketorolac can be used in the recovery room after surgery and can be administered in the muscle or in a vein. There also is an oral form of the drug that can be used by one for pain management.

Motrin, Advil, and Nuprin are trade names for ibuprofen. These drugs are approved for the use in pain management. Nalfon can also be used strictly for pain management in situations where noninflammatory pain is present. If one suffer from fibromyalgia, for example, which is not an inflammatory disease, some of the NSAIDs are approved for pain control.

Dolobid and Naproxen are two brand-name drugs that one can use for pain control. Diflunisal (Dolobid) has a longer duration of action than aspirin and longer than many of the other NSAIDs. It is effective for pain management and has a longer duration of action than the ibuprofen drugs or the fenoprofen drugs. Naproxen has also been successfully used for generalized pain. One should be reminded that these drugs can cause gastrointestinal upset and should not be used long term. They are excellent medications for one to use for three to four weeks.

Prostaglandins can cause one to have a fever. NSAIDs can be effective in decreasing a fever. NSAIDs do affect the smooth muscle of the uterus as well. Prostaglandins can also relax the muscle in the lungs. Some prostaglandins inhibit gastric acid secretion in the stomach and make mucus secretion, which is another protective mechanism in the stomach. Other prostaglandins can increase gastrointestinal motility. The "good" prostaglandins can regulate the blood flow to the kidneys as well as sodium/potassium exchange. The "bad" prostaglandins can sensitize nerve endings to pain.

NSAIDs are not without potential serious problems, especially in elderly patients. These drugs can also cause fewer serious effects such as peptic ulcer disease as well as gastritis and belching. NSAIDs can also cause one to experience diarrhea. NSAIDs should not be used if one has a fractured bone. The use of NSAIDs may delay healing of a bone fracture. NSAIDs may affect cartilage repair in joints if a patient suffers from osteoarthritis.

The older NSAID drugs such as ibuprofen (Advil) inhibit both the COX-1 and COX-2 enzymes. The new classes of NSAIDs called COX-2-specific inhibitors include Celebrex. Because the COX-1 enzyme is necessary for normal functioning of the body, it is essentially preserved by using a COX-2 inhibitor. The development of the COX-2 enzyme inhibitor is a significant development from the older nonsteroidal anti-inflammatory drugs, which inhibit COX-1 and COX-2 enzymes.

NSAIDS are contraindicated for the treatment of perioperative pain in coronary artery bypass graft surgery; in patients who have demonstrated allergic-type reactions to sulfonamides; or in patients who have experienced asthma, urticaria, or allergic-type reactions after taking aspirin or other NSAIDs. A patient must only take the lowest effective dose for the shortest duration consistent with individual patient treatment goals.

Non-steroidal anti-inflammatory drugs (NSAIDs) are one of the most commonly used medications in the elderly. They have been widely studied as possible preventive agents against cognitive decline because of the properties of anti-inflammatories, which sustain cerebral blood flow and mitigate the neurotoxicity of microglial cells. A recent published meta-analysis of prospective cohort studies indicates that NSAID use may be associated with a decreased risk of cognitive decline.[5]

Non-steroidal anti-inflammatory drugs (NSAIDs) may enhance resistance training induced gain in skeletal muscle mass and strength, but it is unknown if NSAIDs affects muscle loss during periods of inactivity in elderly individuals. A recent study concluded that NSAID treatment does not significantly influence muscle mass in elderly patients.[6] On the other hand, despite decreasing Helicobacter pylori prevalence, the prevalence of peptic ulcer disease is increasing in the aged population, mainly due to increasing use of NSAIDs to manage pain and inflammation.[7]

In a recent study up to 40% of patients with chronic pain in patients aged 75 to85 years suffered from neuropathic pain.[8] However, only a few elderly people with chronic pain used medications specifically for chronic pain, which may be due to side effects or non-willingness to experiment with these drugs. Elderly people with chronic pain rated their health and mobility to be worse and felt sadder, lonelier and more tired but were not less satisfied with their lives than those without chronic pain.

As with all NSAIDs, any one of them can lead to the onset of new hypertension or worsening of pre-existing hypertension, either of which may contribute to the increased incidence of cardiovascular events. A patient's blood pressure should be monitored closely with all NSAIDs.

References

1. Jones MR, Ehrhardt KP, Ripoll JG, et al. Pain in the Elderly. Curr Pain Headache Rep. 2016;20(4):23.

2. Tahara T, Shibata T, Kawamura T, et al. Telomere length in non-neoplastic gastric mucosa and its relationship to H. pylori infection, degree of gastritis, and NSAID use. Clin Exp Med. 2016;16(1):65-71.

3. Mackey AL, Rasmussen LK, Kadi F, et al. Activation of satellite cells and the regeneration of human skeletal muscle are expedited by ingestion of nonsteroidal anti-inflammatory medication. FASEB J. 2016;30(6):2266-2281.

4. Risques RA, Vaughan TL, Li X, et al. Leukocyte telomere length predicts cancer risk in Barrett's esophagus. Cancer Epidemiol Biomarkers Prev. 2007;16(12):2649-2655.

5. Wang W, Sun Y, Zhang D. Association Between Non-Steroidal Anti-Inflammatory Drug Use and Cognitive Decline: A Systematic

Review and Meta-Analysis of Prospective Cohort Studies. Drugs Aging. 2016.

6. Dideriksen K, Boesen AP, Kristiansen JF, et al. Skeletal muscle adaptation to immobilization and subsequent retraining in elderly men: No effect of anti-inflammatory medication. Exp Gerontol. 2016;82:8-18.

7. Shim YK, Kim N. [Nonsteroidal Anti-inflammatory Drug and Aspirin-induced Peptic Ulcer Disease]. Korean J Gastroenterol. 2016;67(6):300-312.

8. Rapo-Pylkko S, Haanpaa M, Liira H. Chronic pain among community-dwelling elderly: a population-based clinical study. Scand J Prim Health Care. 2016;34(2):159-164.

14. Anticonvulsants

Many elderly patients suffer from nerve pain as a result of diabetes, thyroid disease, and spine disease. Arm or leg nerve pain, facial pain, etc. are examples of nerve (neuropathic) pain. Anticonvulsant drugs have been used for the management of neuropathic pain since the 1960s. These drugs interfere with the total number of pain signals that travel to the brain.

Telomere length, considered a measure of biological aging, is linked to morbidity and mortality. Psychosocial factors associated with shortened telomeres are also common in chronic pain. Patients with shorter telomeres were more sensitive to evoked pain and had less gray matter in brain regions associated with pain processing. This data supports a relationship between pain and telomere length.[1] Another study demonstrated that cellular aging may be more pronounced in older adults experiencing high levels of perceived stress and chronic pain.[2]

This type of drug seems to be especially effective for managing sharp, shooting and lancinating pain. It is possible that anticonvulsant drugs stabilize excitable nerve membranes, limit neural hyper excitability, and inhibit trans synaptic neuronal impulses in the CNS. Gabapentin a GABA-mimetic medication, is the anticonvulsant used most widely in North America in the treatment of RSD. Pregabilin is however becoming very popular for pain control.

Gabapentin binds to the outer layer of the brain. The anticonvulsant effects of gabapentin may be mediated by increasing the release of GABA. When GABA is released in the spinal cord, pain signals going toward the brain are decreased. Gabapentin has both analgesic and antianxiety effects. In mice, gabapentin selectively blocks pain signals associated with inflammation, suggesting a central site of action, perhaps by blocking the sensitization of dorsal horn neurons in your spinal cord that occurs during inflammation.

Gabapentin appears to differ from the other anticonvulsants in its mechanism of action. Gabapentin is not metabolized by the liver and can be safely be given with other anticonvulsants. It is well tolerated and has few adverse effects (drowsiness, fatigue and dizziness). These side effects tend to decrease with continued usage.

The clinical impression of these drugs is that they are useful for chronic neuropathic pain, especially when the pain is lancinating or burning. Pain is usually the natural consequence of tissue injury resulting in approximately forty million medical appointments per annum. In general, following most injuries, as the healing process commences, the pain and tenderness associated with your injury will usually resolve. Unfortunately, some individuals experience pain without an obvious injury or they may suffer pain that persists for months or years after their initial injury. This pain condition is neuropathic in nature and accounts for a large number of patients presenting to pain clinics with chronic pain.

In neuropathic pain, the peripheral or central nervous systems are malfunctioning and become the cause of the pain. In other words, after a nerve has healed, the central nervous system may still transmit pain signals to the brain. An example is a car alarm. The alarm will sound if a vehicle is being tampered with. This is normal. Now imagine that the alarm sounds when no one is near the car. Somehow, there is a short circuit. The same occurs within the nervous system.

Neuropathic pain is a complex, pain state that usually is accompanied by nerve injury. With neuropathic pain, the nerve fibers themselves may be damaged, dysfunctional or injured. These damaged nerve fibers send incorrect signals to other pain nerves. The impact of nerve injury includes a change in nerve function both at the site of injury and areas around the injury. Symptoms may include: shooting and burning pain as well as tingling and numbness.

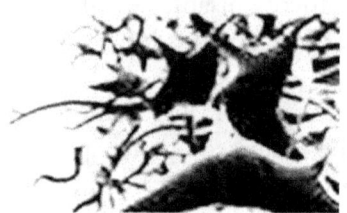

Figure 1. When nerves become hyperactive, a patient may experience nerve pain.

In order to understand the effects of anti-seizure drugs, one needs to be aware that these drugs can block the ion (calcium and sodium) channels that are present throughout the nervous system. Ion channels are pore-forming proteins that help to establish and control a small electric gradient between the inside and outside of your nerve cells. When ions flow in and out of a neuron, this electric gradient ceases and pain signals subsequently cease to be transmitted to the brain. Calcium and sodium channel anticonvulsant drugs block the pores or channels. When these drugs drop off of these channels, a patient will experience recurrent pain.

Anti-seizure drugs are frequently used in pain management. It is not known exactly how anticonvulsants work to reduce pain. They may block the flow of pain signals from the brain and spinal cord. Some anticonvulsant drugs may work better than others under certain conditions. Neuropathic pain is a form of chronic pain caused by an injury to or a disease of the peripheral or central nervous system. It does not respond well to traditional pain therapies like opioids or nonsteroidal anti-inflammatory drugs.

In neuropathic pain, it has shown that a number of pathophysiological and biochemical changes take place in the nervous system as a result of an insult to a nerve. This property of the nervous system to adapt to external stimuli plays a crucial role in the onset and maintenance of pain symptoms.

Carbamazepine (Tegretol), the first anticonvulsant studied in clinical trials, probably alleviates pain by decreasing conductance in sodium channels and inhibits ectopic nerve discharges. Results from clinical trials have been positive in the treatment of trigeminal neuralgia, painful diabetic neuropathy and post herpetic neuralgia with this medication.

Gabapentin (Neurontin) and pregabilin (Lyrica) have the most clearly demonstrated analgesic effects for the treatment of neuropathic pain, specifically for the treatment of painful diabetic neuropathy and post herpetic neuralgia. Based on the positive results of these studies and its favorable adverse effect profile, gabapentin or pregabilin should be considered the first choice of therapy for neuropathic pain. Evidence for the efficacy of phenytoin as an antinociceptive agent is, at best, weak to modest. Lamotrigine (Lamictal) on the other hand, has a good potential to modulate and control neuropathic pain.

There is potential for phenobarbital, clonazepam, valproic acid, topiramate, pregabalin and tiagabine to have antihyperalgesic and antinociceptive activities based on results in animal models of neuropathic pain, but the efficacy of these drugs in the treatment of human neuropathic pain has not yet been fully determined in clinical trials. The role of anticonvulsant drugs in the treatment of neuropathic pain is evolving and has been clearly demonstrated with gabapentin and carbamazepine. Further advances in our understanding of the mechanisms underlying neuropathic pain syndromes and well-designed clinical trials should further the opportunities to establish the role of anticonvulsants in the treatment of neuropathic pain.

The clinical impression is that the anticonvulsant drugs are applicable for the treatment of chronic neuropathic pain, especially when the pain is lancinating or burning. There are seven drugs that are useful in neuropathic (nerve injury) pain; pregabilin (Lyrica), gabapentin (Neurontin), carbamazipine (Tegretol), valproic acid (Depakote), clonazepamm (Klonopin), phenytoin (Dilantin), zonisamide (Zonegran)) and lamotrigine (Lamictal).

Neurontin is an effective drug for the treatment of neuropathic pain but Lyrica is becoming widely used as previously mentioned in the management of many pain syndromes. It has fewer side effects than other anticonvulsant drugs. These drugs can be useful for the treatment of shingles, diabetic neuropathy and fibromyalgia. Reflex Sympathetic Dystrophy, diabetic neuropathy migraine headaches, sciatica, radiculitis, and pain associated with multiple sclerosis may respond to either of these drugs. Severe postherpetic neuralgia and other neuropathic pain syndromes have been reported to be alleviated by topical gabapentin.[3]

If a patient experiences sharp shooting pain, these drugs may be helpful in decreasing the pain. If a patient experiences side effects from either drug, other anticonvulsant medications are available. Oxcarbazepine (Trileptal), lamotrigine (Lamictal), topiramate (Topamax), and zonisamide (Zonegran) may also be effective in reducing pain caused by diabetic neuropathy and postherpetic neuralgia. Lyrica is now recently FDA approved for the treatment of fibromyalgia, shingles, diabetic neuropathy and spinal cord injury pain.

Anticonvulsant drugs are effective in the treatment of chronic neuropathic pain as well as the management of postoperative pain. However, similar to any nerve injury, surgical tissue injury is known to produce neuroplastic changes leading to spinal sensitization and the expression of nerve induced pain. Gabapentin (Neurontin) may decrease post-surgical pain.

The pharmacological effects of anticonvulsant drugs, which may be important in the modulation of these postoperative neural changes, include suppression of sodium channel, calcium channel and glutamate receptor activity at peripheral, spinal and supraspinal sites. Gabapentin and pregabalin reduce pain and opioid consumption after surgery in confront with placebo.[4] Postoperative administration of pregabalin effectively reduced postthoracotomy pain.[5]

Preoperative pregabalin administration significantly reduces postoperative opioid consumption and mechanical hyperalgesia after transperitoneal nephrectomy[6] The perioperative administration of gabapentin and pregabalin are effective in reducing the incidence of chronic post-surgical pain.[7]

Anticonvulsant drugs are effective in the treatment of chronic pain but may also as previously stated be useful for acute pain management following surgery. Similar to any nerve injury, surgical tissue injury is known to produce changes leading to spinal cord sensitization, which can cause one to have pain after surgery even after the wound has healed.

Pregabilin is effective for the treatment of diabetic neuropathy and shingles. Pregabilin binds to calcium channels of nerves, which results in a reduction of one's pain. Some health insurance plans do not pay for Lyrica because it is new and relatively expensive. However, it has been shown to be more cost-effective than gabapentin. In other words, it is more effective than gabapentin for RSD pain control.

Pregabilin drug can cause dizziness, blurred vision, drowsiness, weight gain and swelling of the legs. Pregablin has been reported to be effective administered rectally in an elderly male with neuropathic pain. 8 Oral pregabilin was not effective and it was decided to start pregabalin administered by the rectal route. The patient responded positively to rectal pregabilin. One should be aware that pregabilin may be a cause of acute liver failure reported previously in an elderly patient.[9]

A randomized controlled trial of pregabalin and opioids in 65 consecutive patients aged 65 years or older who had chronic low back pain (LBP).10 Each agent was administered randomly in different phases. Pregabalin was effective for LBP with neuropathic pain, whereas opioids were effective for non-neuropathic pain. Pregabalin was effective for LBP in patients with lower limb symptoms, whereas opioids were effective for those without lower limb symptoms.

Pregabilin may be more expensive than other anticonvulsant medications. However, cost analysis was done at two Veterans Affairs facilities. The analyzed population included all patients receiving pregabalin for pain whose dosing was converted from three times a day to twice daily pregabalin dosing during a one-year period. The primary endpoint was the economic impact of the conversion.

The costs associated with pregabalin therapy differed significantly between the preconversion and post conversion periods. A savings of $115,867 was realized from this conversion for both facilities combined over the course of one year. In patients receiving pregabalin for pain, conversion from three to twice-daily dosing resulted in substantial cost savings while having little effect on clinical outcomes.[11]

Gabapentin is effective for the management of oral phantom pain following a tooth extraction. Gabapentin binds to nerve calcium channels. Gabapentin has a mild effect on pain in CRPS. It can significantly reduce a sensory deficit in the affected limb. A subpopulation of CRPS patients may therefore, benefit from gabapentin. Gabapentin is useful for the management of CRPS pain as well as facial RSD. The drug is useful in most nerve injury pain disorders.

An average dose is 300 mg taken three times a day. A rare side effect has been reported with gabapentin use. A 35-year-old woman suffered a traumatic injury to her right sciatic nerve. She developed a complex regional pain syndrome and was treated with gabapentin for pain control. Three months after the initiation of gabapentin therapy (1800 mg/day), the patient reported complete cessation of her menses. The patient was weaned off the gabapentin over six days with return of her menses two weeks later. It concluded that gabapentin has the potential to cause cessation of periods with return of menses occurring after discontinuation of the drug.

Tegretol is a drug that is chemically related to amitriptyline. It prevents repetitive discharges of sensory nerves. This medication works on sodium channels in the painful nerves. Inhibition of these sodium channels can decrease pain sensations. An average dose is 200 mg every day. Side effects include dizziness, drowsiness, blurred vision and nausea. This medication can cause various forms of anemia and liver damage. Tegretol is rarely used today for RSD pain because of the side effects associated with this drug.

Tegretol has been shown to be effective for the treatment of trigeminal neuralgia. Some physicians use this drug for RSD pain relief. Depakote is given in a dose of 250 mg twice a day. This medication can cause one to have liver failure. This medicine is used when the other anti-convulsion medications have been tried but failed to provide pain relief. Side effects of this drug include nausea, vomiting loss of appetite and diarrhea. Tremors and sedation may also be associated with this medication.

Klonopin may be useful for the treatment of pain associated with the burning mouth syndrome. Klonopin is applicable also for the treatment of lancinating pain associated with the phantom limb syndrome. The drug may also be useful for migraine headache prophylaxis and for the treatment of trigeminal neuralgia. The usual dose is 1 mg per day. Side effects include mood disturbances and delirium. Lethargy and sedation may also be seen. This drug has a significant sedative effect. It should be initially only taken at bedtime. It is prescribed by some physicians for RSD pain.

Dilantin alters sodium, calcium and potassium channels in nerves. An average dose is 300 mg three times a day. The number of side effects associated with this drug is significant. Liver damage can occur and the drug can decrease folic acid levels in the bloodstream. A decrease in folic acid blood levels may actually cause a patient's nerves in the extremities to have burning sensations.

Zonegran's mechanisms of action suggest that it may also be effective in controlling neuropathic pain symptoms. It can therefore, be efficacious in the management of CRPS pain. It also decreases sodium channel activity on the sodium channels of nerves. Side effects can include a decrease in blood sodium levels, kidney stones, visual difficulties and secondary angle-closure glaucoma. A typical dose of this medication is 300 mg per day. Side effects related to this drug include agitation, anxiety, ataxia, confusion, depression, difficulty concentrating, headache, difficulty sleeping, memory problems, stomach pain as well as liver pathology. This medication may also cause weight loss. A dry mouth and flu like syndrome may also be associated with this drug.

Lamictal also exerts its effects on sodium channels. This drug decreases the release of some pain-causing chemical from the ends of nerves. The reason why a patient develops chronic pain after having acute nerve injury pain remains unclear. However, it is believed that Lamictal in addition to some of the other drugs mentioned may prevent this transformation. A typical dose will be 200 mg twice a day after starting at a low dose and going to 200 mg slowly. Adverse effects related to this drug include headaches, dizziness, blurred vision and nausea and vomiting. This medication may be of benefit for the treatment of pain associated with Reflex Sympathetic Dystrophy as well.

Lamictal also can be effective for many kinds of neuropathic pain, including that which comes from CRPS, AIDS and central brain pain as a result of a stroke. Lamictal is a seizure medicine that acts as a sodium channel blocker as previously mentioned but may exhibit some calcium channel blockade. In one study with patients who had severe refractory neuropathic pain who had failed at least two other treatments, resulted in an average 70% decrease in their pain in 14 of 21 patients.

In early studies where lower doses of 200 mg a day or less were used, the effects were marginal. Doses of 200 to 400 mg a day divided through the day are more effective for some kinds of pain. The most troublesome side effect is a rare rash (called Stevens - Johnson syndrome), which can be fatal.

Post-herpetic neuralgia is a painful condition and its prevalence increases with age. It is a burden for older patients and the association of age-related pharmacokinetic and pharmacodynamic changes, high co-morbidity and polypharmacy leads to the risk of adverse drug reactions and interactions. Shingles is a painful rash that results from reactivation of latent varicella zoster virus in the dorsal root ganglia or cranial nerves. The most effective way to prevent post-herpetic neuralgia and its consequences is the prevention of herpes itself.[12] A live attenuated vaccine has been available for several years, and is approved in adults aged 50 years old. Post-herpetic neuralgia is associated with significant distress and morbidity.

The management of acute neuritis and/or post-herpetic neuralgia can be particularly difficult. A multidisciplinary approach is required. A team consisting of the primary care physician, pain specialist, neurologist, geriatrician, pain psychologist, psychiatrist, and a physiatrist with an integrated approach will provide the best results. Early interventional therapy with sympathetic nerve blocks may significantly decrease the need for long-term opioid therapy, as well as long-term use of anticonvulsants, antidepressants, or membrane stabilizers.

Early referral to a multidisciplinary pain center may furthermore decrease the behavioral trauma and family disruption associated with this painful condition.[13] Gabapentin has been shown to be equally efficacious but is better tolerated compared to nortriptyline and can be considered a suitable alternative for the treatment of post-herpetic neuralgia.[14]

Persistent pain in older adults is common, and associated with substantial morbidity. Optimal management starts with assessment, including pain presence, intensity, characteristics, and interference; painful conditions; pain behaviors; pain-related morbidity; pain treatments; and coping style. Treatment incorporates analgesics demonstrated to decrease pain and improve a patient's sense of well-being. The World Health Organization's 3-step pain ladder is widely accepted and adopted for selecting analgesics among elderly patients with non-cancer pain.[15]

In summary, chronic pain, whether arising from nerve or any other tissue or structure, is, more often than commonly thought, the result of a mixture of pain mechanisms, and therefore, there is no simple formula available to manage chronic complex pain states. The analgesic recommendations for difficult-to-treat pain syndromes include gabapentin or pregabalin in addition to an opioid or antidepressant.

References

1. Hassett AL, Epel E, Clauw DJ, et al. Pain is associated with short leukocyte telomere length in women with fibromyalgia. J Pain. 2012;13(10):959-969.

2. Sibille KT, Langaee T, Burkley B, et al. Chronic pain, perceived stress, and cellular aging: an exploratory study. Mol Pain. 2012;8:12.

3. Hiom S, Patel GK, Newcombe RG, Khot S, Martin C. Severe postherpetic neuralgia and other neuropathic pain syndromes alleviated by topical gabapentin. Br J Dermatol. 2015;173(1):300-302.

4. Dauri M, Faria S, Gatti A, Celidonio L, Carpenedo R, Sabato AF. Gabapentin and pregabalin for the acute post-operative pain management. A systematic-narrative review of the recent clinical evidences. Curr Drug Targets. 2009;10(8):716-733.

5. Yoshimura N, Iida H, Takenaka M, et al. Effect of Postoperative Administration of Pregabalin for Post-thoracotomy Pain: A Randomized Study. J Cardiothorac Vasc Anesth. 2015;29(6):1567-1572.

6. Bornemann-Cimenti H, Lederer AJ, Wejbora M, et al. Preoperative pregabalin administration significantly reduces postoperative opioid consumption and mechanical hyperalgesia after transperitoneal nephrectomy. Br J Anaesth. 2012;108(5):845-849.

7. Clarke H, Bonin RP, Orser BA, Englesakis M, Wijeysundera DN, Katz J. The prevention of chronic postsurgical pain using gabapentin and pregabalin: a combined systematic review and meta-analysis. Anesth Analg. 2012;115(2):428-442.

8. Doddrell C, Tripathi SS. Successful use of pregabalin by the rectal route to treat chronic neuropathic pain in a patient with complete intestinal failure. BMJ Case Rep. 2015;2015.

9. Kowar M, Friedrich C, Jacobs AH. [Pregabalin as a rare cause of liver disease]. Dtsch Med Wochenschr. 2015;140(23):1759-1760.

10. Sakai Y, Ito K, Hida T, Ito S, Harada A. Pharmacological management of chronic low back pain in older patients: a randomized controlled trial of the effect of pregabalin and opioid administration. Eur Spine J. 2015;24(6):1309-1317.

11. Okolo C, Malmstrom R, Duncan K, Lopez J. Conversion from thrice- to twice-daily pregabalin dosing for pain: Economic and clinical outcomes in a veteran population. Am J Health Syst Pharm. 2015;72(17 Suppl 2):S74-78.

12. Calvo-Mosquera G, Gonzalez-Cal A, Calvo-Rodriguez D, Primucci CY, Plamenov-Dipchikov P. [Pain in herpes zoster: Prevention and treatment]. Semergen. 2016.

13. Ackerman WE, 3rd, Ahmad M. Multidisciplinary approach for the management of post-herpetic neuralgia in elderly patients. J Ark Med Soc. 1999;95(12):528-531.

14. Chandra K, Shafiq N, Pandhi P, Gupta S, Malhotra S. Gabapentin versus nortriptyline in post-herpetic neuralgia patients: a randomized, double-blind clinical trial--the GONIP Trial. Int J Clin Pharmacol Ther. 2006;44(8):358-363.

15. Malec M, Shega JW. Pain management in the elderly. Med Clin North Am. 2015;99(2):337-350.

15. TENS unit

For many elderly people with chronic pain increasing the level of drugs to deal with the pain may not be the best solution. Pain relief for elderly patients may be obtained by electrical current and is now based on transcutaneous or percutaneous nerve stimulation, deep stimulation, posterior spinal cord stimulation, and transcutaneous cranial stimulation.

Transcutaneous electrical nerve stimulation (TENS) is effective in con-trolling pain associated with nerve and muscle pain. Transcutaneous electrical nerve stimulation however, is only effective if it acts on neurogenic pain/neuropathic pain, only if the nerve pathways to be stimulated are superficial and only if the conduction pathways between the area of stimulation and the superior centers are intact.

The most common form of electrical stimulation used for pain control is the transcutaneous electric nerve stimulation (TENS) therapy, which provides short-term pain relief. Electric nerve stimulation and electro thermal therapy are used to relieve pain associated with various pain conditions. TENS is the acronym for Transcutaneous Electric Nerve Stimulation. A TENS unit is a pocket-size portable, battery-operated device that sends electrical impulses to certain parts of the body to interfere with pain signals going to your brain.

The electrical currents produced are mild, but can prevent pain messages from being transmitted through the brain and may raise the level of endorphins produced by the brain. A TENS unit is sometimes of value in an effort to break the pain cycle. Adhesive patches which are electrodes are attached to your skin, and small electrical impulses are delivered to underlying nerve fibers. This works in two ways.

The first way is through endorphins. The body has its own mechanisms for suppressing pain. The body releases natural chemicals called endorphins in the brain, which act as pain relieving substances. TENS units can activate this mechanism. Secondly, the electrical stimulation of the nerve fibers through the electrodes can actually block a pain signal from being carried all the way to the brain. If it is blocked, the pain is not felt. Patients who use TENS units may experience significant pain relief, while at the same time engaging in a therapy that is drug-free.

TENS units have not helped significantly with all cases of pain because the electrode placement is sometimes difficult and there is no carryover relief from TENS treatment, which means that when the unit is turned off, the pain returns. Treatment is directed to the relief of pain so the patient can begin more progressive rehabilitation caused by the disease itself.

Stimulation of the spinal cord and nerve endings by electrical current is done to relieve pain. TENS provides a beneficial adjunct for the treatment of cancer pain in elderly patients, especially when utilized as a goal-directed therapy.[1,2] TENS units may furthermore, be useful for the management of phantom limb pain as well.[3]

Interferential stimulation, which is another form of electric therapy and has been used for pain relief, has the benefit of extending pain relief post-treatment. Because the units are large, expensive, and require greater amounts of electric energy, the patient would have to go to a facility for treatments. There are some interferential units that are portable and are powered by an AC adapter or by batteries for home use. The patient can self-treat as needed. The carryover relief period seems to extend over longer periods of time as more treatments are done.

Interferential current therapy involves the placement of two electrodes to the skin at a painful area or the spinal nerve root associated with an aching region. Alternating currents of medium frequency are applied through the electrodes to the area. The currents rise and fall at different frequencies. It is theorized that the low frequency of the interferential current causes inhibition or habituation of the nervous system, which results in muscle relaxation, suppression of pain and acceleration of healing. It uses a medium-frequency of alternating currents to incite tissues of injured muscles and joints.

The medium-frequency is carried by the two independent circuits of paired electrodes. Interferential stimulation is believed to reduce pain, decrease swelling or edema in tissues and increases blood circulation in damaged tissues, thus stimulating repair and health. Some pain syndromes can cause decreased blood flow in affected muscles. This modality may provide some relief.

Treatments using neuromuscular stimulators, on the other hand, create involuntary muscle contractions that minimize the degenerative changes in muscles that usually occur following immobilization or partial denervation. Neuromuscular Stimulation is indicated for use in conditions that may result in disuse atrophy (muscle wasting). These devices can be combined with TENS units as well.

Electronic Muscle Stimulation is called EMS. This type of electrical stimulation is characterized by a low volt stimulation targeted to stimulate motor nerves to cause a muscle contraction. contraction/relaxation of muscles has been found to treat a variety of musculoskeletal and vascular conditions.

Most common uses of EMS are to prevent or retard disuse atrophy, strengthening programs, reeducation of muscles and reduction of muscle spasms. EMS differs from TENS in that it is designed to stimulate muscle motor nerves, while TENS is designed to stimulate sensory nerve endings to help decrease pain.

The elderly, terminally ill patient often experiences physical, emotional, and spiritual pain. While pharmacology remains the cornerstone of pain management, non-pharmacologic methods can serve as adjuncts for pain relief, and also serve to enhance the overall quality of the patient's life. Neurostimulation, such as TENS unit, acupuncture, and massage, are based on the gate theory of pain control. These treatments can be useful particularly in muscular pain.[4]

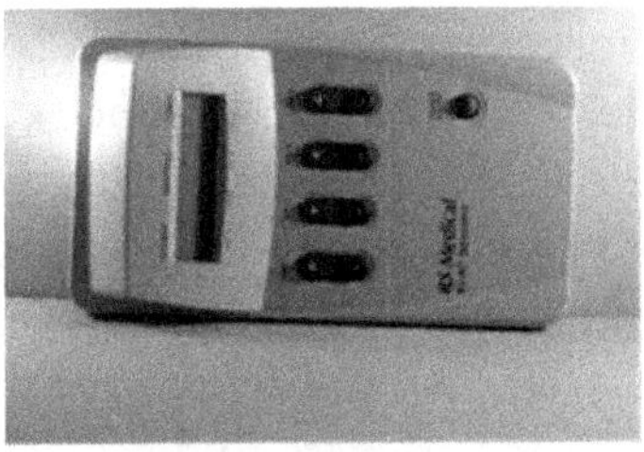

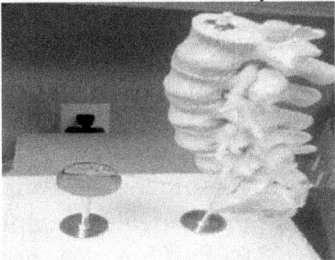

Figure 1. This device is a combination TENS/muscle stimulator. is useful in restoring muscle mass caused by lack of use if muscles in an arm or leg.

If all treatments fail, implantation of a dorsal column stimulator (SCS) may provide pain relief for patients. A trial electrode is placed initially. You will then assess the efficacy of the electrical stimulation. If a patient receives more than 50% pain relief, that patient may be a candidate for surgical implantation of both the battery, as well as the stimulator lead wire.

Figure 2. The battery is on the left side of the picture. A wire connects the battery to the spinal cord lead in the spine.

Spinal cord stimulators are surgically implanted devices, which are de-signed to provide pain relief from chronic intractable pain. Prior to placing an implantable spinal cord stimulator, typically the patients receive a trial of a temporary stimulator to assess the efficacy of stimulation in providing pain relief for that patient.

The surgical procedure involves placing a compact generator in the lower anterior abdomen wall and connecting a wire to a strip of electrodes placed next to the to the rear part of the spinal cord. Through low-voltage electrical stimulation of the electrodes, the normal pain signals which travel in the posterior parts of the spinal cord are altered to provide partial or complete pain relief from conditions such as cancer pain, post-spinal cord injury pain, RSD pain and pain from back or neck surgery.

Modern spinal cord stimulators are programmable so that once implanted; the signal can be adjusted for optimal pain relief. All neuro stimulation systems use low intensity electric impulses to keep the pain signals from reaching the brain. These electrical impulses produce a tingling or massaging sensation known as paresthesia. When patients are selected care-fully and the systems' electrodes are positioned properly, neurostimulation can be a successful therapy on certain types of neuropathic pain.

Neurostimulation systems typically consist of three components designed to work together: 1. Leads are very thin cables, or wires, with small electrodes that deliver the electrical impulses to the nerves. 2. The generator is the power source that sends electrical energy to the electrodes. 3. The programmer allows the patient to change programs and turn the stimulation up or down. Three types of neurostimulation systems are used: radiofrequency (RF), conventional implantable pulse generator (IPG), or rechargeable IPG systems. The use of radiofrequency systems which utilize an outside battery has decreased dramatically since the introduction of rechargeable technology. Electrostimulation over time can lessen telomere length.[5,6]

The proportion of patients with intractable pain successfully managed with spinal cord stimulation. However, this treatment remains disputed by some investigators. The merits of the systems are often debated, and the efficacy of each can vary from one patient to another, from one body area to another, and from one disease state to another. Additionally, research is still needed to determine whether incisions made when implanting the system can result in the spread of RSD/CRPS to other parts of the body.

RSD/CRPS is sometimes a migrating or progressive disease: pain may begin in one area or extremity, only to spread and involve other extremities. This progres-ion can significantly increase the power and electrode requirements for RSD/CRPS patients. Patients also should be aware that, because the systems contain metal, if they receive an implanted system, they cannot be exposed to magnetic resonance imaging.

Pain relief with SCS appears to decrease over time. Despite the diminishing effectiveness of SCS over time, 95% of patients with an implant would repeat the treatment for the same result. Although life-threatening complications was sustained in those patients who continued to use the stimulator for several years. Most patients who received a dorsal column stimulator would choose to receive an electrical stimulator again. A rigid selection protocol can maximize the proportion of patients with intractable pain who are successfully treated with SCS. Strict neurosurgical technique eliminates infection risk. Hardware selection minimizes the incidence of malfunction.

For selected patients who have not obtained adequate relief with medical management, SCS for phantom limb pain can prove an effective intervention.[7] Spinal cord stimulation (SCS) can be used in cases to control resistant deafferentation pain resulting from causalgia, phantom limb, plexus and nerve root avulsion, postherpetic neuralgia, reflex sympathetic dystrophy and amputation.[8] SCS appears to be an effective long-term treatment for neuropathic visceral pain related to chronic pancreatitis.[9] Spinal cord stimulation might be an option in the management of refractory knee pain following total knee replacement as well.[10]

While pharmacology remains the cornerstone of pain management, non-pharmacologic methods can serve as adjuncts for pain relief, and also serve to enhance the overall quality of the patient's life. Neurostimulation, such as TENS unit, acupuncture, and massage, are based on the gate theory of pain control. These treatments can be useful particularly in muscular pain.[4]

References

1. Loh J, Gulati A. The use of transcutaneous electrical nerve stimulation (TENS) in a major cancer center for the treatment of severe cancer-related pain and associated disability. Pain Med. 2015;16(6):1204-1210.

2. Searle RD, Bennett MI, Johnson MI, Callin S, Radford H. Transcutaneous electrical nerve stimulation (TENS) for cancer bone pain. J Pain Symptom Manage. 2009;37(3):424-428.

3. Carabelli RA, Kellerman WC. Phantom limb pain: relief by application of TENS to contralateral extremity. Arch Phys Med Rehabil. 1985;66(7):466-467.

4. Urba SG. Nonpharmacologic pain management in terminal care. Clin Geriatr Med. 1996;12(2):301-311.

5. Omura Y, Chen Y, Lermand O, Jones M, Duvvi H, Shimotsuura Y. Effects of transcutaneous electrical stimulation (1 pulse/sec) through custom-made disposable surface electrodes covering Omura's ST36 area of both legs on normal cell telomeres, oncogen C-fosAb2, integrin alpha5beta1, chlamydia trachomatis, etc. in breast cancer & alzheimer patients. Acupunct Electrother Res. 2010;35(3-4):147-185.

6. Omura Y, Lu DP, Jones M, et al. New clinical findings on the longevity gene in disease, health, & longevity: Sirtuin 1 often decreases with advanced age & serious diseases in most parts of the human body, while relatively high & constant Sirtuin 1 regardless of age was first found in the hippocampus of supercentenarians. Acupunct Electrother Res. 2011;36(3-4):287-309.

7. Viswanathan A, Phan PC, Burton AW. Use of spinal cord stimulation in the treatment of phantom limb pain: case series and review of the literature. Pain Pract. 2010;10(5):479-484.

8. Sanchez-Ledesma MJ, Garcia-March G, Diaz-Cascajo P, Gomez-Moreta J, Broseta J. Spinal cord stimulation in deafferentation pain. Stereotact Funct Neurosurg. 1989;53(1):40-45.

9. Vergani F, Boukas A, Mukerji N, Nanavati N, Nicholson C, Jenkins A. Spinal cord stimulation for visceral pain related to chronic pancreatitis: report of 2 cases. World Neurosurg. 2014;81(3-4):651 e617-659.

10. Lowry AM, Simopoulos TT. Spinal cord stimulation for the treatment of chronic knee pain following total knee replacement. Pain Physician. 2010;13(3):251-256.

16. Spinal fluid opioid therapy

Some elderly patients, especially those with cancer may benefit from a "morphine pump." Narcotic drugs like morphine, baclofen, a muscle relaxant and a snail toxin called Prialt can be administered into the spinal fluid for pain control. A long term spinal fluid morphine therapy is a useful treatment option for patients with intractable severe pain who have failed other therapies and remain markedly disabled.

Drugs are administered via a pump system from a pump placed in the abdominal area with a tube that goes to the spinal fluid. The spinal infusion pump, commonly known as a "morphine pump," is a specialized device, which delivers concentrated small amounts of medication into the spinal fluid space via a small catheter.

The intrathecal space is the sac that contains the spinal fluid. The spinal infusion pump is also identified as an intrathecal infusion pump. Spinal infusion pump implants are offered to patients with chronic and severe pain, who have not adequately responded to other, more conservative, treatments. Usually these patients cannot be easily con-trolled on oral pain medications. As a result, to control their pain, these patients may benefit from a continuous spinal infusion of a pain medication, like morphine. Patients have to meet certain screening criteria before a spinal infusion pump is implanted.

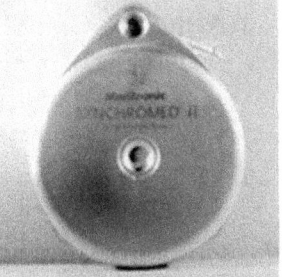

Figure 1. Spinal pump. The center of the pump has a hole where a drug can be placed to give continual pain relief. The pump is battery driven, and the dose of drug administered is controlled by a hand held programmer.

The spinal infusion pump delivers concentrated amounts of medication into the spinal fluid, thus continuously bathing the pain receptors on the spinal cord with pain medication. This allows the patient to eliminate or substantially decrease the need for oral medications for pain control.

The pump system delivers medication around the clock, consequently eliminating or minimizing breakthrough pain and other symptoms. The implantation of a spinal infusion pump is a surgical procedure. The patient procedure involves inserting an introducer needle through skin and deeper tissues. So, there is some pain involved.

However, the skin and deeper tissues are numbed with a local anesthetic using a very thin needle before inserting the larger introducer needle. Almost all the patients have anesthesia or also receive deep intravenous sedation that makes the procedure easy to tolerate. The spinal infusion catheter is inserted in the midline at the lower back. The infusion pump is then placed on the side of the abdomen in a pocket under the skin.

The pump is usually activated while a patient is still on the operating table. There will typically be some swelling over the pump site and tenderness or pain from the incisions. However, in many patients, this surgical pain and tenderness is controlled by the morphine infusion and may not require additional pain medications. The medication contained within the pump will last about 1 to 3 months depending on the concentration and amount infused. It is then refilled via a tiny needle inserted into the pump chamber. This is done in the office or at your home, and it takes only a few minutes.

The batteries in the pump may last 3 to 5 years. The batteries cannot be replaced or recharged. The pump must be replaced at that time. It is sometimes difficult to predict if a spinal infusion pump will indeed help you or not. For that reason, a trial of different doses of morphine injection into the spine is carried out to determine if a permanent pump would be efficient to relieve your pain or not. To find out whether a morphine pump is going to be effective, a trial with a temporary catheter connected to an externalized pump is often performed.

The Synchromed system is very expensive, and a patient, therefore, want to know if the spinal drug system provides pain relief. The trial is performed as an in-patient. A narrow gauge temporary catheter is inserted into the intrathecal space in the operating theatre using local anesthetic and intravenous sedation. This catheter is then tunneled around to the front of the abdomen and fixed in place with a nurse-proof and patient-proof dressing.

The catheter is then attached to an ambulatory battery operated infusion pump, which contains the preservative-free intrathecal (IT) morphine. During the first 24 hours, the morphine-containing oral drugs are slowly stopped, while the intrathecal morphine infusion is gradually increased to the point where the only morphine received is via the intrathecal route.

All other painkillers which do not contain morphine like drugs may be continued as normal, e.g. NSAIDs, amitriptyline, gabapentin, etc. Mobilization is encouraged the day after the procedure, and is combined with IT morphine dose adjustments to achieve reasonable relief while fully ambulant. A successful trial is one where there is obvious improvement in pain relief during a full range of normal activities, e.g. walking, sitting, dressing, bending, etc. At the end of the trial, the temporary catheter is removed, after noting the 24-hour dose of IT morphine. This helps the implanting surgeon start at the correct dose immediately post procedure.

Other types of spinal trials have been described. A single shot injection of spinal morphine may be administered. The effect of the morphine lasts only 24 hours and does not allow an adequate trial of full mobilization. Spinal headaches can also occur. Extradural infusions may be tried.

Achievement with an epidural infusion does not guarantee success with an IT infusion and vice versa. A patient should be aware that MRIs, if necessary, can be performed with a spinal infusion catheter and infusion pump in place. Special protocols for pump patients can be given to the MRI technicians and radiologists.

Prialt, (ziconotide) a snail toxin may help control pain from RSD as well as other neuropathic pain. This is a new drug used in the spinal drug-delivery systems. Of the patients who experienced substantial improvement in pain, edema, skin abnormalities, and/or mobility with ziconotide therapy, some patients have discontinued ziconotide and are pain free. Other patients experienced marked reversal of both edema and advanced skin trophic changes. Adverse events included urinary retention, depression, anxiety, and hallucinations.

Adverse events generally resolved spontaneously, with treatment, or with zicononotide discontinuation/dose reduction. Ziconotide holds promise as an effective treatment for RSD/CRPS as well. In general, the dose selection for an elderly patient should be cautious, usually starting at the low end of the dosing range, reflecting the greater frequency of decreased hepatic, renal or cardiac function, and of concomitant disease or other drug therapy.

Use of intrathecal admixtures is widespread, but compounding these is sometimes challenging and may result in errors and complications causing super-potency or sub potency adverse events in patients or malfunctions in the pump itself. Prospective assays provide benefits in ensuring accuracy of intrathecal mixture compounding and in preventing overdosing or sub dosing, most notably concerning Ziconotide.[1]

Loss of opioid tolerance due to delayed pump refill may subject patients to the development of severe respiratory depression. A meticulous approach should be employed when refilling pumps in these patients when their pumps are completely empty.[2] Intrathecal infusion with a low-concentration multidrug mixture could be considered as an alternative modality for intractable pain relief in older adults or in malignancies.[3]

In conclusion, spinal fluid drug delivery can provide excellent relief in some situations where other modalities have failed. There is no data to date that describes telomere effects.

References

1. Dupoiron D, Devys C, Bazin C, et al. Rationale for Prospective Assays of Intrathecal Mixtures Including Morphine, Ropivacaine and Ziconotide: Prevention of Adverse Events and Feasibility in Clinical Practice. Pain Physician. 2015;18(4):349-357.

2. Ruan X, Couch JP, Liu H, Shah RV, Wang F, Chiravuri S. Respiratory failure following delayed intrathecal morphine pump refill: a valuable, but costly lesson. Pain Physician. 2010;13(4):337-341.

3. Abdolmohammadi S, Hetu PO, Neron A, Blaise G. Efficacy of an intrathecal multidrug infusion for pain control in older adults and in end-stage malignancies: A report of three cases. Pain Res Manag. 2015;20(3):118-122.

17. Topical analgesics

Patients may turn to topical analgesics as a way to obtain relief with minimal adverse effects. Pain relievers that can be applied directly to the skin are available for the control of a variety of pain syndromes. These topical pain relievers are a noninvasive and convenient method for delivering pain-relieving medication to a patient. Topical analgesics have many advantages over systemically administered analgesics, including the ability to provide effective analgesia with reduced systemic drug levels, a factor particularly beneficial to the elderly.

Topical analgesics differ from transdermal delivery systems in that the latter's goal is to deliver systemic rather than local effects. Currently, the common topical analgesics include capsaicin cream 0.75%, lidocaine/prilocaine (EMLA), and the 5% lidocaine patch (Lidoderm). This is especially important and beneficial if you are not able to take medications by mouth. Topical pain relievers include complementary and alternative medications as well as conventional medications.

Ointments, creams, gels, and skin patches can help relieve pain. Often this is more effective than oral medications because they will have fewer side effects and fewer drug interactions. Topical analgesics can be used to relieve minor pain from muscle soreness to major pain from cancer. While the stronger versions of topical analgesics are prescription only, a patient can buy mild topical analgesics over-the-counter.

Topical forms of analgesics, or pain relievers, have been used throughout human history. The use of ointments for medicinal purposes is mentioned in the Bible on many occasions. The purpose of a topical analgesic is to transmit a medication through the skin for the effect of pain relief.

The amount of drug that actually gets through the skin is determined by the amount of pressure applied rubbed over the skin, the area of skin covered by the drug, the way in which the drug is dissolved, and the use of dressings over the skin. Analgesics are available in ointments, creams, and gels. They also may be placed in patches that may be applied to the skin as well.

The advantage of topical analgesics is that they can be placed on the skin over the site of the pain. When compared to oral medications, a patient will have a lower blood level of the drug and will have fewer side effects and fewer drug interactions.

Ointments are semisolid preparations that melt at body temperature and spread easily. Ointments are not routinely used for the practice of pain medicine unless the ointment is specially compounded by a pharmacy. Ointments are defined in three categories based on the skin penetration. One type of ointment does not penetrate beyond the external layer of the skin called the epidermis.

Ointments of this class can be used in the treatment of sunburn. A second type of ointment penetrates to the internal layer of your skin called the dermis. The third type of ointment actually goes through the skin to the nerves and ligaments and in some instances into the bloodstream.

Substances applied on the skin can evaporate. A pharmacist will add substances such as glycerin to the ointment to keep this evaporation from happening. Ointments can be prepared by a pharmacist or purchased over the counter or by prescription; ointments should be packaged in tubes. Some ointment preparations will contain absorption enhancers. Absorption enhancers make it easier for the drug to be absorbed through the skin. Azone and DMSO can both enhance the absorption of ointments through the skin.

Creams are opaque, thick, liquid substances that consist of medications dissolved in a cream base that usually vanishes through the skin. They are less of a liquid consistency than ointments. The term cream is used to describe a soft type of preparation that is less affected by body temperature than ointments. The therapeutic difference between creams and ointments is that creams penetrate deeper than ointments.

Pain-relieving creams, also called topical analgesics, applied to the skin over the joints can provide relief of minor arthritis pain. They are available over the counter and can often be used in conjunction with oral medications. Examples include capsaicin (Zostrix), salicin (Aspercreme), methyl salicylate (Bengay), and menthol (Flexall).

Gels are a drug-delivery system that usually contain penetration enhancers and are usually used for administering anti-inflammatory medications. The anti-inflammatory medication must be absorbed through the skin to provide pain relief. Gels are useful treatment methods if one has arthritic and/or muscle pain. Gels usually are thicker than creams or ointments and are usually clear, unlike creams and ointments. The concentration of medication in gels is usually no greater than 2 percent.

For example, lidocaine, which is a numbing medicine for the control of pain, is dispensed as a 2 percent gel. However, the cream is available in a 5 percent concentration. This is because medications are usually absorbed through the skin better if used in gel form. Gels typically have clarity and sparkle. They maintain their thickness even with an elevated body temperature. Some gels have been developed to be given nasally.

Voltaren Gel (diclofenac topical) gives patients the ability to apply something topically, which will not give significant blood levels, but will penetrate the skin and help reduce pain. This gel should not be used in combination with oral NSAIDs or aspirin because of the potential for adverse effects. The Voltaren gel is used for pain caused by osteoarthritis. Gels are usually dispensed in tubes or squeeze bottles.

Many elderly patients can't take oral NSAIDs because they have stomach or heart risk factors. The new Voltaren Gel gives aging patients the ability to apply something topically, which will not give significant blood levels, but will penetrate the skin and help reduce pain.

A new form of NSAID delivery is Pennsaid, which comes in a liquid application. Osteoarthritis of the knee is a chronic condition requiring long-term therapy for elderly patients. Studies have suggested that topical NSAIDs may present a safer GI alternative to oral therapy because of their low systemic exposure to the active NSAID molecule.

Diclofenac systemic exposure from PENNSAID application (four times daily for one week) was calculated to be 3.3%. Although NSAIDs have been shown to inhibit platelet aggregation, PENNSAID had no effect on platelet aggregation after maximum clinical use for seven days.

Another delivery system for analgesics is a transdermal patch, which contains medication that is transmitted directly through the skin. A patch containing a medication is placed on the skin and remains there for a specified time so that the drug within the patch can be delivered through the skin to the bloodstream.

Local anesthetics such as lidocaine, capsaicin cream, and fentanyl, a potent opioid medication, are some of the medicines that can be delivered through the skin using a transdermal drug delivery system. These patches should be applied only to areas on the skin that have no blisters or open areas such as a cut.

The patches are made of adhesive materials. A patient should not use the patch if the patient is allergic to some adhesives. With respect to the patches, the amount of drug that is absorbed from the patch is directly related with the length of the application of the patch, as well as the area of the skin to which it is applied.

Topical 5% lidocaine medicated plasters represent a well-established first-line option for the treatment of peripheral localized neuropathic pain (LNP). The 5% lidocaine medicated plaster is efficacious and safe in LNP and may have particular clinical benefit in elderly and/or medically compromised patients because of the low incidence of adverse events.[1]

A nonsteroidal patch called the Flector patch (diclofenac) has become popular in the treatment of arthritis. It is used in acute pain situations. The Flector topical patch is a nonsteroidal anti-inflammatory drug (NSAID). It may cause an increased risk of serious and sometimes fatal heart and blood vessel problems (e.g., heart attack, stroke, blood clots). The risk may be greater if a patient has heart problems, or if a patient uses the Flector topical patch for a long time. Elderly patients may be at greater risk of these side effects.

The advantage of the patch is that it gives a patient a continuous flow of analgesic medications. When a patient takes a pill, after it leaves the stomach or intestine and enters into the bloodstream, a patient receives a high concentration of the drug initially. As the drug is distributed in other tissues in the body, the blood level of the drug will decrease.

Once the body breaks down the drug, a patient will no longer have an analgesic effect of that particular drug. However, when using a patch, a patient will have a continuous release of the drug from the patch into the bloodstream. A patient will have constant pain relief without the peaks and valleys of the drug concentration in the bloodstream associated with oral medications.

Topical analgesics represent a promising area for future drug development. Their use has grown to a $150 million dollar industry. Elderly women use these medications more than men. However, there have been no good studies comparing the effects of topical analgesics on men as compared to women. As new topical analgesics are being developed, it is anticipated that a gender analysis will be a part of the topical analgesic drug study.

Topical aspirin (ASA) may be an effective analgesic in patients with acute herpetic neuralgia and post herpetic neuralgia. Patients with excellent pain relief showed a trend towards higher ASA skin concentrations. The analgesic effect can be obtained only after topical administration, because by this route the skin levels of ASA are much higher than after oral administration.[2]

The mechanism is exclusively local. There are no active drugs in plasma after topical administration. Furthermore, peppermint oil (containing 10% menthol) applied to the skin, resulted in an almost immediate improvement in acute herpetic neuralgia and post herpetic neuralgia pain.[3]

The 5% lidocaine medicated plaster is a topical treatment for peripheral neuropathic pain symptoms (e.g. burning, shooting and stabbing pain) and is registered for the treatment of post herpetic neuralgia. A study has demonstrated that 5% lidocaine medicated plaster provides sustained pain relief over long-term treatment in patients with neuropathic pain of various causes and is well tolerated.[4]

Evidence-based treatment guidelines recommend the 5% lidocaine (lignocaine) medicated plaster or pregabalin as first-line therapy for relief of peripheral neuropathic pain. 5% lidocaine medicated plaster treatment was associated with similar levels of analgesia in patients with PHN or DPN but substantially fewer frequent adverse events than pregabalin.[5]

Natural compounds such as herbs or leaves and roots also can be used to treat pain topically. Aloe Vera can be used to decrease pain if a patient has sunburn. Use of this natural topical product for the treatment of various medical conditions was discovered in 1935. This drug is effective in the treatment of skin inflammation as well as minor burns. There are no side effects nor are there are any known drug interactions.

Capsaicin is a drug that has been extensively studied in both the clinical and laboratory settings. Capsaicin is the active component of chili or red peppers. Capsaicin can be put on the skin over a patient's joints if he/she has joint pain. The capsaicin first stimulates the small pain-transmitting fibers by depleting them of the neurotransmitter substance P.

After the substance P has been depleted, a patient will have a block of the pain fibers that cause burning pain sensations. Observations in Hispanic individuals demonstrated that they did not have mouth or stomach pain after ingesting red peppers. The reason is the depletion of the substance P in the nerve endings in these areas following continuous exposure to red peppers.

Topical non-steroidal anti-inflammatory drugs (NSAIDs) are recommended in international and national guidelines as an early treatment option for the symptomatic management of knee and hand osteoarthritis, and may be used ahead of oral NSAIDs due to their superior safety profile.[6]

Substance P also is present in a patient's joints throughout the body. For this reason, capsaicin can be an effective pain reliever for the treatment of pain associated with osteoarthritis and rheumatoid arthritis. It may take a week to feel the pain-relieving effects of capsaicin.

As substance P is being depleted from nerve endings, a patient's nerve endings still manufacture substance P. As a result, it will take several days to deplete enough of the substance P to provide pain relief. Once a patient discontinues use of this cream, the nerves will replenish substance P, and the pain may return.

Some studies have shown that if a patient has a neuropathy related to diabetes a patient could have significant pain relief with topical capsaicin.

Some pain-medicine physicians have used topical capsaicin to relieve the pain associated with shingles. A patient may have a brief burning sensation following the use of capsaicin. A patient should be warned to avoid contact with the eyes and genital areas. It is recommended that a patient use rubber gloves when applying the capsaicin cream.

A patient should use the capsaicin cream no more than three times a day. Various concentrations of capsaicin exist. Begin with a small concentration that contains 0.025 percent capsaicin. A patient may eventually increase ther capsaicin dose to 0.075 percent capsaicin.

Menthol is oil that is one component of peppermint oil. This oil as a cream base can significantly decrease pain. When one places a menthol preparation on the skin, the menthol will feel cold to a patient's nerve endings. While a patient feels the cold sensation, the pain-stimulating nerves will be depressed. Following the initial cool sensation, a patient will feel a period of warmth. Menthol products can be used for the treatment of pain associated with arthritis, muscle pain, and tendonitis.

Application of a menthol-containing cream may be of benefit to a patient if he/she suffers from tension headaches. It can be rubbed around the neck muscles just below the skull. It can be an extremely effective method in the treatment of headaches. Allergic reactions with menthol have been reported.

It is recommended that a patient test a small amount of menthol on the skin before applying it extensively to assure that he/she is not allergic to it. A patient should not use the menthol preparation more than three times a day. Do not use a heating pad or a cold pack over the area of the skin where the menthol substance was placed.

Some natural herbs and vegetables can be used as a topical analgesic. One example is an onion. It is reported by some doctors that spreading the juice of a sliced onion over one of painful areas could reduce pain.

A tincture can be made by putting 100 grams of minced onions in 30 grams of ethanol for a 70 percent solution. There are no hazards or side effects associated with the topical administration of an onion. However, frequent contact with the onion over time could possibly lead to an allergic reaction.

Poplar tree bark also can be used for relieving pain. The bark is dried and placed in capsules or chemicals are extracted, for example, as in a tea. The bark can be used for control of pain over a patient's joints or nerves, or if a patient has rheumatoid arthritis. A patient should not use the bark if he/she is allergic to aspirin. When externally applied using the poplar bark and leaves, a patient should use no more than five grams of the drug per day.

When using these topical natural products, a patient must follow the directions for the use of these medicines that are contained either on the outside of the package or from an insert that may be placed in a box that holds a tube of any of these substances. A patient should remember that although these are natural products, they can have side effects like any other medication.

Another topical medication used to decrease pain is EMLA cream. It is used as a numbing agent more than it is used for reducing pain. This is a cream consisting of lidocaine and prilocaine, which are both numbing agents. This local anesthetic combination is packaged in tubes. There also is an EMLA cellulose disc that can be applied over painful areas.

The purpose of this medication is to provide pain relief over the area on the skin. It is used in children to reduce the pain of starting intravenous lines. Some pain-management doctors advocate its use to decrease the pain associated with reflex sympathetic dystrophy or the pain associated with shingles. This cream should be placed on an intact skin area.

The EMLA should be applied with a bandage for at least 60 minutes to provide relief over the painful area of the skin. This cream is not recommended if a patient has an allergy to lidocaine or prilocaine. If a patient has the blood disorder methemoglobinemia, a patient should not use this cream. A patient should not exceed the recommended dose prescribed by a physician.

The problem with this cream as opposed to the Lidoderm patches is that it does provide pain relief for the skin. This means that a patient has block of all sensations on the skin treated with this cream. A patient should avoid causing any trauma to the area, including scratching the skin or rubbing or exposing the skin to extreme hot or cold temperatures until a patient has a complete return of sensation to the skin. It is recommended that a patient not use this medication if the patient is taking heart medication. The local anesthetics in this cream can interact with some heart medicines.

If a patient develops a rash with use of this cream, the must stop using it. There have been reports of blistering on skin following application of the EMLA cream. You may experience itching as well. The problem with this topical analgesic is that it is hard to control and regulate the dose of medication that a patient receives. A patient must refer to the insert supplied by the drug company. This can be found in the box that contains the tube of the cream.

Another analgesic cream that is available is a combination of methyl salicylate and menthol. This is a cream that is effective for the temporary relief of arthritis and pain in muscles. A patient should not use this medicine if a patient is sensitive to the oil of wintergreen. A patient should apply this cream around the sore areas on the body. A patient should not apply this cream more than three times a day. A patient should not place this cream over areas on the skin that are broken because it will cause extreme discomfort to that area.

Steroid creams are sometimes used in the treatment of joint pain. Topical steroids are anti-inflammatory agents. Pramoxine hydrochloride is a topical anesthetic agent that sometimes is combined with steroids to attempt to manage pain. This cream provides a temporary relief from pain. Adjuvant analgesics, topical analgesics, anesthetic techniques and interventional techniques are all valid methods to help in the difficult management of pain and BTP in elderly patients with cancer.[7]

Nonsteroidal anti-inflammatory agents (NSAIDS) that are commonly taken by mouth for the treatment of bone, joint, and muscle pain may be placed into a cream by your pharmacist. For these drugs to give you pain relief, they must penetrate the skin and enter the bloodstream.

These creams should not be used more than three times a day. Side effects with the nonsteroidal anti-inflammatory creams are the same as with the NSAIDs taken by mouth. However, the side effects of the topical NSAIDS are less than the oral NSAIDS. The side effects of any NSAID can include stomach upset and allergic reactions. If the dose is high enough, it could affect the liver and kidneys.

These NSAIDs can be very effective for the management of pain when applied over the skin. The use of a ketoprofen gel (Ketoprofen Gel) and a diclofenac gel, both NSAIDs, were compared at painful sites in a four-week study. The ketoprofen gel gave positive results for the treatment of knee pain and was shown to be better at relieving pain than the diclofenac gel. Aspirin creams also may provide you with some pain relief when applied over the painful joints or muscles as well.

Amitriptyline, which is an antidepressant, has recently been shown to have pain-relieving properties when applied topically. Amitriptyline cream may be advantageous if one does not want to take amitriptyline pills by mouth. The amitriptyline cream will not help a patient if a patient is suffering from significant depression, but can be helpful in decreasing pain.

Some people complain of being tired while taking amitriptyline. However, amitriptyline can contribute to pain relief in fibromyalgia and the topical application may be a way of avoiding significant side effects that can be associated with oral use. There is ongoing research in this area.

Current research is being done at a cancer center using a combination of lidocaine and morphine administered topically. This combination showed greater pain-relieving effects than the topical opioids or topical local anesthetics by themselves. Studies demonstrate a potent interaction between the morphine and the lidocaine that can offer potential advantages in the clinical management of the pain if it is severe. Again, follow the development of this drug combination. This combination is currently only under investigation for cancer patients.

Another way of delivering medication is through a patch placed on the skin over the site of the pain. Research is promising in the area of skin patches that relieve pain. Because analgesic patches have fewer side effects and fewer drug interactions than some oral medications, a patient may find that a patch will work better.. The transdermal fentanyl patch system has become popular since it was introduced in the 1980s.

This strong opioid medication was used initially for cancer pain management and then for non-cancer, chronic pain management. The fentanyl is able penetrate the skin easily. Fentanyl is 70 times more potent than morphine. It produces less histamine release from cells in the bloodstream and causes less itching than morphine. The fentanyl patch is primarily used for chronic or cancer-related pain. A fentanyl patch can be used for most moderate to severe pain syndromes.

In the fentanyl patch, the medication exists as a gel in a drug reservoir. Between this reservoir and the skin is a release membrane that has various-size holes that regulate the amount of fentanyl that is delivered to the skin. The larger the size of the holes, the more fentanyl that is distributed to the skin and eventually through the skin.

The adhesiveness around the patch keeps it in place. When the fentanyl patch is placed on the skin, the drug diffuses through the holes in the release membrane to the surface of the skin. It then goes to the outer layer of the skin and is deposited in a storage area. From the storage area, it is gradually absorbed into the bloodstream.

This is the reason that it takes at least an hour before the fentanyl has begun to enter the bloodstream. A patient will probably not notice any pain-relieving effects from this drug-delivery system for about six hours. The patch is usually removed every three days. After the patch is removed, a patient will still have some drug that remains in the storage area under the skin. If a patient removes the patch and does not replace it, a patient will still receive Fentanyl for hours after the patch has been removed.

Fentanyl patches come in different concentrations (12, 25, 50, 75 and 100 micrograms). The concentrations correlate with the area on the skin to which they are applied. The effectiveness of the patch is not affected by placing it on the chest, back, or upper arm. An increase in temperature will cause however, cause the medication to be rapidly delivered from the patch to the bloodstream.

A patient's skin thickness also can affect the amount of fentanyl that is absorbed through the skin. The thicker the skin, the slower the rate of delivery of the fentanyl will be. The patch on the other hand should not be applied over broken skin because the blood level of fentanyl can be significantly raised. The patch can cause a decrease in breathing and even death if a patient receives a significantly high dose of the fentanyl.

If a patient has significant vomiting associated with severe pain, a patient cannot keep oral medications in the stomach. Therefore, they are not absorbed into a patient's bloodstream, and the patient receives no pain relief from the medicine. If this is the case, a doctor may prescribe the fentanyl patch for pain control.

There is no upper limit as to the number of fentanyl patches that can be worn at one time. Some cancer patients require more than one patch at a time. Side effects of the patches containing fentanyl include nausea, constipation, and sleepiness. The patch can cause reactions to the skin related to the adhesive used in the patch if a patient is allergic to adhesives.

Occasionally, an oral medication can be taken for treatment of any breakthrough pain. Elderly patients can be at risk for harm if they do not properly use the patches. The FDA said patients also accidentally overdose by using the patches wrong, such as putting on more than prescribed, replacing them too frequently or getting them too hot.

Another popular patch that is readily available by prescription is the lidocaine containing patch called Lidoderm. The Lidoderm transdermal drug-delivery system exerts a significant amount of its pain-relieving effects by releasing a small amount of lidocaine into the bloodstream.

There also is an effect upon the nerves under the skin that are transmitting pain. This patch is used for the treatment of post-herpetic neuralgia, a long-lasting pain that is a result of shingles. Approximately, 1 million people develop shingles every year. Twenty percent of these individuals will develop post-herpetic neuralgia, which is an extremely painful syndrome.

The U.S. Food and Drug Administration has approved the use of the Lidoderm patch for the treatment of the severe pain following the onset of shingles. Shingles is an infection caused by the chicken pox virus. A patient may have had chicken pox as a child. However, the virus remains inactive in the nervous system for many years. At some time in a patient's life, this virus can become reactivated and travel via nerves to certain areas on the skin, causing a patient to have severe pain.

When the virus reaches a patient's skin, he or she may develop blisters that can be severely painful as well. After the blisters have disappeared, a patient may have persistent pain. This pain is called post-herpetic neuralgia. In many instances, there is no cure for this pain. The Lidoderm patch has been demonstrated in clinical studies to significantly decrease pain following the outbreak of shingles.

The Lidoderm patch contains five percent lidocaine. The lidocaine penetrates the skin just enough to reach the nerve endings that are transmitting the pain. As a result, there are minimal side effects from the use of this patch other than from the adhesive layer of the patch. The amount of the lidocaine that is absorbed from the Lidoderm is related with the length of application over the skin.

The patch should be used for 12 hours over the painful area and then removed for 12 hours. If an irritation or a burning sensation occurs around the adhesive aspect of the patch, one should discontinue the use of the patch. None of the patches mentioned in this chapter should ever be reused.

A patient should not use the Lidoderm patch if the patient is using a heart drug to control the heartbeat. Even though the amount of lidocaine that a patient can absorb is small, it can interfere with some heart medicines. Clonidine is another transdermal medication. This patch is applied weekly to an area of the skin. The clonidine patch inhibits the release of norepinephrine, which is a pain transmitter. The clonidine patch also is used in the treatment of hypertension.

If a patient has neuropathic pain or reflex sympathetic dystrophy, the clonidine patch may provide significant pain relief. It also can be successfully used if a patient has shingles. Clonidine patches are alpha agonists. They work by relaxing blood vessels and decreasing a patient's heart rate, which lowers the blood pressure.

Topical analgesics have many advantages over systemically administered analgesics, including the ability to provide effective analgesia with reduced systemic drug levels which is a factor which may be particularly beneficial to the elderly patient. Anti-aging medicine-oriented groups have intervened on the market with products working on telomerase activation for a broad range of degenerative diseases in which replicative senescence or telomere dysfunction may play an important role.

Since oxidative damage has been shown to shorten telomeres in tissue culture models, the adequate topical, transdermal, or systemic administration of antioxidants (such as, patented ocular administration of 1% N-acetylcarnosine lubricant eye drops in the treatment of cataracts) may be beneficial at preserving telomere lengths and delaying the onset or in treatment of disease in susceptible individuals. Therapeutic strategies toward controlled transient activation of telomerase are targeted to cells and replicative potential in cell-based therapies, tissue engineering and regenerative medicine.[8]

Eye drops may preserve telomere length in cataract patients. Research may eventually demonstrate telomere length in other anatomic areas. Patented ocular administration of 1% N-acetylcarnosine lubricant eye drops in the treatment of cataracts) may be beneficial at preserving telomere lengths and delaying the onset or in treatment of disease in susceptible individuals. Therapeutic strategies toward controlled transient activation of telomerase are targeted to cells and replicative potential in cell-based therapies, tissue engineering and regenerative medicine.[4]

References

1. de Leon-Casasola OA, Mayoral V. The topical 5% lidocaine medicated plaster in localized neuropathic pain: a reappraisal of the clinical evidence. J Pain Res. 2016;9:67-79.

2. Bareggi SR, Pirola R, De Benedittis G. Skin and plasma levels of acetylsalicylic acid: a comparison between topical aspirin/diethyl ether mixture and oral aspirin in acute herpes zoster and postherpetic neuralgia. Eur J Clin Pharmacol. 1998;54(3):231-235.

3. Davies SJ, Harding LM, Baranowski AP. A novel treatment of postherpetic neuralgia using peppermint oil. Clin J Pain. 2002;18(3):200-202.

4. Wilhelm IR, Tzabazis A, Likar R, Sittl R, Griessinger N. Long-term treatment of neuropathic pain with a 5% lidocaine medicated plaster. Eur J Anaesthesiol. 2010;27(2):169-173.

5. Baron R, Mayoral V, Leijon G, Binder A, Steigerwald I, Serpell M. Efficacy and safety of 5% lidocaine (lignocaine) medicated plaster in comparison with pregabalin in patients with postherpetic neuralgia and diabetic polyneuropathy: interim analysis from an open-label, two-stage adaptive, randomized, controlled trial. Clin Drug Investig. 2009;29(4):231-241.

6. Rannou F, Pelletier JP, Martel-Pelletier J. Efficacy and safety of topical NSAIDs in the management of osteoarthritis: Evidence from real-life setting trials and surveys. Semin Arthritis Rheum. 2016;45(4 Suppl):S18-21.

7. Pautex S, Vogt-Ferrier N, Zulian GB. Breakthrough pain in elderly patients with cancer: treatment options. Drugs Aging. 2014;31(6):405-411.

8. Babizhayev MA, Yegorov YE. Tissue formation and tissue engineering through host cell recruitment or a potential injectable cell-based biocomposite with replicative potential: Molecular mechanisms controlling cellular senescence and the involvement of controlled transient telomerase activation therapies. J Biomed Mater Res A. 2015;103(12):3993-4023.

18. Acute post-surgical pain

Pain (chest, stomach, hip, etc.) is the most common symptom encountered in an elderly hospitalized patient. If a patient suffers from chronic pain, a patient could be hospitalized for surgery and subsequently have acute post-surgical pain. The patient still needs the chronic pain medications, but now has additional acute pain in addition to the chronic pain.

A patient's current medications will not help the new severe pain. Although effective pain treatment is available for cancer-related pain and acute post-operative pain, many patients suffer unnecessarily.

Acute pain management is necessary following surgery, in burn patients and in sickle cell disease. The manner in which acute pain is treated can affect the chronic pain occurrence and its management for elderly patients. Acute pain is the pain that a patient experiences after tissue injury from surgery, cancer or trauma. Chronic pain is the pain that continues after the tissue has healed. Pain that is under treated at the hospital can lead to an increase in a patient's blood pressure and heart rate.

If a patient has severe acute pain, a patient can suffer psychological distress as well as demoralization. The treatment of acute pain must be provided on an individualized basis. Under treated acute pain may make the management of chronic pain difficult, as a patient may be skeptical about pain care from other physicians.

A patient may as a result of improperly acute pain management exaggerate symptoms to ensure that the patient receives an adequate dose of pain medications for acute pain management.

The acute pain specialist who is usually the anesthesiologist must be responsive to a patient's needs. Effective pain management is fundamental to quality care, and excellent pain control speeds recovery following surgery.

Advantages of good acute pain management can be shown by increases in patient mobility and cough suppression. Effective relief can be achieved with oral non-opioids and non-steroidal anti-inflammatory drugs. These drugs are appropriate for many post-surgical and post traumatic pains, especially when a patient goes home on the day of the operation.

The optimal treatment of both acute and chronic pain should employ both medications and non-medication approaches. For some chronic or acute pain, an epidural catheter can be placed in a patient to give numbing medications (epidural block). Non opioids, such as nonsteroidal anti-inflammatory drugs, gabapentin, pregabilin and acetaminophen, are used to treat mild pain for minor surgical procedures.

A single low dose of 600 mg gabapentin administered 1 h prior to surgery produced effective and significant postoperative analgesia after total mastectomy and axillary dissection without significant side effects.[1] Perioperative administration of 150 mg of pregabalin decreased opioid consumption in a hospital setting and reduced daily pain scores and adjunct opioid consumption for 1 week after discharge.[2]

Many patients may suffer from neuropathic pain in the early post-surgical period after lumbar discectomy. Gabapentin and pregabalin are anticonvulsant agents that may decrease perioperative central sensitization and early post-surgical neuropathic pain. Gabapentin and pregabalin effectively relieved neuropathic pain and prevented the conversion of acute pain to chronic pain at the 1-year follow-up after lumbar discectomy.[3]

Administration of gabapentin 1,200 mg prior to surgery reduces preoperative NRS anxiety scores and pain catastrophizing scores and increases sedation prior to entering the operating room. These results suggest that gabapentin 1,200 mg may be a treatment option for patients who exhibit high levels of preoperative anxiety.[4]

Gabapentin and ketamine are similar in improving early pain control and in decreasing opioid consumption following surgery. However, gabapentin also prevented chronic pain in the first 6 postoperative months.[5]

Moderate to severe pain after total knee arthroplasty often interferes with postoperative rehabilitation and delays discharge from hospital. Patients who received gabapentin postoperatively used significantly less patient-controlled morphine analgesia at 24 h, 36 h and 48 h. The postoperative gabapentin patients had significantly better active assisted knee flexion on postoperative days 2 and 3, with a trend toward better flexion on postoperative day 4. Patients who received gabapentin postoperatively reported less pruritus than patients who received placebo. There were no differences in pain scores between the groups.[6]

Opioids are recommended for moderate to severe pain. In other words, the patient's pain intensity should determine the choice of medication. Acute pain should be treated early to avoid needless suffering. Patients should be placed on long-acting medications like extended release morphine to control their chronic pain and shorter-acting medications like tramadol to control breakthrough pain.

Some patients may have more breakthrough pain relative to their chronic pain. Their treatment must therefore be individualized. For a patient whose breakthrough pain comes on gradually and lasts 45 minutes to an hour, conventional, shorter acting opioids may suffice.

A patient's perception of pain varies among individuals. A person's first experience with severe pain may be after surgery. At one time post-surgical pain was managed with shots of narcotics into the muscles. Postoperative pain management is now more advanced. The goal of acute pain management is to keep a patient comfortable while avoiding opioid addiction.

Inadequately treated acute pain may result in patient depression and/or anxiety. Depression can decrease a patient's pain tolerance. This means that mild pain may be perceived as severe pain by the depressed patient. There is an ethical and humanitarian need to treat patients suffering from acute pain.

Barriers to effective pain management involve prejudice on the part of the physicians and/or patients and their families. Patients and some physicians are afraid of opioid addiction. Addiction usually does not occur when an opioid is used short term.

When considering the use of opioids for acute pain, the treating physician must consider the risks and benefits of opioid administration. The physician must, however, consider the ethical responsibility of relieving a patient's pain and suffering. For severe acute pain opioids are the first-line treatment.

Intermittent opioid injections can provide effective relief from acute pain. Unfortunately, adequate doses are withheld because of traditions, misconceptions, ignorance and fear. Doctors and nurses fear addiction and respiratory depression.

Addiction is not a problem with opioid use in acute pain. Irrespective of the route, opioids used for people who are not in pain, or in doses larger than necessary to control the pain, can slow or stop breathing. The key principle is to titrate the dose against the desired effect.

There is no evidence that demonstrates that one opioid is better than another. Morphine is commonly used in the treatment of acute pain. Morphine has an active metabolite, morphine-6-glucuronide. Morphine also has a metabolite, morphine-3-glucuronide that does not provide pain relief. In renal dysfunction morphine-6-glucuronide can accumulate in your body and result in a greater effect from a given dose, because it is more active than morphine.

Less morphine will be needed to control a patient's pain. Accumulation of morphine can be a problem with unconscious intensive care patients on fixed dose schedules when renal function is compromised. Opioid adverse effects include nausea and vomiting, constipation, sedation, pruritus (itching), urinary retention and respiratory depression. There is no-good evidence that the incidences of these side effects are different with different opioids.

Aggressive pain management can decrease postoperative recovery time. This aggressive management can decrease the incidence of developing chronic pain. Patient-controlled analgesia is a method of pain relief that allows you to self-administer small amounts of narcotics on demand into your vein. The patient presses a button and receives a pre-set dose of opioid, from a syringe driver connected to an intravenous or subcutaneous needle. This device delivers opioid to the same opioid receptors as an intermittent injection, but allows one to prevent delays for pain treatment.

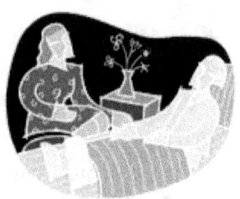

Figure 1. Good acute pain management is important in the hospitalized older patient.

There is little difference in outcome between efficient intermittent injections and patient control analgesia. A patient can select how much medication is necessary to control the pain. This method of pain relief avoids delays in the pain management. A patient has have control over the pain.

This method of pain relief is safe because the drug-delivery machine only allows a patient to get a specific amount of drug each hour. When it is time to discontinue the medicine, a patient will be given an oral medication. A patient will still have access to the drug-delivery machine.

Another method of pain relief is the administration of a drug under the skin (subcutaneous). If a patient's veins are not readily accessible, this method of pain relief can be effective. Epidural analgesia is another method for managing your pain after surgery.

A small tube is placed in a patient's back. A pump is connected to this tube to give pain medicine when needed. This pump can be programmed to give medication not unlike the patient controlled drug delivery system. Narcotics, local anesthetics and muscle relaxants can be placed into the body by this method.

Narcotics can also be placed into a patient's spinal fluid. This is called intrathecal therapy and is used for acute cancer pain management. If a patient is having surgery on an arm or leg for example, a small tube can be placed in the extremity that will give a continuous dose of local anesthetic. A patient can then have physical therapy without pain. Other routes of opioid administration include joint injection, nasal, active transdermal and inhalational administration.

Pre-emptive analgesia is used when patients have established pain prior to surgery. For example, if a patient has severe chronic hand and wrist pain prior to scheduled surgery, the anesthesiologist may do a nerve block to stop the pain prior to hand surgery. The advantage of regional analgesia with a local anesthetic is that it can deliver complete pain relief by interrupting pain transmission from a specific area, so avoiding generalized drug adverse effects. This advantage is more obvious when it is possible to give further doses via a catheter, extending the duration of analgesia.

Established pain is harder to control than new pain. When chronic pain occurs, changes occur in the brain and spinal cord. These changes enhance pain perception after surgery.

Placement of an epidural catheter with the administration of a local anesthetic (numbing medication) can significantly decrease postoperative pain and may decrease the chance of developing chronic pain. Extradural infusion via a catheter can offer continuous relief after trauma or surgery, for the lower limb, spine, abdominal or chest.

The risks of associated with an extradural injection include a spinal headache, infection, bleeding or nerve damage. Some epidural infusions contain local anesthetics. Side effects of local anesthetics include a decrease in blood pressure, motor block of muscles, seizures, and heart rhythm disturbances. If opioids are used, side effects can include nausea and vomiting, sedation, urinary retention, respiratory depression and generalized itching.

References

1. Grover VK, Mathew PJ, Yaddanapudi S, Sehgal S. A single dose of preoperative gabapentin for pain reduction and requirement of morphine after total mastectomy and axillary dissection: randomized placebo-controlled double-blind trial. J Postgrad Med. 2009;55(4):257-260.

2. Clarke H, Page GM, McCartney CJ, et al. Pregabalin reduces postoperative opioid consumption and pain for 1 week after hospital discharge, but does not affect function at 6 weeks or 3 months after total hip arthroplasty. Br J Anaesth. 2015;115(6):903-911.

3. Dolgun H, Turkoglu E, Kertmen H, et al. Gabapentin versus pregabalin in relieving early post-surgical neuropathic pain in patients after

lumbar disc herniation surgery: a prospective clinical trial. Neurol Res. 2014;36(12):1080-1085.

4. Clarke H, Kirkham KR, Orser BA, et al. Gabapentin reduces preoperative anxiety and pain catastrophizing in highly anxious patients prior to major surgery: a blinded randomized placebo-controlled trial. Can J Anaesth. 2013;60(5):432-443.

5. Sen H, Sizlan A, Yanarates O, et al. A comparison of gabapentin and ketamine in acute and chronic pain after hysterectomy. Anesth Analg. 2009;109(5):1645-1650.

6. Clarke H, Pereira S, Kennedy D, et al. Gabapentin decreases morphine consumption and improves functional recovery following total knee arthroplasty. Pain Res Manag. 2009;14(3):217-222.

19. Injection therapy

Various pain-modifying procedures are available to help alleviate pain. Epidural steroid injections (ESI) can decrease pain if it goes from the neck to the arm (cervical ESI), the mid back to the chest (thoracic ESI) or the lower back down the leg (lumbar ESI). If a patient has an injured disc in one of these areas of the spine, some chemicals can leak out and affect one or more of the nerves. These chemicals can cause nerves to swell. When the nerves swell, they may cause pain.

Epidural steroid injections (ESIs) are a common treatment option for many forms of low back pain and leg pain. They have been used for low back problems since 1952 and are still an integral part of the non-surgical management of low back pain and sciatica.

The goal of the injection is pain relief; at times, the injection alone is sufficient to provide relief, but commonly an epidural steroid injection is used in combination with a comprehensive rehabilitation program to provide additional benefit.

Most practitioners will agree that the effects from the injection tend to be temporary. The ESI can provide relief from pain for one week up to one year. An epidural injection can be very beneficial to a patient during an acute episode of back and/or leg pain. Importantly, an injection can provide sufficient pain relief to allow a patient to progress with a rehabilitative stretching and exercise program.

If the initial injection is effective, a patient may have up to three in a one-year period. In addition to addition to low back (the lumbar region), epidural steroid injections are used to ease pain experienced in the neck (cervical) region or in the mid spine (thoracic) region.

An ESI can be done by the transforaminal or route. The transforaminal (TF) approach is preferred by some physicians to the interlaminar (IL) approach because it can deliver injectates directly around nerve root and dorsal root ganglion, which is regarded as main pain sources.

Cervical epidural injection showed favorable results in 2 weeks and moderate results in 8 weeks in patients with axial pain due to cervical disc herniation. IL and TF showed no significant difference in clinical efficacy. Considering TF was relevant to more serious side effects, IL was more recommendable in patients.[1] It is important to know that transforaminal epidural steroid injections can injure nerve roots as well as the spinal cord when done even by the most experienced pain pain management physician.

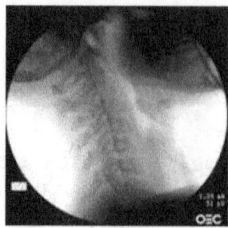

Figure 1. An epidural needle is being placed in the epidural space with X ray guidance.

Although many studies document the short-term benefits of epidural steroid injections, the data on long-term effectiveness are less convincing. Indeed, the effectiveness of epidural steroid injections continues to be a topic of debate. This is accentuated by the lack of properly performed studies. For example, many studies do not include use of fluoroscopy or x-ray to verify proper placement of the medication although fluoroscopic guidance is routinely used today.

Additionally, many studies do not classify patients according to diagnosis and tend to 'lump' different sources of pain together. These methodological flaws tend to make interpretation and application of study results difficult to impossible.

More studies are needed to properly define the role of epidural steroid injections in low back pain and in sciatica as well as pain in the neck and mid back. Despite this, most studies report that more than 50% of patients find measurable pain relief with epidural steroid injections.

They also underscore the need for patients to enlist the services of professionals with extensive experience administering injections, and who always use fluoroscopy to ensure accurate placement. Epidural steroid injections deliver medication directly (or very near) the source of pain generation. With X ray guidance the needle tip can be placed where the discs are disrupted. In contrast, oral steroids go throughout your body may have unacceptable side effects.

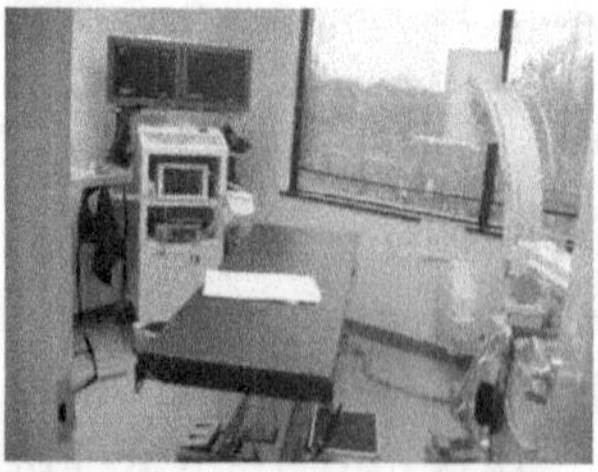

Figure 2. An injection can be performed as an office, surgery center or hospital with an X-ray machine. The heart rate, heart rhythm and oxygen content are routinely monitored.

The effect of the ESI tends to be temporary. ESI is most helpful if a patient have severe pain in the spine and extremity. An ESI can provide sufficient pain relief to allow one to progress to physical therapy. Inflammatory chemicals and immunologic substances can generate pain and are associated with common back problems such as lumbar disc herniation. This condition can cause inflammation that in turn can cause significant nerve root irritation and swelling.

Steroids inhibit the inflammatory response caused by chemical sources of pain. Steroids, furthermore, work by reducing the activity of the immune system to react to inflammation associated with nerve or tissue damage. A typical immune response is the body generating white blood cells and chemicals to protect it against infection and foreign substances such as bacteria and viruses. This response makes the skin red and swollen.

When a patient has an epidural injection, he/she is placed face down on an x-ray table with a small pillow under the stomach. The skin over the back area is cleaned with a surgical scrub solution, and then the skin is numbed with a local anesthetic. Using x-ray a needle is inserted through the skin and directed toward the epidural space.

Once the needle is in the proper position, contrast dye is administered to confirm the needle location. The epidural steroid solution is then injected. Following the injection, a patient is monitored for 15-30 minutes to make sure that one does not have an allergy to the steroid before being discharged home.

A patient will follow-up with the doctor in two weeks after the procedure. If a patient did not have complete pain relief with the injection, the ESI may be repeated two more times until a patient has had three. A patient may have three injections every six months.

Occasionally following an ESI a patient can develop a headache. This is from loss of spinal fluid. This is a complication and is remedied by injection some of a patient's blood into the epidural space to patch up any leak of spinal fluid.

A patient may have facet joint pain. Lumbar facet joints are small located in pairs on the back of the spine. They provide stability and guide motion in the back. If the joints become painful, they may cause pain in areas away from the location of the joints. The facet joint is the moveable joint of the spine that connects one vertebra to another.

A facet injection is a non-surgical treatment that can temporarily relieve pain in the spine from inflammation or irritation of the facet joints in the spine. The procedure has two purposes as it can be used as a diagnostic test to see if the pain is actually coming from the facet joints, and it can be used as a therapy to relieve inflammation and pain. Just like an epidural injection, facet joint pain is temporary.

If these procedures do provide a patient with relief, a long acting, neruo destructive block can be done using heat, chemicals or freezing cold. This procedure is an injection of both steroid and an anesthetic (numbing agent) into a painful facet joint of the spine.

The injection can be placed inside the joint capsule (intra articular) or in the tissue surrounding the joint capsule (median branch nerve block). Steroids reduce inflammation, and they're very effective when delivered directly into the part of the back that is causing pain. Steroids are different than the steroids that athletes use and these steroids will not cause weight gain.

Radiofrequency (RF) denervation, an invasive treatment for chronic low back pain (CLBP), is used most often for pain suspected to arise from facet joints, sacroiliac (SI) joints or discs. The review authors found no high-quality evidence suggesting that RF denervation provides pain relief for patients with CLBP. Similarly, we identified no convincing evidence to show that this treatment improves function. Overall, the current evidence for RF denervation for CLBP is very low to moderate in quality; high-quality evidence is lacking.[2]

When a patient has a facet joint injection, he/she is placed face down on an x-ray table. The skin over the back area is cleansed with a surgical scrub solution, and then the skin is numbed with a local anesthetic. Using x-ray, a needle is inserted through the skin and directed toward the painful facet joint.

Once the needle is in the proper position, contrast dye is administered to confirm that the needle location is accurate. The facet local anesthetic/ steroid solution is then injected. Following the injection, a patient is monitored for 15 minutes to make sure that a patient does not have an allergy to the steroid before being discharged home.

If a patient did not have complete pain relief with the initial injection, the facet injection may be repeated another time until a patient has had two. Usually the painful facet joint and the one above are injected. If a patient's pain persists, one of the long-term facet injections mentioned previously can be done.

About 50% of patients experience some degree of pain relief. The pain may be relieved for several days to several months. It is not unusual to have physical therapy or chiropractic therapy after these injections are performed.

Sacroiliac joint pain is not uncommon as well. This joint is between the backbone and the hip bone. The sacroiliac joint is the largest joint of the lower spine in the buttock region. This joint occasionally becomes painful and inflamed. Steroid medication injected into the joint can reduce the inflammation and thus alleviating the pain.

Sacroiliac (SI) joint injections are commonly used to determine what is causing back pain. Analogous to facet joint injections these injections can be diagnostic and/or therapeutic. These injections eliminate pain by filling the SI joint with a local anesthetic medication as well as a steroid that numbs the joint and deposits steroid within the joint.

Articulation between the L5 transverse process and the sacrum or ilium has been implicated as a cause of low back pain. An anomalous transitional articulation should be considered as a possible factor in the genesis of low back pain in patients who do not have the degenerative lesions classically responsible for this symptom.[3] Local steroid injections should be tried before surgery is considered.

If the SI joint is injected with a numbing medicine and the pain goes away for several hours, it is likely that this joint is causing the pain. These injections are an adjunct treatment, which facilitates participation in an active exercise program and may assist in avoiding the need for surgical intervention. When sacroiliac joint injections are employed, they should be performed with X ray using contrast medium to ensure proper needle and medication placement are done.

Following an injection a comprehensive exercise program should be done. When this procedure is performed a patient will be placed on the stomach on the x ray table. The area over the pain will be cleansed with surgical soap. Once X ray has identified the joint the skin over this area will be numbed with a local anesthetic.

A patient will then receive more local anesthetic and steroid. If a patient has pain relief with several injections but if the pain recurs, a patient can have a rhizotomy of the SI joint. The sacroiliac joint (SIJ) can cause pain after lumbosacral fusion as well.[4]

If a patient has had a whiplash injury and have chronic neck pain and headaches, an occipital-atlanto injection may provide pain relief. The atlanto-axial joint is the joint formed by the uppermost cervical vertebrae. It is a common cause of pain at the base of the scalp that can radiate all the way behind the eye. Treatment of pain from this joint with injection therapy can provide long-term relief of these frequently under diagnosed or misdiagnosed headaches.

The occipital-occipital joint is the joint formed by the joining of the skull with the cervical spine. Although a more unusual cause of headaches, it can be a cause of upper neck pain and headaches that occur with rotation of the head. These injections are performed into the uppermost portion of the spine to treat and diagnose headaches and neck pain. This procedure is performed with x ray.

A patient will be placed on the side or face down on the X ray table. The skin over the upper neck will be scrubbed with surgical soap. A needle will be guided into this joint with x ray. Contract dye will be administered. Once proper needle tip confirmation has been done, a patient will receive a local anesthetic and steroid.

Headaches originating at the base of you're the skull may be seen in arthritis or trauma. A patient might benefit from an occipital nerve block. Occipital nerve blocks may be of benefit in migraine headache treatment. Occipital nerve block is a procedure where local anesthetics are injected near the occipital nerve at the back of the head near the base of the skull from the side of the headache. Facet joint injections and C(2), C(3) spinal rami blocks were shown to be effective and well tolerated for the treatment of cervicogenic headache as well.[5]

If a patient has RSD affecting the arm, a patient may need a stellate ganglion block. The stellate ganglion is part of the sympathetic nervous system. The infiltration of local anesthetic around the ganglion is used to treat reflex sympathetic dystrophy. These injections are frequently performed with X ray. Indications for stellate ganglion blocks include reflex sympathetic dystrophy of the upper extremities, Raynaud's syndrome of the upper extremities, herpes zoster of the face or neck and upper extremity pain due to arterial insufficiency.

For reflex sympathetic dystrophy of the leg, a lumbar sympathetic block can be done. The sympathetic nerves are a chain of nerves that run on the front side of the spinal column. They are part of the autonomic nervous system that controls many bodily functions such as sweating, heart rate, digestion, and blood pressure. Early stellate ganglion blockade, in combination with an antiviral agent, is a very effective treatment modality; it dramatically decreases the intensity of acute pain and shortens its duration and reduces the incidence of postherpetic neuralgia.[6]

A celiac plexus block is a pain treatment procedure used to numb nerves in the upper abdomen if a patient has intolerable abdominal pain. The celiac plexus block procedure is most frequently used if a patient has pancreatic cancer. When doing a celiac plexus block procedure the use of an x-ray is necessary to allow for the precise placement of the needle.

A local anesthetic is administered through this needle. In some instances, two needles may be placed. This block can provide pain relief for the liver, gallbladder, omentum, mesentery, stomach, small intestine, as well as the ascending and transverse portion of the colon.

Kyphoplasty and vertebroplasty are two modalities that may provide a patientwith pain relief if he/she has had a compression fracture involving the spine. Kyphoplasty is a minimally invasive spinal surgery procedure used to treat painful, progressive vertebral compression fractures. A compression fracture is a fracture in the body of a vertebra, which causes it to collapse. A compression fracture may be caused by osteoporosis or by the spread of a tumor to ther vertebral body.

Kyphoplasty is not appropriate for patients with young, healthy bones or those who sustained a vertebral body fracture or collapse in a major accident, patients with spinal curvature such as scoliosis or kyphosis that results from causes other than osteoporosis, patients who suffer from spinal stenosis or a herniated disk with nerve or spinal cord compression and loss of neurologic function not associated with a compression fracture.

Percutaneous kyphoplasty for the treatment of thoracolumbar scoliosis osteoporotic fracture can significantly improve patients spinal deformity.[7]

Kyphoplasty involves the use of a device called a balloon tamp to restore the height and shape of the vertebral body. This is followed by application of bone cement to strengthen the vertebra. The procedure is performed with the patient lying face down on the operating room table and under intravenous sedation. Two x-ray machines are used to show the collapsed bones. To begin the procedure, the surgeon makes two small incisions in the back. A tube is inserted into the center of the vertebral body to the site of the fractured bone. The balloon tamp is then inserted down the tube and inflated. This pushes the bone back to its normal height and shape. Usually a patient has significant pain relief following the procedure.

Vertebrpolasty is another modality used to treat a compression fracture. A hollow needle (trocar) is passed into the vertebral bone and a cement mixture, and a solvent is injected. The physician will monitor the entire procedure on a fluoroscopy imaging screen and make sure that the cement mixture does not back up into the spinal canal.

After vertebroplasty, the cement stabilizes the fracture, which is thought to provide the pain relief. A patient should begin regaining mobility within 24 hours and should be able to reduce the pain medication. Vertebroplasty plays a major role for the management of specific bone weakening vertebral lesions causing, obviating the need for kyphoplasty.

It remains uncertain whether one of these procedures is superior for the treatment of compression fractures. Both procedures reduce the amount of pain in the immediate postoperative period by approximately 50%. Both procedures reduce pain in symptomatic osteoporotic vertebral compression fractures that have failed conservative treatment. Randomized controlled trials are needed to provide definitive data on which procedure is the most effective for vertebral compression fractures.

Spinal cord electrical stimulation is used for pain management in cases of chronic pain following back surgery, reflex sympathetic dystrophy and vascular insufficiency. In this therapy, electrical impulses are used to block pain from being perceived in the brain. Instead of pain, a patient feels a mild tingling sensation from a catheter placed in the back.

Sometimes a neurosurgeon can decrease pain with surgery (cut the nerves, spinal cord or parts of the brain that cause a patient to experience pain). A neurosurgical procedure that is used to relieve pain is by cutting the nerves of the spinal cord responsible for transmitting pain impulses through the nerve pathways. This procedure is done in cancer patients.

Dorsal root entry zone (DREZ) lesioning is used to treat central neuropathic pain in patients with traumatic spinal cord injury. It is commonly done after brachial plexus injuries. Commissural myelotomy disrupts pain-conducting fibers as well as a polysynaptic pain pathway that runs through the center of a patient's spinal cord. Indications for myelotomy include pelvic cancer pain.

The removals of herniated discs are common surgical procedures that are done by neurosurgeons. In 1934 a disc herniation was first recognized as a source of sciatica. This important discovery led to the first surgical removal of a disc. Surgical challenges associated with disc surgery are removal of the bad fragment while leaving the remainder of the good disc intact. A discectomy is done to relieve arm or leg pain and not to decrease neck or back pain. A patient will need back surgery if he/she loses control of the bowel or bladder function, weakness in an extremity or have a foot drop. Disc surgery usually does not totally relieve the back pain.

There are many options available to a patient for pain management. Injection is one option. The treatment should be tailored to the problem and a patient's overall health. A "one size fits all approach" cannot be used when addressing chronic pain problems.

References

1. Lee JH, Lee SH. Comparison of Clinical Efficacy Between Interlaminar and Transforaminal Epidural Injection in Patients With Axial

Pain due to Cervical Disc Herniation. Medicine (Baltimore). 2016;95(4):e2568.

2. Maas ET, Ostelo RW, Niemisto L, et al. Radiofrequency denervation for chronic low back pain. Cochrane Database Syst Rev. 2015(10):CD008572.

3. Avimadje M, Goupille P, Jeannou J, Gouthiere C, Valat JP. Can an anomalous lumbo-sacral or lumbo-iliac articulation cause low back pain? A retrospective study of 12 cases. Rev Rhum Engl Ed. 1999;66(1):35-39.

4. Katz V, Schofferman J, Reynolds J. The sacroiliac joint: a potential cause of pain after lumbar fusion to the sacrum. J Spinal Disord Tech. 2003;16(1):96-99.

5. Zhou L, Hud-Shakoor Z, Hennessey C, Ashkenazi A. Upper cervical facet joint and spinal rami blocks for the treatment of cervicogenic headache. Headache. 2010;50(4):657-663.

6. Makharita MY, Amr YM, El-Bayoumy Y. Effect of early stellate ganglion blockade for facial pain from acute herpes zoster and incidence of postherpetic neuralgia. Pain Physician. 2012;15(6):467-474.

7. Qu HB, Tong PJ, Ji WF, Li J. [Percutaneous kyphoplasty for the treatment of osteoporotic vertebral compression fracture with degenerative scoliosis]. Zhongguo Gu Shang. 2016;29(1):38-40.

20. Cervical spine pain

At any given time, neck pain affects 10 percent of the general population in the United States. Neck pain is common among the elderly. Seniors are not the most likely demographic to suffer chronic neck pain. Neck pain is a frequent reason why patients seek medical attention. Seniors demonstrate the most widespread and verifiable spinal deterioration compared to younger age groups. The spine does not get better with age. It only gets worse.

A reported survey of 10,000 adults in the United States discovered that 34 percent of responding individuals experienced neck pain during the previous year before the survey. Chronic neck pain was reported in 17 percent of women and 10 percent of men in a similar study. Another study evaluated 8,000 adults, and chronic neck pain was identified in 13.5 percent of female respondents as compared to 9.5 percent of males.

Neck pain is common among the elderly. Intrinsic causes of pain in elderly patients arise in the neck bones, arthritis the neck bone joints (facet joints), disc disorders, trauma, tumors, and infection in the cervical musculature, myofascial pain syndrome, and whiplash; and in the spinal cord from tumors. Differentiation of these causes from extrinsic causes of neck pain will enable the appropriate management protocols to be implemented.

Neck pain can range from mild discomfort to severe throbbing and is experienced by everyone at some point in their lives. Neck pain affects many seniors, particularly older females. Loss of bone density can facilitate many problems, including the increase of arthritic processes, vertebral fractures, spinal stenosis and spinal instability. Some cases of osteo arthritis in the spine can be problematic, enacting pain through central canal or foraminal stenosis, bone spur formation or facet joint syndrome.

Degenerative disc disease is the complete loss of hydration from discs in the cervical spine is common in elders, possibly leading to increased arthritic interaction between vertebrae and spinal joints, as well as facilitating possibly symptomatic herniated discs.

Neck pain is caused by conditions that compress nerves or irritate the outer part of discs that are cushions between the bones in the neck. Ligaments in the front and in the back of the bones in the neck can cause pain because they have many pain fibers within these ligaments. These ligaments are called the anterior and posterior longitudinal ligaments.

Where the bones of a patient's the neck stack on top of each other like Lego blocks, they form a joint called a facet joint. The outer capsule of this joint has a rich supply of pain fibers. The outer capsule holds the top and bottom of the facet joint together not unlike a clamshell. If this capsule is pulled or stretched by an injury, the parts about the joint loosen making the joint unstable. This instability can cause spine pain. If the neck becomes misaligned, a patient can also develop significant neck pain.

Over time, the bones and joints in the neck can wear out as well. This is called degenerative disc or joint disease or in medical terms is called osteoarthritis. The disc between the bones can rupture. The facet joints in the neck can deteriorate and be a cause of chronic neck pain. Radiofrequency (RF) denervation, an invasive treatment for chronic back pain, is used most often for pain suspected to arise from facet joints, sacroiliac (SI) joints or discs. No high-quality evidence suggesting that RF denervation provides pain relief for patients with Back pain. Overall, the current evidence for RF denervation for chronic spine pain is very low to moderate in quality.[1]

There are seven separate bone segments in the neck. These bones are held together by ligaments and stack on top of each other and form joints with the analogy of joints formed by Lego blocks. The lining of these joints can wear out. These joints contain a lubricating fluid that helps a patient turn and move the neck up and down. These joints in the neck not only limit the neck motion but also allow the neck to move in many planes. Irritation or injury to muscles or ligaments in the neck as well as the discs and joints in the neck can cause you to have neck pain.

The bones in the neck protect the spinal cord and the nerves that come off of the spinal cord. The nerves that come off of the spinal cord pass through holes in the bones in the neck. If these nerves are compressed by narrowing of the hole where the nerve exits from the bone in the neck, it can cause you to have significant pain. If the nerve is compromised by bones in the neck, you can have weakness as well as pain in the arms.

Neck pain can come not only from the degeneration of discs in the neck or the degenerating facet joints in the neck, but also can arise from infections or tumors of structures in the neck. Neck pain in general does not occur as often as lower-back pain in elderly patients. Therefore, the overall cost of neck pain to society is much less than that of lower-back pain. There are fewer medications prescribed in patients with neck pain as opposed to lower-back pain. A head weighs between 10 and 12 pounds. The bones in the neck are relatively small in comparison to the head. The neck muscles are necessary to hold the head in a proper position.

The bones in the neck that are called vertebral bodies contain many pain fibers. Each bone is wrapped by a tissue called a periosteum. If a patient fractures one of these bones he/she can have severe pain. The tissue wrapper around the bones can be injured. The fracture of a bone in the neck can cause abnormal stress to the ligaments, muscles, and joints around the fracture as well as injury to the periosteum. Osteoporosis, which is a weakening of the bones with a loss of bone density, can cause small, tiny fractures in the bones of the neck and in turn can be a source of pain. Osteoporosis therefore can be a source of severe neck pain.

Discs are cushions between the bones in the neck. These discs act as shock absorbers in between the bones. The cushions are important because without them, the neck bones (vertebra) would stack on top of each other. In the very center of the disc in the neck is a thick fluid like substance called a nucleus pulposus. This fluid ball is surrounded by an outer tough fiber called an annulus. Annulus is Latin for "outer ring." A fluid nucleus acts as a ball bearing when a patient bends his/her head forward and backward or from side to side. It also is a ball bearing when a patient rotates the neck.

The annulus (ring) around the disc acts as a ligament that prevents the neck from having excessive motion. The annulus at its outer layer has many pain fibers.

To find out if pain is coming from the disc in the neck, a doctor can place a needle in the disc. After the needle has been properly placed, fluid can be injected into the disc. If the injected fluid into the disc reproduces the neck pain, this is a good indication that the disc in the neck is the cause of the pain syndrome. This test is called a discogram.

If the neck becomes skewed, a patient can compress a nerve that goes to one of the organs and could affect the function of the organ. For example, a spinal cord injury could affect the diaphragm and make it difficult for a patient to take a breath. A patient's head always needs to be supported in the proper position to allow one to have normal motion.

The discs in the neck have a normal blood supply when a patient is a toddler until he/she becomes a teenager. These discs are nurtured with oxygen and sugar into the bloodstream until the blood supply decreases, which occurs when a patient reaches adolescence. By age 30, the discs in the neck have no blood flow. Therefore, the nutrition to the discs must come from the ends of the bones in the neck. The bones in the neck are like sponges soaked with blood. Pressure gradients will provide the discs with nutrition. When the disc eventually begins to lose fluid, it will deteriorate.

The very center of the disc is called the nucleus pulposus and is 80 percent water. Substances in this liquid environment can attract fluid into the discs to keep the discs well hydrated. Eventually, this hydration will dry up. As a patient gets older, the ends of the bones calcify. When this happens, less blood flow is available for the discs as the blood cannot get out of the vertebrae to hydrate the disc. The disc will essentially dry out. The disk becomes wafer thin and does not provide a nice cushion. As a result, a patient will begin to experience some degree of neck pain.

The outer ring of the disc, called the annulus, will contain the nucleus pulposus within its structure. Think of this anatomy as a jelly doughnut. The jelly in the doughnut is held in place by the outer doughnut ring. Be aware that a basic law of physics states that the nucleus pulposus, which is a liquid, cannot be compressed. Therefore, any pressure applied to the disc at any point can cause the nucleus pulposus to spread outward and even rupture through the outer annular ring.

As an example, a patient can compress a foam pillow to make the pillow smaller during compression. However, compressing a liquid will not decrease its size (volume). The disc jelly will not become smaller in its dimensions under pressure. Consequently, when this liquid mass is attempted to be compressed, it will push through the outer ring of the disc. This is a disc herniation.

The nucleus pulposus material contains acids. When this disc material does come out of the annulus, the surrounding tissues can be become swollen and red from the acidic liquid. This is the reason that a doctor may do a cervical epidural steroid injection. The purpose of this method is to decrease the swelling of the tissue and nerves caused by the acidic nucleus pulposus contents. The acid will make the nerves sensitive to irritability, which will cause a patient to experience pain.

In front of the bones in a patient's neck is a ligament that runs vertically. In the back of the bones in the neck is another ligament that also runs vertically. These ligaments are called longitudinal ligaments. These ligaments run all the way from the base of the skull to the lower back and contain many pain fibers. The ligament in the back of the bones limits the ability to bend the head forward. If a patient bends too far, the ligament transmits pain signals to the brain telling a patient to stop this movement. The front ligament and the joints in the anterior neck keep a patient from bending the neck backward too far. Sometimes the neck can be bent backward following a whiplash injury and can cause a patient to have significant pain.

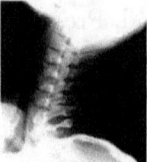

Figure 1. X ray of a neck (cervical spine) looking at the neck from the side.

The holes in the bones in the neck (foramina) allow the nerves from the spinal cord to come out and go to the arms, legs, and organs. Elderly patients can have a decreased opening size of one or more of these holes (stenosis) which can compress the nerves. This can cause an elderly patient to have neck and arm pain.

The spinal cord and the nerves that come off of the spinal cord can be sources of neck pain. When a patient bends the head forward or bend the head backwards, the spinal cord will move up and down a short distance because it is somewhat elastic. This means that the nerves that go through the holes in the cervical spine also move along with spinal cord movements. If the foramina decrease in diameter as is seen in arthritis, movement of these nerves across a small hole can cause irritation in the nerves and make them swell and become extra sensitive to irritability. A patient may then experience pain in the arms.

Sometimes, if a patient has arthritis, the small bony growth in the neck can irritate or compress one of the nerves. This bone growth is called an osteophyte. Osteophytes themselves are not painful. However, when they brush over nerves or ligaments, they can cause a patient to have neck pain. Osteophytes, if they occur, are usually pointed. If one of the nerves brushes up against one of these osteophytes, or if the osteophytes compress the nerves, a patient may experience mild to moderate pain.

Steroid injections in and around a patient's nerves can decrease the swelling of the nerve and decrease the pain. The injection places a tiny amount of steroids at the area of their pain. Oral steroids have to go to the stomach and pass out of the gastrointestinal system to reach the bloodstream. The total amount of the steroid that will reach the swollen nerves will vary. The amount of drug placed at the nerve is more reliable than that given by mouth.

Blood vessels run vertically up to the neck toward the brain. A neck injury with compression can occasionally decrease the blood flow to the brain. If the neck is bent backward for a significant length of time, a patient could possibly lose consciousness. This can be seen occasionally in a syndrome called a beauty shop syndrome.

In people with a poor blood supply to their brains, such as an elderly person, a prolonged extension of the neck could cause that person to have a stroke. This posture could also cause a patient to rupture the discs in the neck. Professional shampoos have previously been implicated in beauty parlor stroke syndrome and salon sink radiculopathy. Individuals with a history of such dizziness with head movement symptoms should probably exercise caution when deciding whether to receive a salon sink shampoo.[2]

The muscles of the neck can be a source of pain. The neck muscles are probably the most common cause of neck pain. There are two groups of muscles in the neck. There is a group that bends the head forward, and there are a group of muscles that extend the head backward. Most of the muscles in the neck are located toward the back of the neck. These are the muscles that bend a patient's head backward. If a patient has poor posture, the muscles at the back to the neck can become longer or can become shorter. When this happens, the short muscles in the neck lose blood flow, causing a patient to have pain.

The muscles at the base of the skull can compress a nerve that comes off of the spinal cord and travels along the top of the head. This is called the occipital nerve. If this nerve is compressed by a tight muscle, a patient can develop a headache called an occipital headache. If a patient put heat over the muscle that is compressing this nerve, it can relax the muscle and relieve the headache.

The nerve roots coming off of the spinal cord that run through the holes (foramina) in the cervical spine s also can be a source of neck pain. Coverings of the facet joints in the neck called facet joint capsules can be a source of pain as well. Electromyography and/or nerve conduction tests consist of needles placed in the muscles and nerves of the upper arms and legs. The electromyography study can determine if a patient has compression of one of the nerves that goes from the spinal cord to the fingers.

When a patient becomes older than 55 years of age, he/she may develop degenerative disc disease in the neck. Degeneration of the neck is called spondylosis. Degenerative disc disease of the cervical spine causes more neck pain and upper-extremity nerve pain than does a disc herniation. Men have a higher incidence of cervical spondylosis than women. In one study, the evidence of spondylosis was noted to be 60 percent in women but 80 percent in men. These findings were before the age of 49 years. However, at age 70 or greater there was a 95 percent incidence of degenerative disc disease both in men and women. With degenerative disc disease, the disk becomes narrow. Think of a normal disc as a jelly donut; a degenerated disc is more like a thin communion wafer.

A diagnosis of spondylosis is made by x-ray but also can be seen on an MRI. As stated previously, there is decreased blood flow to the discs following puberty. A patient's discs normally obtain blood from the spongy vertebral bodies. However, if the end plates are calcified, the discs cannot receive hydration and nutrition. As a result, the discs essentially dry out, also called desiccation.

At this time, the outer ring of a patient's disc called the annulus can deteriorate. Cracks can occur in the outer ring allowing the acidic center of the disc to leak out. This leakage can cause irritation of the nerves, ligaments, and muscles. Epidural steroid injection therapy can sometimes decrease the pain if a patient has leakage of acidic material from the disc. An epidural injection is placement of a needle into a space in the neck that surrounds the spinal fluid.

Surgical intervention for neck and back pain in elderly patients without significant comorbidities can significantly improve a patient's symptoms and quality of life when more conservative therapies fail. Current spine literature strongly supports the paradigm of treating elderly patients with stable, chronic neck or back pain with conservative therapies first in order to optimize the risks and benefits of all available treatment options.[3] If less-invasive methods fail to achieve satisfactory outcomes, more aggressive surgical options can, at that time, typically be implemented with excellent results in elderly patients without significant comorbidities.

If a patient has a severe state of contractions of a muscle in the neck, a patient may have severe pain. This prolonged contraction of a neck muscle is called torticollis. This usually occurs on one side of the neck. A patient's head is usually twisted to one side with the chin pointing to the opposite side. Torticollis usually results from disease or an injury to the brain or spinal cord. Injuries to the muscles of the neck can also be a cause of torticollis as well. Sometimes an injection of botulism toxin into the muscles can provide temporary relief.

The transforaminal (TF) epidural approach is preferred by physician to interlaminar (IL) approach because it can deliver an injectate directly around nerve root and dorsal root ganglion, which is regarded as main pain sources. IL and TF showed no significant difference in clinical efficacy. Considering TF was relevant to more serious side effects, IL was more recommendable in these patients.[4]

Women have more neck pain than men and elderly patients have more neck pain than younger adults. The incidence of neck pain increases with age. Whiplash injuries can cause neck pain as well and are more common in women than in men. Furthermore, repetitive activities in a workplace setting can be a source of neck pain. Unfortunately, a patient can have neck pain for a long time. It is not self-limiting as some other types of pain syndromes are. Neck pain is a symptom of problem processes going on in the neck.

Reports in the United States reveal that neck pain occurs more frequently in women than in men. Older patients, both men and women, have a higher incidence of neck pain. People who have mentally and physically stressful jobs are more prone to have neck pain as well. The reason why smokers have increased neck pain has been studied. Cigarette smoking stops the formation of bone. Smoking interferes with the repair of fractures involving the neck bones. The mechanism of association between smoking and neck pain is still being studied.

Potentially modifiable predictors of chronic neck pain (NP) among employees: workplace bullying, sleep problems, and high body mass index in women, and work-related emotional exhaustion in men. In both genders, previous acute NP and chronic low back pain were predictive of chronic NP.5 Smoking is a risk factor for long-term sick leave due to unspecific back or neck pain.6

Women are more prone to neck pain because they have smaller necks, and it makes them vulnerable to the onset of pain. Remember that the neck must hold a 10- to 12-pound head. A smaller neck receives more stress from the head than a larger neck. It also has been hypothesized that men are more stoic than women and do not report their neck pain as often as women. Because of their smaller necks, women are more prone to suffer severe whiplash injuries than men. Not only do men have larger necks than women, but the overall body mass of the neck is more than a woman's.

Chronic whiplash-associated disorders (chronic WAD) cover a large variety of clinical manifestations that can occur after a whiplash injury. Women have an increased risk of developing chronic WAD, and it is suggested that psychosocial factors are related to long-term pain and functioning following whiplash injury and persistence of chronic pain.[7]

Neck pain is a considerable health problem, affecting elderly individuals. Of particular concern is the negative impact that neck pain may have on the functional ability of the geriatric population, already challenged by decreased mobility and balance associated with aging. Interestingly, the rate of increase for the neck operations is different across the nation. In Idaho, there were more surgeries than in Washington, DC.

The condition most often warranting the surgery was cervical spondylosis with myelopathy, which is a degenerative condition that affects the spinal cord. Fifty-two percent of those elderly patients who had the fusion surgery were men. Of these patients, 88% were white and 41% were between the ages of 65 and 69. With increasing age and advancing disc degeneration, senescent nucleus pulposus chondrocytes increase or accumulate in the NP.

References

1. Maas ET, Ostelo RW, Niemisto L, et al. Radiofrequency denervation for chronic low back pain. Cochrane Database Syst Rev. 2015(10):CD008572.

2. Foye PM, Najar MP, Camme AA, Jr., et al. Pain, dizziness, and central nervous system blood flow in cervical extension: vascular correlations to beauty parlor stroke syndrome and salon sink radiculopathy. Am J Phys Med Rehabil. 2002;81(6):395-399.

3. Kalkanis SN, Borges L. Neck and Back Pain in the Elderly. Curr Treat Options Neurol. 2001;3(3):215-228.

4. Lee JH, Lee SH. Comparison of Clinical Efficacy Between Interlaminar and Transforaminal Epidural Injection in Patients With Axial Pain due to Cervical Disc Herniation. Medicine (Baltimore). 2016;95(4):e2568.

5. Kaaria S, Laaksonen M, Rahkonen O, Lahelma E, Leino-Arjas P. Risk factors of chronic neck pain: a prospective study among middle-aged employees. Eur J Pain. 2012;16(6):911-920.

6. Skillgate E, Vingard E, Josephson M, Holm LW, Alfredsson L. Is smoking and alcohol consumption associated with long-term sick leave due to unspecific back or neck pain among employees in the public sector? Results of a three-year follow-up cohort study. J Rehabil Med. 2009;41(7):550-556.

7. Malfliet A, De Kooning M, Inghelbrecht E, et al. Sex Differences in Patients with Chronic Pain Following Whiplash Injury: The Role of Depression, Fear, Somatization, Social Support, and Personality Traits. Pain Pract. 2015;15(8):757-764.

21. Whiplash injuries

Whiplash injuries can be a devastating experience, especially in an older patient. In 1990, in Quebec, Canada, a group of scientists, including doctors, reviewed the scientific literature and made public policy on the prevention and treatment of whiplash injuries. They described the magnitude of the problem of whiplash injury and presented some strategies to address this entity effectively. The cost of treatment for whiplash injury is high and continues to rise. The problem is that there is considerable inconsistency concerning diagnostic criteria for the diagnosis of whiplash injury.

The term "whiplash injury" was initially described in 1958 by Dr. H. Crowe. Whiplash was described as a sudden speeding up or slowing down of the neck that results in a lash-like effect. A head weighs 10 to 20 pounds and sits on a relatively small neck. If a patient is hit from behind, the body accelerates. The head is left behind. As the body speeds up, the head falls backward, causing trauma to the neck. The term "whiplash" has become a medical and legal term, as well as a social dilemma.

Be aware that the term "whiplash" is not a medical diagnosis. It is a result of muscle, ligament, and joint trauma to the cervical spine. It occurs when a sudden force (e.g., a car accident) causes forward, backward, or sideways movement of the head that is beyond the normal range of motion, or from a sudden jolt. The elderly and patients who have chronic conditions that affect the neck are at increased risk for sustaining a whiplash injury.

The mechanism of a whiplash injury is a result of a sudden speeding up or a unexpected stoppage of the head and neck with respect to the body. The motion of a whiplash injury results in the extensive bending backward of the neck or an excessive forward bending of the neck. Motor-vehicle accidents account for more than 90 percent of all whiplash injuries. However, sports injuries also contribute to whiplash injuries. Be aware that rear-end collisions account for 88 percent of whiplash injuries. Less than 10 percent are from side-to-side collisions.

The classic description of whiplash injury is where a patient is a driver or passenger in a vehicle that is struck by another vehicle. Be aware that the degree of damage to a vehicle involved in the motor-vehicle accident bears little relationship to the size of the force applied to the neck, head, and the remainder of the body. Be appreciative that injuries in which the neck is bent backward usually result in more trauma to the neck than injuries that cause the neck to bend forward.

Whiplash is in the elderly patient is essentially the adult version of a shaken baby syndrome. Some individuals think that whiplash injuries are only caused by rear end motor vehicle accidents. Anything that causes the elderly patient's head to snap forward or backward can cause a whiplash injury. For example, the number of elderly passengers who sustain whiplash in bus-related road traffic accidents is increasing because they often take longer to sit down and get off the bus and are less likely to see items projecting into the aisles.

The symptoms of whiplash injury include pain in the shoulders, arm, dizziness, tinnitus, vertigo, migraines, nausea, headache, irritability, discomfort, back pain and blurred vision. The extent of the whiplash injuries depends on the age of the person who is injured. In the elderly people, the muscles and ligaments would be weaker so the severity of the whiplash injury would be more severe. As a result, Older drivers and occupants that may already have health and mobility challenges can face greater injury and healing time than younger drivers.

The Whiplash Associated Disorder (WAD) is a good example of a medical condition where there is often an apparent disconnect between the magnitude of injury and the magnitude of disability. In addition to neck pain, there may be pain in one or both arms, between the shoulder blades, the face and even the low back. Other symptoms include heaviness or tingling in the arms, dizziness, ringing in the ears, vision changes, fatigue, poor concentration or memory and difficulty sleeping.

Some elderly individuals prefer vehicles that are not low to the ground to allow them easy access in and out of the vehicle. This can be a problem because studies have revealed that those traveling in SUVs, pickups and minivans are more likely to sustain whiplash during rear-end collisions. This is because the seats and headrests in these particular models provide inadequate rear impact protection.

The incidence of whiplash injuries is 3.8 injuries per 1,000 people in the United States. Of these injuries, 20 percent of people develop symptoms in their neck. Note that the incidence in women is 14.5 whiplash injuries per 1,000 women. The discs between the bones in the neck can be compressed, and the joints that are in the back of the neck also can be compressed. The facet joints in the neck can be fractured as well. Women have higher initial pain levels in the acute whiplash injury. Age and ethnicity have less impact on those pain levels.[1]

A patient may have been involved in a front-end collision. With respect to frontal impact injuries, the frontal impact rapidly stops the vehicle. The body continues forward until deceleration, caused by the seat belt or if a patient hits the steering wheel or dashboard. The head continues to move forward until the neck stops the forward movement of the head. At this time, you a patient may sustain an injury to the joint where the head attaches to the neck. After this, movement occurs, the neck recoils with a whip like effect, and the neck is pulled backward.

Whiplash-associated disorders (WAD) are the most common injuries that are associated with car collisions in many Western countries. However, there is no clear evidence regarding the potential risk factors for poor recovery from WAD. Dizziness, numbness or pain in the arms, and lower back pain) had the strongest associations with prolonged treatment for WAD.[2]

Patients with whiplash associated disorders (WAD) may present with physical and psychological symptoms which persist long after the initial onset of pain. Several studies have shown that therapeutic exercise for motor and sensorimotor control combined with manual therapy in a multimodal rehabilitation (MMR) program is effective at improving pain and disability in patients with neck disorders.[3] Sleep disturbances are a common finding in individuals with neck pain and are associated with the intensity of ongoing pain in WAD.[4]

Myofascial trigger points are a primary cause of pain in whiplash injured patients. Pain from trigger points is often treated by needling, with or without injection.[5]

Studies in mathematical models have demonstrated that a frontal impact injury also can cause a patient's head to rotate. A patient can have a neck injury in the absence of a head injury. If you are hit from the side, the neck can flex to one side or the other or possibly even both sides. If a patient is hit on the driver's side of the vehicle, the head may flex to hit the driver-side window and then whip to the opposite side causing injuries to muscles, ligaments, and joints in the neck.

Neck injuries resulting from motor vehicle collisions (MVC), often referred to as whiplash trauma and injury, often demonstrate little or no evidence of significant tissue damage. In rare instances, however, serious injury to the anterior neck organ injuries can result from such trauma.[6] Clinicians should be aware of the potential for significant complications in the whiplash trauma-exposed patient who complains of chest pain, mid-thoracic pain, discomfort in the neck and throat, respiratory distress, or hoarseness. For those forensic specialists involved in whiplash cases these study results highlight the need to consider esophageal injuries as a rare but potential consequence of whiplash trauma.

If a patient suffers a whiplash injury, the spinal cord may be stretched. Sometimes, the area where the nerves from the arms or legs attach to the spinal cord is traumatized. An area where the nerves meet the spinal cord is called dorsal root ganglia. This ganglia can be stretched and/or bruised and can cause a patient to have pain in the neck and arms for a significant length of time.

Many victims of a motor vehicle collision report crippling upper back pain resistant to conservative treatment. Although this pain is often regarded as nonspecific or related to a whiplash type of cervical spine injury, this study demonstrates it may be caused by a thoracic disc herniation.[7]

As the neck excessively bends forward and backward, arteries in the neck that go to the brain can be compressed. This is the reason why a patient could lose consciousness following a whiplash injury. A patient could sustain a concussion, which is a bruise to the brain tissue as a result of trauma. A patient can develop a temporal mandibular joint (TMJ) dysfunction as well.

Whiplash injuries do not affect genders equally. Women appear to experience whiplash injuries more often than men. Studies done in 1995 related that women experienced more whiplash injuries than men because they have slimmer and less-muscular necks. As a result, women are less able to resist the damage in acceleration forces of the head that are generated at the time of motor-vehicle impact. Another reason for gender differences between men and women with respect to whiplash injury complaints is that women are more likely to seek medical attention.

The facet joints in your neck may be significantly damaged if you suffer a whiplash injury. These joints can easily be fractured. A case of a single severe arthritic change in a cervical facet joint was noted after death in a person who had neck pain for many years following a whiplash injury. The pain persisted and became severe, causing the person to become depressed and commit suicide. The single isolated facet joint that was traumatically injured was found on examination after death.

The discs between the bones in the neck are often injured in a whiplash injury. The outer ring of the discs can be torn. The discs could be separated from the bones in the neck. Furthermore, fractures at the ends of the bones in the neck have been reported and can cause significant pain.

A whiplash injury can cause the discs in the neck to degenerate as well as the joints in the neck. The injury accelerates the degeneration of both the discs and the facet joints. If the neck extends too far backward, the liquid nucleus pulposus in the center of the disc can burst through the disk after being compressed by the extended neck.

Studies have shown that approximately 60 percent of whiplash injury pain can come from the cervical facet joints. This information was noted following a study in which different structures of a patient's neck were injected with local anesthetics to determine the exact cause of a patient's neck pain following a whiplash injury. Injections of local anesthetics in other structures in the neck can confirm the cause of the neck pain.

Other structures causing neck pain are muscles and ligaments. These structures can be injected with local anesthetics mixed with steroids. This combination of drugs injected into the joints may stop the pain. If the pain goes away after injecting these structures (guided by x-rays), the exact cause of the pain can be diagnosed and treated.

Muscle tears and sprains have been documented and noted since these types of injuries were published in 1976. Muscle tears have been visualized on ultrasound examinations. Animal studies have been done simulating whiplash injuries. Partial and complete tears and hemorrhage have been noted.

Ligaments in the neck and other soft tissues may be damaged following a whiplash injury. If a patient sustains a ligament injury of the neck, it is difficult diagnosing this type of injury. In animal experiments, tears of the ligaments in the front of the neck bones have been reported. The ligaments in front of the neck bones attach to the discs between the vertebrae.

The top two bones of the neck (C1 and C2) enable the head to rotate and look up and down. A fracture of either or both of these bones can cause death or cause a patient to have a serious neurological injury. Some individuals have become quadriplegic as a result of an injury to one or both of the first two vertebrae in the neck. The first two bones in the neck provide a patient with a wide range of rotational movement about the neck. The two bones are connected by ligaments. If the ligaments have been damaged, the head in relation to the neck may become overly mobile.

Often compressive forces on your cervical vertebrae can compress the vertebral bones downward. This is called a compression fracture. The brain can be injured at the time of a whiplash injury as well. As the head is being whipped around, the brain can be traumatized as the brain hits the inside of the skull. A patient can suffer a concussion. A patient may have headaches for months following an injury. Unfortunately, some brain injuries may go undetected.

Following neck pain, headaches are the most frequent complaint following a whiplash injury. The pain typically begins at the base of the skull. It then progresses to the top of the head. Sometimes the pain can go to the temples on either side of the head. If a patient has sustained a concussion, he/she may have a headache as well. Most headaches following a whiplash injury are from soft tissues in the neck.

If a patient has sustained a whiplash injury, he/she may complain of difficulty with vision. A patient may have problems focusing the eyes. Sometimes the nerves that go to the eyes from the brain (optic nerves) can be damaged. Sometimes the arteries that go to the back of the brain where a patient actually see objects (optic lobe) can be temporarily blocked as the neck is whipped about at the time of impact. This can cause a patient to have temporary loss of vision.

Neuropsychological tests following whiplash injury revealed deficits in areas of attention, concentration, and memory. It is possible that if a patient has decreased attention and memory that it may be due to the severity of the pain as opposed to a direct brain injury. Studies using CT scans and MRI studies in patients who have had whiplash injuries disclosed no significant pathology. Brain wave studies have been done. It has been estimated that approximately 50 percent of patients following a whiplash injury have abnormal electroencephalograms (EEG).

The joint in the jaw that enables a patient to open and close the mouth is called the temporal mandibular joint (TMJ). Injuries to the temporal mandibular joint may occur during a whiplash injury. Frequent pain in the jaw-face can be part of the spectrum of symptoms in chronic WAD. The finding of self-reported numbness in the jaw-face indicates disturbed trigeminal nerve function.[8]

The exact mechanism regarding how the temporal mandibular joint is injured in a whiplash injury remains to be studied. It is believed that the maxilla (the upper jaw bone) compresses with the mandible (the lower jaw bone). This sudden compression can injure the temporal mandibular joint. As a result, a patient may have difficulty opening and closing the mouth and may have chronic pain in this joint.

A patient may suffer prolonged dizziness following a whiplash injury. The exact mechanism by which dizziness occurs following a whiplash injury remains speculative. Again, it is thought that the arteries in the neck that go to the brain are irritated, which compromises the blood flow to the brain. A decrease in the blood flow to the brain can cause people to have disturbances in balance and equilibrium.

There is no good diagnostic test to demonstrate that a patient did have a temporary nerve compression at the time of the neck injury. Furthermore, if a patient sustained a muscle injury and has muscle pain, that particular muscle will be weak. Sensation of tingling and numbness in the hands can occur following a whiplash injury. These symptoms can be attributed to nerve compression. These symptoms usually resolve quickly in one to two months and are normally of no long-term consequence.

A patient may suffer from a loss of concentration as well as memory disturbances following a whiplash injury. Some studies published during the past decade have noted psychological factors in whiplash patients. If a patient has severe persistent pain, over time a patient may develop emotional symptoms such as depression. A whiplash injury may cause a patient to have abnormal psychological distress as well.

There is an increased risk of posttraumatic dissection and cerebrovascular events within 12 months after whiplash injury. An automobile accident is an important risk factor for arterial dissections.[9] A study was to evaluate whether there is injury to the transverse ligament of the atlas in patients with acute whiplash. The results of this study indicate possible involvement of the transverse ligament in whiplash injury.[10]

Although MRI may be helpful to study injury-related changes of anatomic structures, it is not suited for individual diagnosis because the alterations are too small.

Chronic pain patients and brain injured patients frequently exhibit anxiety, depression, perseveration, and fixed ideation about their injuries. Both populations also frequently suffer from decreased attention, impaired concentration, easy fatigability, personality changes, impaired relationships with family and friends, and difficulty maintaining a job.[11] In cases where chronic pain coexists with traumatic brain injury, the brain injury is often obscured. Treatment failure is high in this subgroup of pain patients unless treatment is directed toward the sequelae of both brain injury and chronic pain.

It is hypothesized that people will complain of exaggerated pain and injury in order to secure a financial gain. However, studies have demonstrated that the duration of pain following a whiplash injury is independent of litigation. It is interesting to note that in one study of whiplash patients, after monetary settlement 88 percent of these patients recovered and had no residual symptoms. A problem exists in that there is no real evidence that pretending to be ill or in pain with the hopes of being awarded a large settlement in a court of law contributes in any significant way to the natural history of a whiplash injury.

Studies have shown that the older a person is and an injury-related decrease in attention and memory, and the severity of the initial neck pain are predictive of symptoms that will last beyond six months. If a patient had a history of degenerative disc disease in the neck prior to the injury, for instance, the prognosis for resolution of the pain is poor. Older people do worsen after whiplash injury. The most common abnormal x-ray finding is straightening of the normal curve in the neck. A CT scan can show neck bone dislocations as well as misalignments and fractures but do not demonstrate soft tissue injury. The MRI is useful in assessing soft-tissue injury as well as injury to the bones.

Treatment of a whiplash injury should be personalized specifically for each patient. Personalization is necessary because of the variation in symptoms as well as the degree of severity of soft-tissue injury. In other words, a patient may have a worse injury than another individual who has a whiplash injury. Transcutaneous nerve stimulation (TENS) may help a patient decrease the pain symptoms. Studies have demonstrated that a patient can benefit significantly if he/she begins to move as soon as possible following the injury.

Sometimes a patient needs medications to control the pain. Drugs, however, have a limited role in the management of whiplash injury pain. Drugs, especially narcotic drugs, have a significant potential for misuse and can have potential adverse side effects. Pain medications have their greatest application immediately after injury. Nonsteroidal anti-inflammatory drugs can provide a patient with pain relief as they decrease swelling in the tissues. However, long-term use gives a patient a risk of ulcers.

Muscle relaxants may or may not help a patient with muscle spasms. Studies have shown that morphine could reduce pain following whip-lash injury but did not improve function. Antidepressant drugs can help a patient to rest. Proper sleep is important in the healing process and allows the body to build up chemicals that can decrease the pain. Sometimes following an injury and if a patient has associated chronic pain, he/she can become depressed. Antidepressant medications may not only decrease the pain, they also may decrease the depression if a patient has developed depression post-injury. Patients' psychological problems are reported to be a consequence than a cause of somatic symptoms in whiplash injuries.[12]

Sometimes cervical epidural steroid injections decrease post traumatic neck pain. This epidural space may become swollen following an injury. If a doctor injects a small amount of steroid into the area, the pain may be significantly reduced. If a patient sustained a disc injury in your neck following a whiplash injury, sometimes leakage of this disc material may form small scars in the epidural space, called adhesions. An epidural steroid injection can break up some of these adhesions and decrease the swelling in the nerves.

If a patient has headaches that begin in the base of the skull, the nerve coming out of this area to the top of the head can be treated with local anesthetic and steroid. This nerve is called the occipital nerve, and the name of the headache is occipital neuritis. Sometimes the joint between the top two bones of the neck can become compressed and injured. The administration of a steroid into this joint can provide a patient with significant pain relief as well. Most of the injections mentioned should be done with x-ray needle guidance.

The whiplash injury of the alar ligament is an important reason for chronic neck pain in elderly patients. This causes long-term neck pain and headaches due to alar ligament injury in elderly patients.[13] As previously mentioned, the facet joints in the neck may also be injured. Injection into the joint itself or injection of the nerve that goes into the joint may decrease pain. Injection into any of these joints may provide a patient with good pain relief. If the pain returns, however, surgical removal of the nerve to this joint can be done with either heat or cold application. This procedure is called a facet joint rhizotomy.

A complicated interrelationship of various factors before the collision constitutes a pre-disposing vulnerability that may be triggered by the whiplash trauma and act together with multifactorial maintaining factors after the accident in the course of developing persistent pain and disability after whiplash trauma.[14]

Whiplash injuries usually go away in several months. However, some whiplash injuries can last more than 10 years. Treatment for whiplash generally consists of medications, injections, physical therapy and/or chiropractic therapy.

References

1. Koren L, Peled E, Trogan R, Norman D, Berkovich Y, Israelit S. Gender, age and ethnicity influence on pain levels and analgesic use in the acute whiplash injury. Eur J Trauma Emerg Surg. 2015;41(3):287-291.

2. Oka H, Matsudaira K, Fujii T, et al. Risk Factors for Prolonged Treatment of Whiplash-Associated Disorders. PLoS One. 2015;10(7):e0132191.

3. Chiarotto A, Fortunato S, Falla D. Predictors of outcome following a short multimodal rehabilitation program for patients with whiplash associated disorders. Eur J Phys Rehabil Med. 2015;51(2):133-141.

4. Valenza MC, Valenza G, Gonzalez-Jimenez E, De-la-Llave-Rincon AI, Arroyo-Morales M, Fernandez-de-Las-Penas C. Alteration in sleep quality in patients with mechanical insidious neck pain and whiplash-associated neck pain. Am J Phys Med Rehabil. 2012;91(7):584-591.

5. Tough EA, White AR, Richards SH, Campbell JL. Myofascial trigger point needling for whiplash associated pain--a feasibility study. Man Ther. 2010;15(6):529-535.

6. Uhrenholt L, Freeman MD, Jurik AG, et al. Esophageal injury in fatal rear-impact collisions. Forensic Sci Int. 2011;206(1-3):e52-57.

7. Cornips EM. Crippling upper back pain after whiplash and other motor vehicle collisions caused by thoracic disc herniations: report of 10 cases. Spine (Phila Pa 1976). 2014;39(12):988-995.

8. Haggman-Henrikson B, Gronqvist J, Eriksson PO. Frequent jaw-face pain in chronic Whiplash-Associated Disorders. Swed Dent J. 2011;35(3):123-131.

9. Hauser V, Zangger P, Winter Y, Oertel W, Kesselring J. Late sequelae of whiplash injury with dissection of cervical arteries. Eur Neurol. 2010;64(4):214-218.

10. Ulbrich EJ, Eigenheer S, Boesch C, et al. Alterations of the transverse ligament: an MRI study comparing patients with acute whiplash and matched control subjects. AJR Am J Roentgenol. 2011;197(4):961-967.

11. Anderson JM, Kaplan MS, Felsenthal G. Brain injury obscured by chronic pain: a preliminary report. Arch Phys Med Rehabil. 1990;71(9):703-708.

12. Radanov BP, Begre S, Sturzenegger M, Augustiny KF. Course of psychological variables in whiplash injury--a 2-year follow-up with age, gender and education pair-matched patients. Pain. 1996;64(3):429-434.

13. Chen J, Wang W, Han G, Han X, Li X, Zhan Y. MR investigation in evaluation of chronic whiplash alar ligament injury in elderly patients. Zhong Nan Da Xue Xue Bao Yi Xue Ban. 2015;40(1):67-71.

14. Carstensen TB. The influence of psychosocial factors on recovery following acute whiplash trauma. Dan Med J. 2012;59(12):B4560.

22. Joint pain

Aging is associated with a number of pathologies involving various organs including the skeleton. Age-related bone loss and resultant osteoporosis put the elderly population at an increased risk for fractures and morbidity.[1]

Osteoarthritis is the most common form of arthritis, affecting millions of people worldwide. It occurs when the protective cartilage on the ends of your bones wears down over time. Although osteoarthritis can damage any joint in your body; the disorder most commonly affects joints in your hands, knees, hips and spine. CD8 T cells with markers of replicative senescence are correlated with increased osteoporotic fractures in the elderly.

Thus, senescent CD8 T cells are associated with a variety of deleterious health-related outcomes, suggesting that these cells may exert pleiotropic negative effects on both immune and non-immune organ systems during ageing.2 Osteoarthritis occurs when the cartilage or cushion between joints breaks down leading to pain, stiffness and swelling.

Muscle pain can occur when muscles are stretched beyond their normal elastic limits. When this happens, it is called a strain. A scar can develop within an injured muscle. An area in this scar can be a source of pain. The scar can be very tender to touch. The tender areas in muscles are called trigger points, and these cause a myofascial pain syndrome.

A patient also has cartilage which is a substance that exists between bones and can be compressed. This compressive ability makes the cartilage act as a shock absorber in some joints. Cartilage allows bones of joints to slide over each other. If a patient does not have the cartilage, one bone will not easily slide over another bone.

A patient would have increased friction applied to bones in a joint if the cartilage is gone, which could cause significant pain. A patient can also stretch and injure a tendon, which is called a sprain. An acute sprain is a stretch of a ligament at the time of an injury.

A tendon is composed of a group of fibers that attaches your muscles to your bones. A tendon is composed of tough fibers. A tendon injury can take a long time to heal. Muscle injuries, on the other hand, can heal faster than tendon injuries. A tendon injury can be potentially serious because if it does not heal properly a patient can be prone to re-injury. This inflammatory process is called tendonitis.

Some people have bursitis of their shoulders, whereas others may have a bursitis in their hips. A bursa is a sac that is filled with fluid. This fluid-filled sac is placed between either a tendon or a bone or between a ligament and a bone. A bursa allows a tendon to glide over the bone of the shoulder or hip. The fluid is a lubricant.

The covering over a muscle is called a fascia. The fascia is a tissue that covers muscles and separates one muscle from another. The fascia is present throughout the body. This fascia enables one muscle to slide smoothly over another muscle.

The elbow is a complex joint designed to withstand a wide range of dynamic exertional forces. The location and quality of elbow pain can generally localize the injury to one of the four anatomic regions: anterior, medial, lateral, or posterior.[3] An injury to the elbow is usually in the tendons of the muscles that attach to the bones about the elbow.

In tennis elbow, the pain runs to the outer elbow. A patient may also have pain about the inner elbow. This usually occurs when playing golf. Tennis elbow was named because it affected tennis players. Inner elbow pain is called golfer's elbow. The pain usually starts several days after doing an activity. The treatment for golfer's elbow is the same as that for tennis elbow. A patient may also develop pain in the elbow joint or bursitis in the elbow.

Plain radiography is the initial choice for the evaluation of acute injuries and is best for showing bony injuries, soft tissue swelling, and joint effusions. Magnetic resonance imaging is the preferred imaging modality for chronic elbow pain. Musculoskeletal ultrasonography allows for an inexpensive dynamic evaluation of commonly injured structures.[3]

The knee is made up of the femur and tibia and fibula. Ligaments hold bones about the knee together. There is a ligament on either side of the knee. These ligaments provide a knee with stability. A knee also contains cartilage, which coats bones. Cartilage allows bones to slide over each other with ease. If the cartilage wears out, it can cause arthritis.

Muscles that control knee range of motion are called the quadriceps and hamstring muscles. When your quadriceps muscles contract, they make the knee straighten. Lower extremity muscular strength is associated with mobility, morbidity and mortality. When the hamstring muscles contract, the knee and lower leg pull backward at the knee joint. Findings indicate that cellular aging may be more pronounced in older adults experiencing high levels of perceived stress and chronic pain.[4]

Chronic inflammation is a profound systemic modification of the cellular microenvironment which could affect survival, repair and maintenance of muscle stem cells.5 There is age-related modulation of the skeleton involving intrinsic factors such as genetics, hormonal changes, levels of oxidative stress, and changes in telomere length, as well as extrinsic factors such as nutritional and lifestyle choices.[1]

Telomere length and telomerase activity are important indicators of cellular senescence and replicative ability. Loss of telomerase is associated with ageing and the development of osteoarthritis.[6]

To cushion the knee, there are several bursas in the knee. The ligaments about the knee give the knee stability while the meniscus is a cushion for the knee. Without the meniscus, one would have bone rubbing on bone that would be painful. A patient can have several areas of pain within the knee including the joint and kneecap. An injury to any one of these anatomic structures can cause one to have knee pain.

With increasing age, the prevalence of osteoarthritis increases and the efficacy of articular cartilage repair decreases. Chondrocyte senescence contributes to the age-related increase in the prevalence of osteoarthritis and decrease in the efficacy of cartilage repair.[7]

The initiation/progression factors of osteoarthritic (OA) cartilage degeneration and the involved biological mechanisms remain rather enigmatic. One core reason for this might be a cellular senescence-like phenotype of OA chondrocytes, which might show a fundamentally different behavior pattern unexpected from the biological mechanism established in young cells.[8]

The quantification of ultra-short telomeres, stress a role of telomere shortening in human OA. Telomere shortening is associated with a number of common age-related diseases. A role of telomere shortening in osteoarthritis (OA) has been suggested, mainly based on the assessment of mean telomere length in ex vivo expanded chondrocytes.[9]

Hip pain is a common problem, and its source of pain can be confusing because there are many causes. It is important to make an accurate diagnosis of the cause of symptoms so that appropriate treatment can be directed at the underlying hip problem. Arthritis is among the most frequent causes of hip pain. Evidence for linkage in a family suggests that a gene for susceptibility to hip osteoarthritis exists on chromosome 16p. This represents an independent identification of a susceptibility locus previously reported for hip osteoarthritis.[10]

A trochanteric bursitis is an extremely common problem that causes inflammation of the bursa over the outside of the hip joint. A steroid injection into the knee can provide pain relief. Tendonitis can occur in any of the tendons that surround the hip joint. A nonsteroidal anti-inflammatory medication may provide pain relief.

Ostonecrosis is a condition that occurs when blood flow to an area of the hip bone is restricted. If an inadequate amount of blood flow reaches bone, the cells will die and the bone may collapse. One of the most common places for osteonecrosis to occur is in the hip joint. Hip fractures are most common among elderly patients. These fractures usually require surgery. A disc herniation in the lower back may refer pain to the hip as well. Osteonecrosis is most often found in the hips, knees, shoulders, and ankles.

A patient may have osteonecrosis in one or more bones. In people with healthy bones, new bone is always replacing old bone. This process keeps bones strong and also happens when children grow or if a bone is injured. In osteonecrosis, bone breaks down faster than the body can make enough strong, new bone.

If a patient does not get treatment, the disease worsens and the bones in the joints break down. Osteonecrosis is most common in people in their thirties, forties, and fifties. Osteonecrosis is caused when the blood flow to the bone decreases. Known causes of osteonecrosis are: steroid medications, alcohol use and injury.

An ankle sprain is a partial tear of the ligaments of the ankle joint. In a Grade I sprain the ligament is intact. In a Grade II, a ligament is partially torn and in a Grade III tear, a ligament is completely torn. Ligaments can be pulled away from the location where they attach to bones. A sprain can be classified as acute, recurrent, or chronic. In an acute injury, range of motion about the ankle will be limited.

Advancing age is a well-known risk factor for tendon disease. Energy-storing tendons e.g., human Achilles, equine superficial digital flexor tendon are particularly vulnerable and it is thought that injury occurs following an accumulation of micro-damage in the extracellular matrix.11 An x-ray will not help in the diagnosis of an Achilles tendonitis. An MRI scan will help in the diagnosis.

A patient has a bursa about the Achilles tendon as well. This bursa can become inflamed. X-rays are not helpful in the diagnosis of a bursitis in this area. Usually the diagnosis is made if a patient has pain immediately above the heel. An injection of local anesthetic in this area can confirm the diagnosis. Advancing age is a well-known risk factor for tendon disease. Energy-storing tendons e.g., human Achilles, equine superficial digital flexor tendon are particularly vulnerable and it is thought that injury occurs following an accumulation of micro-damage in the extracellular matrix.[11]

A patient may also sustain a rotator cuff tendon tear if one falls on an outstretched arm, or if one frequently using the arm for vigorous activity.

This tendon attaches a muscle to the bone in the humerus. A tear in this tendon can cause weakness and pain in the shoulder.

Excessive pushing and pulling can cause tears as well. These tears usually respond to stretch exercises as well as nonsteroidal anti-inflammatory medications. Injections with steroids are commonly done for the following musculoskeletal disorders. Injection of the subacromial space for treatment of rotator cuff tendinitis and shoulder impingement syndrome is a common and useful injection. This technique also can be used diagnostically to differentiate between the shoulder joint and cervical spine pain. The long head of the biceps tendon often is irritated by overuse. Anesthetic injection of the peritendinous space can help confirm the diagnosis of biceps tendinitis.

The pes anserine bursa is located along the medial aspect of the knee joint about 2 cm below the medial joint line. It is a common site of irritation that results in painful tendinitis or bursitis. The prepatellar bursa often becomes irritated. It is superficial to the patella and easily palpable when swollen. Aspiration of a swollen bursa can provide symptomatic relief and is required for fluid analysis. Intra-articular aspiration or injection into the knee is indicated to obtain fluid for analysis, treat painful osteoarthritis, or relieve a tense effusion. Pes Anserine Bursitis is an underdiagnosed cause of knee pain in overweight women.

Greater trochanteric pain syndrome (GTPS) is a commonly diagnosed regional pain syndrome with a wide spectrum of etiologies, reflecting the anatomy of the structures outside the hip joint capsule. There are five muscle tendons that insert on to the greater trochanter and three bursae in the region of the greater trochanter. The term GTPS includes tendinopathies, tendinous tears, bursal inflammation and effusion.[12]

There are a range of treatments and therapies depending on the specific diagnosis and severity of the condition. MRI can be very helpful in the further investigation of patients in whom there is diagnostic uncertainty as to the cause of lateral hip pain and in whom specialist orthopedic referral is being considered.

De Quervain's tenosynovitis is a painful condition of the thumb and wrist that can be treated with a corticosteroid injection. Injection is indicated for treatment of the carpal tunnel syndrome when fewer invasive treatments are unsuccessful. A dorsal ganglion of the wrist that has become painful or irritated may be aspirated and injected. Lateral epicondylitis may be treated by injection when less invasive treatments have failed. Injection has been shown to provide short-term relief.

Treatment of olecranon bursitis with aspiration and injection closely parallels treatment of prepatellar bursitis. Bursitis of the greater trochanter on the femur is painful and often responds well to corticosteroid injection. An anesthetic injection also is useful to differentiate between local pain and referred pain. Plantar fasciitis of the foot may be treated by an injection as well. Trigger point injections may be used to treat many painful soft-tissue conditions a well.

It is possible that telomerized/rejuvenated presenescent osteoblasts may be used in the development of tissue engineering or cell-based therapy for bone regeneration and repair in the future.[13] the quantification of ultra-short telomeres; stress a role of telomere shortening in human OA. A role of telomere shortening in osteoarthritis (OA) has been demonstrated.[9] The research goal is to stop telomere shortening. The exogenous expression of telomerase may represent a way to expand human OA chondrocytes while allowing maintenance of the chondrocyte-specific phenotype. These cells have the potential to be used for restoration of the articular cartilage defects occurring in this disease.[14]

References

1. Syed FA, Ng AC. The pathophysiology of the aging skeleton. Curr Osteoporos Rep. 2010;8(4):235-240.
2. Effros RB. Replicative senescence of CD8 T cells: effect on human ageing. Exp Gerontol. 2004;39(4):517-524.
3. Kane SF, Lynch JH, Taylor JC. Evaluation of elbow pain in adults. Am Fam Physician. 2014;89(8):649-657.
4. Sibille KT, Langaee T, Burkley B, et al. Chronic pain, perceived stress, and cellular aging: an exploratory study. Mol Pain. 2012;8:12.
5. Duijnisveld BJ, Bigot A, Beenakker KG, et al. Regenerative potential of human muscle stem cells in chronic inflammation. Arthritis Res Ther. 2011;13(6):R207.
6. Wilson B, Novakofski KD, Donocoff RS, Liang YX, Fortier LA. Telomerase Activity in Articular Chondrocytes Is Lost after Puberty. Cartilage. 2014;5(4):215-220.
7. Martin JA, Buckwalter JA. The role of chondrocyte senescence in the pathogenesis of osteoarthritis and in limiting cartilage repair. J Bone Joint Surg Am. 2003;85-A Suppl 2:106-110.
8. Rose J, Soder S, Skhirtladze C, et al. DNA damage, discoordinated gene expression and cellular senescence in osteoarthritic chondrocytes. Osteoarthritis Cartilage. 2012;20(9):1020-1028.

9. Harbo M, Bendix L, Bay-Jensen AC, et al. The distribution pattern of critically short telomeres in human osteoarthritic knees. Arthritis Res Ther. 2012;14(1):R12.

10. Ingvarsson T, Stefansson SE, Gulcher JR, et al. A large Icelandic family with early osteoarthritis of the hip associated with a susceptibility locus on chromosome 16p. Arthritis Rheum. 2001;44(11):2548-2555.

11. Thorpe CT, McDermott BT, Goodship AE, Clegg PD, Birch HL. Ageing does not result in a decline in cell synthetic activity in an injury prone tendon. Scand J Med Sci Sports. 2016;26(6):684-693.

12. Chowdhury R, Naaseri S, Lee J, Rajeswaran G. Imaging and management of greater trochanteric pain syndrome. Postgrad Med J. 2014;90(1068):576-581.

13. Yudoh K, Nishioka K. Telomerized presenescent osteoblasts prevent bone mass loss in vivo. Gene Ther. 2004;11(11):909-915.

14. Piera-Velazquez S, Jimenez SA, Stokes D. Increased life span of human osteoarthritic chondrocytes by exogenous expression of telomerase. Arthritis Rheum. 2002;46(3):683-693.

23. Myofascial pain

Myofascial pain is pain related to muscle injury or overuse resulting in taut bands and palpable areas of pain which is referred to other areas of a body. The most common chronic nonmalignant pain conditions that affect older adults are: myofascial pain, generalized osteoarthritis, chronic low back pain, fibromyalgia, and peripheral neuropathy. Chronic myofascial pain (CMP), also called the myofascial pain syndrome, is a painful condition affecting the muscles and the sheath of the tissue called the fascia that surrounds the muscles. CMP can involve a single muscle or a group of muscles.

Myofascial pain syndrome (MPS) refers to pain and presumed inflammation in the body's soft tissues or muscles. Myofascial pain is a chronic, painful condition that affects the fascia (connective tissue that covers the muscles). Myofascial pain syndrome might involve either a single muscle or a muscle group. The term myofascial pain syndrome is presently used in a vague and indeterminate way to denote any regional musculoskeletal pain syndrome without regard to its source or cause.

the existence of endogenous mechanisms allowing for telomere regulation in skeletal muscle with ongoing cycles of degeneration and regeneration and a model where regulatory factors are possibly involved in the protection of skeletal muscle telomeres.[1] Measuring the DNA telomere length of skeletal muscle in experienced endurance runners may contribute to our understanding of the effects of chronic exposure to endurance exercise on skeletal muscle.[2] Chronic endurance running may be seen as a stressor to skeletal muscle.

Myofascial trigger points are classified into active and latent trigger points. An active trigger point is one with spontaneous pain or pain in response to movement that can trigger local or referred pain. A latent trigger point is a sensitive spot with pain or discomfort only elicited in response to compression.

The myofascial trigger points (active or latent) follow common clinical characteristics such as pain on compression. This may elicit local pain and/or referred pain that is similar to a patient's usual clinical complaint or may aggravate the existing pain.

Snapping palpation (compression across the muscle fibers rapidly) may elicit a local twitch response, which is a quick contraction of the muscle fibers in or around the taut band. Restricted range of stretch, and increased sensitivity to stretch, of muscle fibers in a taut band may cause tightness of the involved muscle.. The muscle with a trigger point may be weak, but usually no atrophy can be noticed. Patients with trigger points may have associated localized autonomic phenomena, including vasoconstriction, pilomotor response and hypersecretion.

The problem with a myofascial pain syndrome is it can present with pain symptoms that are similar to other muscle pain syndromes such as fibromyalgia. Fibromyalgia is a disorder characterized by pain in the fibrous tissue of muscle. Chronic myofascial pain is a painful condition affecting the muscles and the sheath of the tissue called the fascia that surrounds the muscles. Muscle strains and ligament sprains can cause pain in muscles and can contribute to the onset of the myofascial pain syndrome.

Pain related to myofascial pain syndrome can be as severe as that caused by a heart attack or by kidney stones. On the other hand, a patient need to realize that myofascial pain is not life threatening. However, the pain can be severe enough to cause a patient to lie in bed until the pain is gone.

Myofascial pain can decrease activities of daily living. The existence of endogenous mechanisms allowing for telomere regulation in skeletal muscle with ongoing cycles of degeneration and regeneration and a model where regulatory factors are possibly involved in the protection of skeletal muscle telomeres.[1]

In 1942, Dr. Travell emphasized that referred pain to areas away from the trigger point was evident if a patient had a myofascial pain syndrome. It was not until 1973 that scientists took biopsies of muscle tissues from areas of myofascial trigger points. Researchers reported abnormalities in the muscle tissue.

Because it is known that there is an abnormality in a muscle tissue if a patient have muscle pain syndrome, and that palpation of these areas causes a patient to have referred pain, the term "myofascial trigger points" is now used to define painful areas throughout a body.

The diagnosis of a myofascial pain syndrome is made by a health-care provider's history and physical examination and expertise. No laboratory tests are useful for the diagnosis of this syndrome.

If a patient has the myofascial pain syndrome, a patient will complain of localized muscle pain and tenderness as well as the referred pain. To make a diagnosis of myofascial trigger points, a patient must have the presence of painful areas on examination. These painful areas must be nodular and must be reproducible.

Trigger points are classified as either active or latent. An active trigger point causes a patient to have pain at the time of palpation. The latent trigger point on the other hand, does not cause a patient to have pain at rest but can cause a patient to have a restriction of movement about a certain part of a body and will cause weakness of the muscle that has the trigger point. Only the active trigger points cause a patient pain. The latent trigger points, if they do become active, cause a patient to suffer some degree of pain. Myofascial pain is usually not symmetrical on either side of a body. However, medical conditions that cause muscle pain such as fibromyalgia are symmetrical.

A patient's myofascial pain will outlast any precipitating traumatic event. The pain duration is longer in duration than the muscle strain duration. The problem exists that when a patient were injured, a patient's muscles have developed a way of trying to prevent further pain. In doing so, these other muscles will cause a patient's injured muscle to be protected. Eventually, a patient's active trigger points will become latent. If a patient rest a patient's muscle and use a splint or an elastic bandage, a patient's active trigger point may revert to become a latent trigger point. Occasionally, a patient may do an activity that will activate a patient's latent trigger point.

In one study, in the healthy volunteers, most of the patients with lumbosacral radiculopathy had gluteal trigger point, located at the painful side. Further studies are required to test the hypothesis that specific gluteal trigger point therapy could be beneficial in these patients. Dry needling reduces pain and changes myofascial trigger point status. Change in trigger point status is associated with a statistically and clinically significant reduction in pain. Reduction of pain is associated with improved mood, function, and level of disability.

Many of a patient's muscles around a patient's active trigger point can decrease their function, causing a patient's muscles to become weak. If enough of a patient's muscles lose a significant portion of their function, a patient can develop weakness. When a patient is lying in bed, a patient may have some pressure on a patient's body in the area of the trigger points from a mattress. This pressure from a patient's bed can cause a patient to have pain. On the other hand, be aware that sleep disturbances can cause a patient's muscles to contract and become stiff and can worsen a patient's myofascial pain syndrome.

If a patient's health-care provider does not notice spasms of a patient's muscle, this individual may snap a patient's muscle to see if a patient truly has a myofascial trigger point. This essentially amounts to pinching and pulling a patient's muscle up. When this happens, usually a patient's muscle will demonstrate a visible muscle twitch. This muscle response can also be seen if a patient has latent trigger points.

A patient can have pain in the skin over a patient's painful muscle. When a patient's doctor attempts to roll a patient's skin over a patient's painful area, a patient may have significant pain. If a patient's health-care provider is knowledgeable in the pathology of trigger points, a patient's health-care provider will know that this is an infrequent observation but can occur. Furthermore, it does not mean that a patient have a psychological problem.

No blood tests show any abnormalities attributed to a myofascial pain syndrome. X-rays, MRI images, and CT scans have not demonstrated any changes that can be associated with myofascial trigger points either active or latent. There have been no reported electromyographic (EMG) changes when a patient has a myofascial pain syndrome. However, the needle tip can touch a trigger point that can elicit a twitch which will be manifest on the EMG screen.

There is conflicting information on temperature changes associated with myofascial trigger points. Some investigators have noted that a patient's temperature can be decreased over the area at the trigger point. However, for some reason, other investigators have noted increased temperature in the area of a patient's trigger points. The reason for the discrepancy in these findings remains unknown at present.

Further studies have demonstrated that the greatest number of trigger points occur between ages 31 and 50. When a patient is over 50 years old, maximum activity will cause a patient to suffer from myofascial pain. As a patient continue to age and reduce a patient's activity as a result of pain, a patient's range of motion as a result of latent trigger points will become manifest. Many health-care providers are aware of myofascial trigger points.

Following his PT boat injury in World War II, John F. Kennedy, who went on to become president of the United States, was treated by Dr. Travell. John F. Kennedy had significant neck and back pain as a result of commanding a PT boat that was struck by an enemy ship. John F. Kennedy sustained muscle injuries as well as other injuries as a result of this accident.

Dr. Travell noted that John F. Kennedy had areas throughout his body that when touched or when pressed upon caused him to have significant pain. She first reported that he was suffering from "tender points" throughout his body. However, as time progressed, she noted that his condition was chronic. She also noted that if she pressed deeply into his muscle tissue that he would have pain that was referred to other areas about his body.

Eventually the term "tender points" was changed to "trigger points" because palpation of the muscle would elicit referred pain elsewhere in the body. Dr. Travell went on to publish a book with another author that outlines the referred patterns of myofascial trigger points in areas all over the body. These doctors published a book titled Travell & Simons' Myofascial Pain and Dysfunction: The Trigger Point Manual (Lippincott, Williams & Wilkins, 1999).

If a patient suffers from the myofascial pain syndrome and if a patient is receiving adequate treatment for this syndrome, a patient will know that the diagnosis of myofascial pain syndrome needs to be accurate for a patient to receive the appropriate treatment.

A detailed history must be obtained from a patient by a patient's doctor in order to make an accurate diagnosis. Because other painful syndromes such as fibromyalgia can cause muscle pain, a patient must keep a pain diary of how the pain occurred, where the pain is located, and how severe it is.

The central sensitization syndrome encompasses disorders with overlapping symptoms in a structural pathology spectrum ranging from persistent nociception to an absence of tissue injuries such as the one presented in fibromyalgia and myofascial pain syndromes.[3]

Although adult skeletal muscle is composed of fully differentiated fibers, it retains the capacity to regenerate in response to injury and to modify its contractile and metabolic properties in response to changing demands.[4]

Studies have demonstrated that although the regenerative program can also be impaired by the limited proliferative capacity of satellite cells, this limit is not reached during normal aging, and it is more likely that the restricted muscle repair program in aging is presumably due to missing signals that usually render the damaged muscle a permissive environment for regenerative activity.

Telomeres play an essential role in maintaining chromosomal integrity in the face of physiological stressors. Although the age-related shortening of telomere length in highly proliferative tissue is predominantly due to the replication process, the mechanism for telomere shortening in skeletal muscle, which is minimally proliferative.[5]

Chronological age does not affect the cellular aging of skeletal muscle, but reveals that physical inactivity, probably mediated by free radicals, has a profound effect upon this process.

Measuring the DNA telomere length of skeletal muscle in experienced endurance runners may contribute to our understanding of the effects of chronic exposure to endurance exercise on skeletal muscle.[1]

New insights suggest the existence of telomere regulatory mechanisms in several adult tissues. This suggests the existence of endogenous mechanisms allowing for telomere regulation in skeletal muscle with ongoing cycles of degeneration and regeneration and a model where regulatory factors are possibly involved in the protection of skeletal muscle telomeres.1

Primary questions are related to physiological "health outcomes" including the influence of physical activity versus sedentary behavior on the function of a number of critical physiological systems (aerobic capacity, skeletal muscle metabolism and function, telomeres/genetic stability, and cognitive function).

Studies of sedentary behavior, including that of sitting time only, should focus on the physiological effect of a "lack of human movement" in contradistinction to the effects of physical movement and that new models or strategies for studying sedentary behavior-induced adaptations and links to disease development are needed to elucidate underlying mechanism(s).6

A study was done that aimed to demonstrate the effect of self-exercise with a therapeutic inflatable ball (SEIB) in elderly patients with myofascial pain syndrome. SEIB for 4 weeks has an effect for desensitizing myofascial pain and increasing joint flexibility.[7] High accessibility and low cost would make SEIB a practical self-treatment method in elderly patients with myofascial pain syndrome.

Myofascial trigger points may be considered as a trigger factor that can facilitate the onset of migraine or also can potentially also be a promoting factor for pain once the migraine attack has started and hence may contribute to related-disability.[8]

A patient must remember that in myofascial pain, a patient will have a history of a sudden onset of pain following a stressful event to a muscle. A patient can have a gradual onset if a patient is doing repetitive chronic manual lifting. A patient will have tight ropelike bands in muscles if a patient has myofascial pain but will have normal muscle tone if a patient has fibromyalgia.

Long-term endurance training and higher aerobic exercise capacity are associated with improved survival, and dynamic effects of exercise are evident with aging. Although adult skeletal muscle is composed of fully differentiated fibers, it retains the capacity to regenerate in response to injury and to modify its contractile and metabolic properties in response to changing demands.[4]

Chronological age does not affect the cellular aging of skeletal muscle, but reveals that physical inactivity, probably mediated by free radicals, has a profound effect upon this process[5] Although the age-related shortening of TL (telomere length) in highly proliferative tissue is predominantly due to the replication process, the mechanism for telomere shortening in skeletal muscle, which is minimally proliferative, is unclear. Chronological age does not affect the cellular aging of skeletal muscle, but reveals that physical inactivity, probably mediated by free radicals, has a profound effect upon this process.

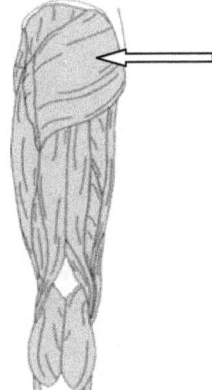

Figure 1. A patient can have a myofascial trigger point in any of a patient's muscles like the hip muscle in the figure above.

Different types of treatment can be used to treat a patient's myofascial pain syndrome. As with other tissues throughout a patient's body, the muscles in a patient's injured area go through different changes. If a patient's muscle has direct trauma to it, it can develop some scar tissue around a patient's injured muscle. These developing scars will limit a patient's muscle's ability to either contract further or relax. This phenomenon can result in a shortened, weakened muscle. If a patient sustained a sprained ankle, a patient may have been placed in a brace. A patient will then have disuse of a patient's muscles, which can cause a patient's muscles to shrink in size, called atrophy.

If a patient had a fracture of one of a patient's bones, a patient may have been placed in a cast by a patient's doctor for six to eight weeks. The muscles about the injured joint under the cast will become weak. As a patient attempt to regain strength to the muscles, a patient may experience the onset of trigger points.

A technique called spray and stretch is sometimes used to decrease myofascial pain. The spray-and-stretch technique involves stretching painful muscle while using a cold spray. This cold spray is a vapocoolant and decreases the pain conduction in muscles from the pain fiber nerve endings. Furthermore, this vapocoolant helps muscles to relax. This form of therapy can provide a patient with immediate relief of a patient's pain. This type of therapy is used for mildly painful myofascial pain. The vapocoolant releases a jet stream of a substance. The vapocoolant is applied in sweeps in different directions about the entire length of a patient's muscle. It is directed toward the area of a patient's referred pain.

Trigger point injections administered by a patient's doctor into a patient's muscles can relax a patient's muscles. The volume of fluid that goes into a patient's muscle tissue is anywhere from one to three milliliters. This volume of fluid can disrupt the scar that has formed around and within a patient's muscles. Some doctors do not inject any local anesthetic or steroid into a patient's muscle. They use what is called a dry-needle technique. They think that insertion of the needle into a patient's muscle can break up some of the scar about the muscle itself. Injection therapy into a patient's trigger points can provide a patient with significant relief.

The procedure is usually done with a patient in a lying position. The procedure consists of using a small needle about the size of an acupuncture needle. A patient's skin is cleansed with alcohol prior to injection therapy. The small needle is injected into a patient's trigger point. At that time, a patient receives a small volume of local anesthetic.

Some doctors mix a local anesthetic with a steroid. The numbing medicine relaxes a patient's muscle and decreases the pain so that a patient's physical therapist can spray and stretch the muscle back to its original length. The steroid works to take the inflammation out of a patient's muscle cells.

Sometimes a muscle trigger point injection can relieve the pain caused by a trigger point. When carpal tunnel syndrome is suspected clinically, physicians must be aware of trigger points in the infraspinatus muscles as a possible cause of the symptoms.

Biomechanical and soft tissue pathologies are common in older adults with low back pain, and many can be assessed reliably using a brief physical examination. Their recognition may save unnecessary healthcare expenditure and patient suffering.

Acupuncture is a method that can be extremely valuable for the treatment of a myofascial pain syndrome. Acupuncture does not use numbing medicines or steroids. The acupuncture needle tip can break up some of the scar around muscle tissues.

Furthermore, placement of the acupuncture needle can stimulate a production of endorphins and other natural chemicals that a patient have stored within a body to decrease pain. Acupuncture therapy has been shown to be an extremely viable treatment of a myofascial pain syndrome.

Unfortunately, myofascial pain often goes unrecognized in elderly patients, is frequently misdiagnosed, or mistreated, leading to unnecessary pain, suffering, and disability. When treated properly, the myofascial pain syndrome has an excellent prognosis.

References

1. Ponsot E, Echaniz-Laguna A, Delis AM, Kadi F. Telomere length and regulatory proteins in human skeletal muscle with and without ongoing regenerative cycles. *Exp Physiol.* 2012;97(6):774-784.

2. Rae DE, Vignaud A, Butler-Browne GS, et al. Skeletal muscle telomere length in healthy, experienced, endurance runners. *Eur J Appl Physiol.* 2010;109(2):323-330.

3. Caumo W, Deitos A, Carvalho S, et al. Motor Cortex Excitability and BDNF Levels in Chronic Musculoskeletal Pain According to Structural Pathology. *Front Hum Neurosci.* 2016;10:357.

4. Barberi L, Scicchitano BM, De Rossi M, et al. Age-dependent alteration in muscle regeneration: the critical role of tissue niche. *Biogerontology.* 2013;14(3):273-292.

5. Venturelli M, Morgan GR, Donato AJ, et al. Cellular aging of skeletal muscle: telomeric and free radical evidence that physical inactivity is responsible and not age. *Clin Sci (Lond).* 2014;127(6):415-421.

6. Thyfault JP, Du M, Kraus WE, Levine JA, Booth FW. Physiology of sedentary behavior and its relationship to health outcomes. *Med Sci Sports Exerc.* 2015;47(6):1301-1305.

7. Kim M, Lee M, Kim Y, Oh S, Lee D, Yoon B. Myofascial Pain Syndrome in the Elderly and Self-Exercise: A Single-Blind, Randomized, Controlled Trial. *J Altern Complement Med.* 2016;22(3):244-251.

8. Ferracini GN, Florencio LL, Dach F, et al. Myofascial Trigger Points and Migraine-related Disability in Women with Episodic and Chronic Migraine. *Clin J Pain.* 2016.

24. Headaches

Headaches in the elderly can be caused by many different conditions.[1] Most headaches are caused by emotional stress or fatigue, but some headaches are a symptom of a disease within the brain. Of the many pains that one can feel throughout the body, pain in the head region is usually the most distressing. Stress has obvious and not so obvious side effects. Headaches and sleeplessness are common, but so are unseen effects like shortened telomere lengths.

Pain in the head can arise in the head or can be referred from the neck as well. Although the prevalence is lower in the elderly than in young adults, headache is a common complaint in the aged population. The prevalence of headaches at different ages in women and men, respectively, is as follows: 21 to 34 years, 92% and 74%; 55 to 74 years, 66% and 53%; and after age 75, 55% and 22%. Many disorders and disabilities are higher in the elderly people who live alone; also there is a difference in the health status of elderly people who live alone, according to their gender.[2]

A headache is pain anywhere in the region of the head or neck. It can be a symptom of a number of different conditions. The brain tissue itself is not sensitive to pain because it lacks pain receptors. The pain is caused by disturbances of the pain-sensitive structures around the brain.

Several areas of the head and neck have these pain-sensitive structures, which are divided in two categories: within the cranium (blood vessels, meninges, and the cranial nerves) and outside the cranium (the periosteum of the skull, muscles, nerves, arteries and veins, subcutaneous tissues, eyes, ears, sinuses and mucous membranes).

A primary headache disorder, one in which no underlying disorder or trauma exists. It accounts for about ninety percent of all headaches. Primary headache disorders may generally be distinguished as being either episodic, such as migraine or cluster headache, or chronic, such a chronic tension-type headache. Secondary headache disorders are caused by trauma to the head, neck or face, flu or sickness with fever, or infection inside the skull, teeth, eyes or face.

Older persons have fewer headaches than younger ones. There is a decreasing prevalence of migraine with older age. Past the age of 70 years, only 5% of women and 2% of men have migraine headaches. There are many causes of new-onset headaches in the elderly, some of which can be particularly worrisome. The risk of serious secondary disorders in persons older than 65 years is 10 times higher than that in younger persons.

There is an independent association between headache and psychological factors in elderly subjects, particularly in women.[3] The findings of this study indicated an independent association between headache and psychological factors in elderly subjects, particularly in women.

Some pain receptors exist outside the skull, and other pain receptors exist within the skull. Structures outside the skull that can cause headaches and include the skin and scalp over the head, muscles about the head and neck, and the outer wrapper of the bone of the skull called the periosteum. Sinuses can also cause head pain. Veins can cause pain as well if they become engorged.

Headache classification in the elderly can be divided into primary and secondary headache disorders as mentioned previously. The primary headache disorders consist of free standing conditions such as migraine, cluster headache, and tension-type headache. Secondary headache disorders reflect underlying organic diseases such as giant cell arteritis, intracranial mass lesion, or metabolic abnormality. Although 90% of headaches in younger patients are of the primary type, only 66% of headaches in the elderly are primary.

Those with migraine headaches usually want to be left alone and typically seek a quiet, dark place. Those with cluster headaches find no relief in any position; they try many positions while attempting to eliminate their headaches and usually end up pacing the floor. Migraine as one of the most common types of headache is known to cause serious intervention with routine activities of affected individuals due to the devastating nature of attacks.4

Emotional disorders can cause headaches. Skull x-rays can prove useful for the diagnosis of a fracture, cancers, bone destruction, or some shift of the structures of the brain. Blood flow studies may be done to determine if there is any compromise in the blood flow going to the brain. A decrease in blood flow can cause significant headaches. Shorter telomere length is associated with a low cortisol state in both depressed and healthy group.

A CT scan may determine whether there is swelling, trauma or a brain abscess. An electroencephalogram (EEG) study is sometimes needed to determine whether if a patient has a seizure disorder or a sleep problem. An MRI scan of the brain can be done to see whether there is a loss of myelin in the brain. With loss of myelin, a patient may develop neurological symptoms that include memory loss and difficulty concentrating.

Occasionally, a spinal tap is done to investigate whether a patient has an infection. At the time that the spinal tap is done, a pressure monitor can be used to determine if a patient has increased pressure in the central nervous system. A loss of consciousness could indicate seizures or a hemorrhage into the brain.

Tumors can cause headaches with neurological abnormalities such as forgetfulness and dizziness. If a patient has a headache that first begins after age 50, the pain may be coming from degeneration of the discs in the neck. Hormonal changes that occur with the decreased function of the thyroid gland can cause headaches as well. Depression also can cause headaches. An MRI can usually reveal problems in structures that could cause a headache. Be aware that headaches are the most common pain syndrome in middle-aged adults.

A common type of headache is the classic migraine headache. By definition, a migraine headache is a headache that returns and varies widely in its intensity and frequency of the attacks and the duration. Usually the headaches occur on one side and are associated with nausea, vomiting, and a loss of appetite. Sometimes a patient may have visual problems associated with this headache.

Some migraines occur without an aura. If a patient has migraines with an aura, usually one has visual disturbances. This type of visual disturbance is seen in 90 percent of patients who have migraine headaches with an aura. Migraine headaches can be triggered if a patient has an abnormal response to stress.

Migraine is a debilitating disorder affecting 6-28% of the population. Studies on the mechanisms of migraine have demonstrated genetic causes but the pathophysiology and subcellular effects of the disease remain poorly understood. Shortened telomere length is associated with age-related or chronic diseases, and induced stresses. Migraine attacks may impart significant stress on cellular function, thus this study investigates a correlation between shortening of telomeres and migraine.

A significantly shorter relative telomere length was observed in the migraine group compared with the control group. No association was observed between relative telomere length and the severity and frequency of migraine attacks and the duration of migraine. Telomeres are shorter in migraine patients and there is more variation in telomere length in migraine patients.[5]

Seventy percent of people inherit the tendency to have migraine headaches. If a patient has migraine headaches, he/she usually have less than two attacks per month. However, 10 percent of patients have attacks every week. Another type of migraine headache can occur that does not have changes in sensation that can forewarn one of an impending headache. This type of headache is called a migraine headache without an aura. Sometimes these headaches occur on both sides of the head. Migraine is a highly prevalent disease that can significantly affect quality of life. Age, sex, education level, depression, congestive heart failure, chronic obstructive pulmonary failure and hypertension are all associated with migraine headaches.[6]

Treatment of migraine headaches can be divided into acute treatment of the attack as well as treatment to prevent the onset of headaches. Whenever possible, the factors that cause the headaches should be avoided. A patient should stay away from foods that could trigger a migraine headache.

Cheese, chocolate, red wine, and some Chinese foods that contain the additive MSG are commonly considered migraine headache triggers. Nonsteroidal anti-inflammatory drugs can also be used to treat this type of headache. Telomeres are shorter in migraine patients and there is more variation in telomere length in migraine patients.[5]

Migraine, tension-type headache and medication-overuse headache are disabling lifelong illnesses. Headache had negative impacts on different aspects of life: education, career and earnings, family and social life.[7]

Ibuprofen is commonly used to treat headaches and can be purchased without a prescription. If a patient has nausea and vomiting associated with the migraine headache, he/she may need to take a nonsteroidal anti-inflammatory drug by the rectal route. New drugs called triptans have been developed and can decrease a headache within a significant time after its onset. Sumatriptan was the first triptan drug to be used for the treatment of migraine headaches. Triptans are much better tolerated than the older caffeine-ergotamine medications. Stronger drugs such as Percocet have been prescribed for the treatment of migraine headaches on occasion.

Medications can be helpful in preventing headaches, but a patient should not become dependent on these drugs to solve any emotional problems that one may have. Avoid an overly busy schedule. Have one hour per day of free time to relax from a busy workday. Attempt to take one afternoon off per week and even one day off from work per month. When you have this time free, do whatever you feel like doing.

Aspirin can prevent the onset of headaches. Benadryl has been used to prevent the onset of migraine headaches as well. Antihypertensive medications such as Nadolol and Verapamil have been used to prevent the onset of migraine headaches. Amitriptyline, an antidepressant, also has been demonstrated to prevent the onset of migraine headache.

Telomeres are shorter in migraine patients and there is more variation in telomere length in migraine patients.[5] Telomeres are shorter in migraine patients and there is more variation in telomere length in migraine patients. Migraine headaches appear to be hormonally related.

They are more common in women until age 60 when the incidence is about equal to men. Migraine headaches commonly occur with the onset of menses in women. These headaches may also occur in the first trimester of pregnancy. The headaches can disappear following a complete hysterectomy.

After the onset of menopause, migraine headaches may disappear or at least decrease in intensity and frequency. However, if a patient receives hormone therapy at the time of menopause, this can prolong headache symptoms. Sometimes migraine headaches can worsen when a patient begins using oral contraceptives. Concern exists about the use of oral contraceptives by those who suffer migraine headaches, because they run a higher risk of stroke. The risk of a stroke is further increased if one smokes.

Another type of headache called a tension-type headache. This also is called a muscle contraction headache or a psychogenic headache. The term "tension type" is used to imply that muscle tension plays a role in the onset of the headache. The headaches should last from 30 minutes to 7 days. A patient will usually have a headache on both sides of the head.

Be aware that some individuals have chronic daily tension-type headaches. Migraine headaches and tension-type headaches are experienced more in women than men. Studies have been done that indicated that tight muscles of the scalp and neck can cause tension-type headaches. Studies used to objectively identify muscle tension have been done and have validated muscle tension as a cause of tension-type headaches.

Muscle tension-type headaches can start at any age. Tension-type headaches can begin in childhood if a child is physically and emotion-ally abused. A family history of tension-type headaches is not as common as with migraine headaches. The treatment for this type of headache is the avoidance of stress. Biofeedback as administered by a psychologist can decrease muscle tension and, therefore, decrease the headaches.

Another type of headache is called a cluster headache. Usually the headache is on one side of your head and can be above your eye or in the temple. In the largest case series of cluster headache published in the literature, age of onset varies between 29.6 and 31.6 years.[8] Usually the headache lasts 15 minutes to 3 hours if untreated.

Usually a patient will have tearing of the eye as well as nasal congestion on the side of the cluster headache. A patient's pupil may be extremely small, and the upper eyelid may droop. The overall incidence of cluster headaches is extremely rare. Less than 10 percent of the population suffers from cluster headaches. Cluster headaches are associated with cigarette smoking and trauma to the head.

The cluster headache occurs more frequently in men than in women. There is a 5:1 man-to-woman ratio of cluster headaches. To treat a cluster headache attack, some doctors suggest inhalation of 100 percent oxygen using a face mask. Usually the headache will settle in 15 minutes. If this does not work, an injection of sumatriptan (Imitrex) may decrease the pain. Some studies have even recommended the use of local anesthetics on a cotton swab placed in the nose. Steroids in high doses can sometimes be used to decrease the onset of cluster headaches. Nonsteroidal anti-inflammatory drugs may be effective to decrease the headaches.

If a patient has had a history of head trauma, he/she may develop headaches. These headaches continue for more than eight weeks after trauma to the head. The headache is often severe and is throbbing. Nausea and vomiting associated with this headache. One's memory may be temporarily impaired. A headache following trauma can be made worse with physical exercise.

A post-traumatic headache differs from migraine symptoms in that a chronic post-traumatic headache is usually generalized and permanent. However, it can be made worse by physical or mental strain. Usually this type of headache subsides in 8 to 10 weeks. Post-traumatic headache is reported more often in women than men. The incidence of a post-traumatic headache can be 40 percent following a head injury.

Treatment of this headache is with anti-inflammatory drugs or mild pain relievers such as Tramadol. A patient may have chronic headaches associated with trauma to the head if the injury occurred when he/she were older than 40. If a patient has a low educational level as well as a low intelligence, the headache could be chronic. Furthermore, a history of previous head trauma or a history of alcohol abuse can predispose one to have post-traumatic headaches for a prolonged duration.

If a patient is over 60 years old, he/she could develop a headache associated with temporal arteritis. This usually occurs after a fever. A patient will have a burning pain caused by inflammation of the temporal artery on the side of the head. It is usually accompanied by a throbbing headache. A patient may have a burning pain about the scalp. Temporal arteritis headaches are worsened by jaw movement such as chewing.

This type of headache can be accompanied by loss of vision, which is a medical emergency. The diagnosis sometimes has to be made with a biopsy of the arterial tissue. The location of the headache is variable and may be on one side or on both sides. One may experience pain associated with talking or eating. Steroids are usually the treatment of choice for this pain. Although 90% of headaches in younger patients are of the primary type, only 66% of headaches in the elderly are primary.

Morning headache is associated with an obstructive sleep apnea syndrome.9 However, obstructive sleep apnea syndrome patients present with various characteristics of morning headache, and they often do not fulfil the International Classification of Headache Disorders (ICHD)-2 criteria for "sleep apnea headaches".

Studies are currently being done to examine the effects of different types of opioids on the treatment of severe migraine headaches. One of the opioids that can be used for the management of severe migraine headaches is butorphanol (Stadol). This drug is administered nasally. Some doctors advocate the use of this drug for the treatment of head-aches. This drug is believed to work better in women than in men.

Women show a greater analgesic response to kappa-stimulating opioids. The other types of opioids are mu-stimulating opioids and include morphine and Demerol. These mu-stimulating opioids have been shown to work better in men than in women. For this reason, studies are being done and more studies need to be done that can evaluate the effects of these drugs for the treatment of severe headaches.

The link between stress and telomere shortening is growing stronger. The current findings suggest that cortisol levels may be a contributor to this process, but it is not yet clear whether telomere length has significance beyond that of a biomarker.

References

1. Forderreuther S. [Headaches in the elderly can be caused by many different conditions]. MMW Fortschr Med. 2015;157(19):63, 65-66.

2. Mouodi S, Bijani A, Hosseini SR, Hajian-Tilaki K. Gender differences in the health status of elderly living alone compared to those who are not alone: Evidence of the AHAP study, North of Iran. Caspian J Intern Med. 2016;7(2):126-132.

3. Ahmadi Ahangar A, Hossini SR, Kheirkhah F, Bijani A, Moghaddas Z. Associated factors of headache in an unstudied cohort of elderly subjects. Caspian J Intern Med. 2016;7(2):120-125.

4. Rabiee B, Zeinoddini A, Kordi R, Yunesian M, Mohammadinejad P, Mansournia MA. The Epidemiology of Migraine Headache in General Population of Tehran, Iran. Neuroepidemiology. 2016;46(1):9-13.

5. Ren H, Collins V, Fernandez F, Quinlan S, Griffiths L, Choo KH. Shorter telomere length in peripheral blood cells associated with migraine in women. Headache. 2010;50(6):965-972.

6. Wang X, Xing Y, Sun J, et al. Prevalence, Associated Factors, and Impact on Quality of Life of Migraine in a Community in Northeast China. J Oral Facial Pain Headache. 2016;30(2):139-149.

7. Allena M, Steiner TJ, Sances G, et al. Impact of headache disorders in Italy and the public-health and policy implications: a population-based study within the Eurolight Project. J Headache Pain. 2015;16:100.

8. Manzoni GC, Taga A, Russo M, Torelli P. Age of onset of episodic and chronic cluster headache - a review of a large case series from a single headache centre. J Headache Pain. 2016;17:44.

9. Suzuki K, Miyamoto M, Miyamoto T, et al. Sleep apnoea headache in obstructive sleep apnoea syndrome patients presenting with morning headache: comparison of the ICHD-2 and ICHD-3 beta criteria. J Headache Pain. 2015;16:56.

25. Spinal deterioration and back pain

Spinal deterioration is one of the most implicated of all back pain causes and in the elderly. Back pain however has many causes in elderly patients. In general, a patient could be experiencing pain in the back as a result of injury, stress, poor posture, or even aging. As people grow older, loss of bone strength from osteoporosis can lead to fractures, and at the same time, muscle elasticity and tone decrease.

Current evidence implicates intervertebral disc degeneration as a major cause of low back pain[5] Numerous characteristic features of disc degeneration mimic those seen during ageing but appear to occur at an accelerated rate.

The intervertebral discs begin to lose fluid and flexibility with age, which decreases their ability to cushion the vertebrae. The risk of spinal stenosis also increases with age. Human degenerative disc disease is characterized by progressive loss of human nucleus pulposus (HNP) cells and extracellular matrix, in which the massive deposition are secreted by HNP cells.[6]

Many older people experience back pain, and there are treatment methods available that could help ease that pain. The lumbar spine is composed of a large number of bones called vertebrae that are separated from one another by discs. These discs act as shock absorbers. Between each bone in our spine, the bones stack on top of each other like Lego blocks and form joints called facet joints.

The purpose of the bones in the spine is to protect the spinal cord from injury. There are foramina, which are holes in each vertebra. The nerves off of the spinal cord go through these holes and go to the arms, legs, and organs within the body. In addition to muscles, a patient has ligaments that attach each bone in the spine to both the one above and the one below. Ligaments also are necessary to give the back stability. The ligaments contain pain fibers and can be a source of back pain.

Most people with chronic back pain do not need surgery. It is usually used for chronic back pain if other treatments do not work. You may need surgery if you have: A herniated disk which occurs when one or more of the disks that cushion the bones of the spine are damaged, the jelly-like center of the disk leaks out, causing pain. Spinal stenosis causes the spinal canal to become narrow. Spondylolisthesis occurs when one or more bones of the spine slip out of place. Vertebral fractures can be caused by a blow to the spine or by crumbling of the bone due to osteoporosis.

Most of the lower-back pain and any associated disability associated with the lower back are usually mechanical in nature. This means that there is usually an abnormal alignment of the bones and/or joints that can cause a patient to have significant lower-back pain. You have five bones in your lower back that are called lumbar vertebrae. The spine functions to support one when a patient is standing, walking, bending, pushing, and pulling.

Back pain is the most expensive and common industrial or work related injury. Back pain is the most common cause of disability for workers younger than age 45. In 90 percent of working people, back pain limits working activity for usually less than 30 days. Five percent of people who have back pain have weakness, loss of sensation, or loss of reflexes in a leg.

Two percent of people with back pain may end up needing surgery. Back pain is the most common cause of activity limitation in the working population between ages 18 to 55 in the United States. Back pain is responsible for 15 percent of work absenteeism in developed countries. Approximately, 5 percent of the work force is disabled by back pain yearly. Attempts to prevent back pain have not been proven to be effective.

The rates for surgery in the United States have increased over the past 20 years. The rate of surgery for back pain in the United States is greater than in most other countries. The reason for this finding is probably due to the large number of surgeons in the United States when compared to other countries.

If a patient is over 50 years of age, he/she can expect to have problems with the back and also have limitations in activity due to back pain. Back pain from heavy physical work is common by age 50. Back pain is an unavoidable part of your life. Even people who have not done heavy physical work can begin experiencing increased back pain by age 50. The muscles in the back must be strong in order to support the back. This is the reason that a patient must do regular exercise activity.

The lower back is made up of five bones called lumbar vertebrae. The lower part of the back below these bones is called the sacrum. It is made up of five fused bones. The tailbone is called a coccyx. Cushions that are called discs are located between the bones in the back. These discs are prone to injury as well as to wear and tear. As one grows older, the discs lose their elastic properties, and they become thinner and can become wafer thin. As the discs in the back decrease in height, the overall body height decreases.

As discs begin to shrink, pressure from the bones above and below can cause the discs to press outward. This is called a disc bulge. Sometimes a disc bulge can press on one of the nerves. A disc bulge is not a disc rupture. If the pain persists and a patient develops numbness, he/she may ultimately have to have surgery to remove a portion of this bulge off of the nerve.

In the very center of a disc is a thick acidic liquid. Liquids cannot be compressed. If one bends a certain way or attempts to lift a heavy object in an awkward position, the fluid inside of your disc can burst through the outer ring of your disc. This is called a disc herniation or rupture and can cause significant pain. The liquid material that bursts outside of the disc is highly acidic. This acid content can cause the nerves, ligaments and muscles to become swollen and inflamed, and can cause severe pain.

Discography is a way of diagnosing whether or not that a patient has disc-related pain. An MRI and CT scan can show a disc herniation. However, these imaging studies cannot define pain. A discogram is an injection of material into a disc. The pressure in the disc is then measured. A patient should have a relatively high pressure when material is injected into the center of the disc. If the disc leaks injected material, the leakage of the acidic nucleus pulposus can cause pain.

Sciatica is pain that is felt in the back and the outer side of the thigh, leg, and foot. It is usually caused by degeneration of one of the discs between the back bones. When the disc protrudes laterally off to the side, it can compress the nerves in the lower back. Usually the last two or three nerves are compressed on the side of the pain. The onset of sciatica can be sudden.

People who have sciatica usually have stiff backs and have pain when they attempt any movement. A patient may have numbness in the leg as well as weakness associated with sciatica. Where the backbone and pelvis meet, they form a joint called the sacroiliac joint. The sacroiliac joint can be a source of back pain. This joint has a thick capsule that has strong ligaments both in the front and the back of the joint. Other ligaments also help to form and support this joint. The joint is C shaped.

As one becomes older, the cartilage that attaches to the pelvic bone degenerates faster than the cartilage in the sacrum. As a result, this joint can become unstable. It can be a cause of pain as well. Related to hormone changes that occur during pregnancy, the ligament becomes loose. This is the reason that many pregnant women experience pain in their sacroiliac joint that can last after the birth of their baby until the ligament becomes stronger.

A bone scan is helpful in diagnosing sacroiliac arthritis. During this procedure, a very small dose of a radioactive dye is injected into a patient's vein. After the radioactive dye has had time to go to the joints, pictures are taken with a camera of the sacroiliac joint. If a patient has an arthritic, there will be darkened areas in the joints that will show up on the scan.

If joint pain does persist, destruction of the nerves that goes to the joint can be done with either heat or cold. This is called a rhizotomy. Occasionally, a surgeon may have to stabilize the joint surgically. Nonsteroidal anti-inflammatory medications also can be very helpful for the management of pain in the sacroiliac joint. If a patient has a disc herniation, the disc herniation can be diagnosed by a CT scan or an MRI.

A patient can lose muscle strength all over the body with aging. Ligaments can become lax and weak and the joints can become stiff from degeneration. Changes in the architecture of the discs and joints which are due to wear and tear is called osteoarthritis. This is the most common form of arthritis, and it affects approximately 21 million Americans. Arthritis can cause the diameter of the spinal column to decrease. The hole in which the spinal cord is placed can narrow and can eventually put pressure on the spinal cord, which can cause significant pain.

With osteoarthritis, the holes in which the nerves emerge from the spinal cord can decrease in diameter. When this happens, one or more of the nerves can be compressed, which can cause pain, numbness, and weakness. Osteoarthritis (OA), the disease characterized by joint pain and loss of joint form and function due to articular cartilage degeneration, is not an inevitable consequence of aging, but a strong association exists between age and increasing evidence of OA.

Aging changes in articular cartilage that increase the risk of articular cartilage degeneration include fibrillation of the articular surface, decrease in the size and aggregation of proteoglycan aggrecans, increased collagen cross-linking and loss of tensile strength and stiffness.[7] These alterations are most likely primarily the result of aging changes in chondrocyte function that decrease the ability of the cells to maintain the tissue including decreased synthetic activity, synthesis of smaller less uniform aggrecans and less functional link proteins and decreased responsiveness to anabolic growth factors. These changes may be a result of erosion of telomere length.

The incidence of osteoarthritis is a disease characterized by joint pain and loss of joint form and function due to articular cartilage degeneration, is directly correlated with age.[8] The senescence associated enzyme beta-galactosidase, erosion of chondrocyte telomere length and mitochondrial degeneration due to oxidative damage causes the age related loss of chondrocyte function.

After the age of 30, bones gradually lose calcium. The loss of calcium can decrease bone mass, especially in the vertebral bodies. This is called osteoporosis. Osteoporosis is seen more commonly in women than men. In females, the loss of the female hormone called estrogen, which occurs at menopause, will accelerate this bone loss. The loss of calcium in bone mass in vertebral bodies can collapse them and cause a fracture of the vertebrae. These fractures are called compression fractures. Leukocyte telomere length (LTL) and bone mineral density are associated with health and mortality. Because osteoporosis is an age-related condition and LTL is considered to be a biomarker of aging.[9]

Osteoporosis can be very painful. Some doctors are now putting a hardening substance into the bones of the back of patients with osteoporosis and have compression fractures. This technique is referred to as vertebroplasty. A kyphoplasty entails placement of a balloon into the bone, which will expand the bone followed by placement of a hardening substance.

In addition to degenerative changes in the back and joints as being common causes of back pain, the most common cause of back pain is muscle tension in the lower back. Approximately, 80 percent of people living in the United States will experience one incident of an aching back at some time in their lives.

The vertebrae and sacrum are common areas for back pain. Slouching puts more excessive pressure and stress on the discs than does any other posture. Slouching can, therefore, decrease the blood flow to the discs and cause the discs to lose their height and begin to calcify, which is called degeneration. This condition can cause chronic pain. Slouching in a chair and at a desk also can cause chronic pain by compressing the nerves that come off of the spinal cord and go to the legs.

The lower back has a natural C curve at the lower end of the back. This normal curve is called a lordotic curve. Chronic slouching can straighten this normal C curve in the back. This misalignment will affect the discs, muscles, ligaments, and joints.

Be aware that as a person ages one of the first consequences of aging is unfortunately in the discs. Changes usually occur in one of both two lower discs in the back. The evaluation and management of back pain in older patients are more complex and challenging than in younger patients. Low back pain in the elderly has a much wider range of possible diagnoses, including a higher incidence of malignant causes.

Acute causes: (pain less than six weeks): lumbar strain/sprain, vertebral or pelvic fracture, abdominal aortic aneurysm. Subacute (6 weeks to 12 weeks, and chronic (greater than 12 weeks) elderly back pain can be caused by: degenerative disk and joint disease, malignancy, fibromyalgia, polymyalgia rheumatica, Parkinson's disease and Paget's disease and spinal canal stenosis. The senescence associated enzyme beta-galactosidase, erosion of chondrocyte telomere length and mitochondrial degeneration due to oxidative damage causes the age related loss of chondrocyte function.[5]

The lower discs in the lumbar spine essentially do not have a blood supply from arteries to the discs after age 12. The blood supply of the discs must come from the ends of the vertebral bodies. Most of the oxygen and sugar that go to the discs come from the ends of the vertebral bodies as well. After the discs have begun to age, the joints in the vertebral bodies will degenerate as well.

As a disc narrows as a result of degeneration, the space between the discs narrows as well. This causes o compression of the discs. This compression causes the discs to wear out faster. The facet joints in the spine work to stabilize the spine. As these joints deteriorate, a patient will lose motion of the lower back. For some reason, the development of loss of lower back range of motion is slower in women than in men.

Spondylolisthesis can be another cause of your back pain. This occurs when one of your bones slips upon the one below it. This is usually hereditary in origin. However, when one bone slips over the other, it can cause pain in the facet joints, and sometimes it can compress the nerves coming off of the spinal cord.

Usually surgery is not needed for this slippage. Osteoporosis is more prevalent in women and can be a significant cause of chronic back pain. Compression of the bones in the lower back can cause fractures and is more common in postmenopausal women because their hormones have significantly declined after menopause.

Age can affect the incidence of back pain. For example, it was published in 1988 that back pain prevalence was higher among women than men at younger ages, but around age 45 the rate for back pain among men exceeded that of women. When people reach 65 years of age or over, the incidence of back pain was similar for both men and women. It is interesting to note that there is a decrease in the prevalence of back pain in women between the ages of 70 to 79 but not in men.

The population of senescent disc cells has been shown to increase in degenerated or herniated discs. However, the mechanism and signaling pathway involved in the senescence of nucleus pulposus (NP) chondrocytes are unknown.[10] The prevention or reversal of the senescence of NP chondrocytes can be a novel therapeutic target for human disc degeneration.

Observed restored telomerase activity, maintained telomere length, delayed cell senescence, and increased cell proliferation rate in transduced nucleus pulposus cells. One study has suggested that lentiviral vector might be a useful gene delivery vehicle for nucleus pulposus cell therapy to treat degenerative disc disease.[6]

Body mass index (BMI), bone mineral density (BMD), and telomere length are phenotypes that modulate the course of aging. Over 40% of their phenotypic variance is determined by genetics.[11] It is normal for a patient to have back pain as one ages.

Studies have demonstrated that in certain parts of the world, back pain is considered a normal part of life. It is, therefore, less debilitating. In Japan, for example, few individuals complain of back pain when compared to the United States.

As a result, disability related to back pain is less. Lower education levels, smoking, obesity, and inactivity contribute to the prevalence of back pain in the United States. Prevention or reversal of the senescence of nucleus pulposus chondrocytes can be a novel therapeutic target for human disc degeneration.[10]

Chiropractic therapy can be an alternative method to significantly decrease lower-back pain. If all conservative methods fail to provide a patient with pain relief, injections of numbing medicines and steroids can be performed in muscles, the epidural space, around nerves going to the spinal cord, and in the facet joints.

Injection therapies usually provide pain relief for a limited duration but if and when the pain returns, the pain intensity is less.

References

1. Le Maitre CL, Freemont AJ, Hoyland JA. Accelerated cellular senescence in degenerate intervertebral discs: a possible role in the pathogenesis of intervertebral disc degeneration. *Arthritis Res Ther.* 2007;9(3):R45.

2. Wu J, Wang D, Ruan D, et al. Prolonged expansion of human nucleus pulposus cells expressing human telomerase reverse transcriptase mediated by lentiviral vector. *J Orthop Res.* 2014;32(1):159-166.

3. Martin JA, Buckwalter JA. Roles of articular cartilage aging and chondrocyte senescence in the pathogenesis of osteoarthritis. *Iowa Orthop J.* 2001;21:1-7.

4. Martin JA, Buckwalter JA. Aging, articular cartilage chondrocyte senescence and osteoarthritis. *Biogerontology.* 2002;3(5):257-264.

5. Nielsen BR, Linneberg A, Bendix L, Harboe M, Christensen K, Schwarz P. Association between leukocyte telomere length and bone mineral density in women 25-93 years of age. *Exp Gerontol.* 2015;66:25-31.

6. Kim KW, Chung HN, Ha KY, Lee JS, Kim YY. Senescence mechanisms of nucleus pulposus chondrocytes in human intervertebral discs. *Spine J.* 2009;9(8):658-666.

7. Lill CM, Liu T, Norman K, et al. Genetic Burden Analyses of Phenotypes Relevant to Aging in the Berlin Aging Study II (BASE-II). *Gerontology.* 2016;62(3):316-322.

26. Fibromyalgia

Fibromyalgia syndrome (FMS) is a chronic disorder characterized by widespread pain and tenderness, accompanied by disturbed sleep, chronic fatigue and multiple additional functional symptoms.[1] FMS continues to pose an unmet need regarding pharmacological treatment and many patients fail to achieve sufficient relief from existing treatments. Fibromyalgia can affect multiple sites throughout your body and interrupt one's daily living. Fibromyalgia is a chronic pain syndrome that affects soft tissue, tendons, and fascia. Anyone can get fibromyalgia, including men and women, children and the elderly. Also referred to as fibromyositis, it affects about 5 percent of the population, 90 percent of which are women of child-bearing age.

Compared to patients under the age of 60, seniors with fibromyalgia syndrome experience unique symptoms. While younger fibromyalgia patients cite pain as the most severe of their fibromyalgia symptoms, seniors are most affected by fatigue, soft tissue swelling, as well as fibromyalgia-related depression.

Early-life adversity increases the risk of developing a number of disorders, such as chronic pain, fibromyalgia, and irritable bowel syndrome.[2] Greater understanding of the impact of early-life stress may inform the development of personalized treatments for chronic pain in later life and strategies to prevent its onset in susceptible individuals.

Fibromyalgia is a heterogeneous condition. Subgrouping of fibromyalgia patients is highly recommendable, since these subgroups show diverse clinical pictures and therefore treatment options should be individually tailored to their specific profile.[3]

Telomere length, considered a measure of biological aging, is linked to morbidity and mortality. Psychosocial factors associated with shortened telomeres are also common in chronic pain. Telomere length was also related to pain threshold and pain sensitivity, as well as gray matter volume, such that patients with shorter telomeres were more sensitive to evoked pain and had less gray matter in brain regions associated with pain processing. There is a relationship between pain and telomere length.[4]

In addition, the above study found that while participants over the age of 60 experienced similar symptoms of fibromyalgia as participants under the age of 60, the former groups were more likely to complain of headaches, anxiety, tension and symptoms aggravated by external factors, such as physical activity (i.e. fatigue). Fibromyalgia in the elderly often occurs in the presence of other musculoskeletal disorders where it is often unsuspected. There is no proven prevention for this disorder. However, over the years, the treatment and management of this disease have improved.

The new criteria keep the requirements that other causes be ruled out and that symptoms have to have persisted for at least 3 months. They also includes 2 new methods of assessment, the widespread pain index (WPI) and the symptom severity (SS) scale score. The WPI lists 19 areas of the body and a patient tells where the pain was in the last week. A patient gets 1 point for each area, so the score is 0-19. Type B constitutes a minor but important component of FM that probably has a marked impact on the patient's perceived illness severity and quality of life. Further, WPI probably is the most important single indicator of disease severity and quality of life in FM.[5]

For the SS scale score, the patient ranks specific symptoms on a scale of 0-3. These symptoms include: fatigue, waking unrefreshed, cognitive symptoms, somatic symptoms in general (such as headache, weakness, bowel problems, nausea, dizziness, numbness/tingling, hair loss). The numbers assigned to each are added up, for a total of 0-12.

Fibromyalgia causes a patient to have muscle pain throughout the body, joint stiffness, and fatigue. One also may experience sleep disturbances and depression. It can cause many places in the body to become extremely tender. The diagnosis of fibromyalgia in seniors is different than that of younger patients. Furthermore, seniors experience different degrees of fibromyalgia symptoms than do individuals under the age of 60 who also have fibromyalgia.

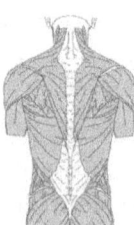

Figure 1. With fibromyalgia, a patient will have symmetric tender areas about the body.

The acupuncture at the acupoints selected from the affected meridians based on the location differentiation and the heavy moxibustion at painful points are safe and effective in the treatment of fibromyalgia syndrome and present the better persistent effect as compared with the combined medication of tramadol sustained release tablets and amitriptyline.[6]

Results reinforce the understanding of fibromyalgia as a heterogeneous condition. Subgrouping of fibromyalgia patients is highly recommendable, since these subgroups show diverse clinical pictures and therefore treatment options should be individually tailored to their specific profile. The combination of 1990c and the m-2010c is potentially useful to identify subgroups of fibromyalgia patients.[3]

The pathogenesis of fibromyalgia has not been clearly elucidated, but central sensitization, which plays an important role in the development of neuropathic pain, is considered to be the main mechanism.[7] The cutaneous silent period which is a spinal reflex mediated by A-delta cutaneous afferents, is useful for the evaluation of sensorimotor integration at the spinal and supraspinal levels.

Multiple tender points are common in the population and, in studies of mid-life adults, are strongly associated with high levels of psychological distress. Whether this relationship occurs in older adults is unclear.[8] Clinical features of primary Sjogren's syndrome overlap with those of fibromyalgia. Fibromyalgia has been shown to be prevalent in primary Sjogren's syndrome.

It is more common for women to have fibromyalgia than men. Because of this, researchers are trying to find gender-specific causes of fibromyalgia. In general, the amount of pain that women can withstand is lower than the amount of pain that men can withstand. Some researchers think that the differences in hormones between men and women can cause the differences in the amount of pain they can each withstand. Fibromyalgia is seen mostly in women between 20 and 50 years of age. However, it can affect children and elderly people as well.

The exact cause of fibromyalgia remains unknown. Studies of muscle tissue in people with fibromyalgia have shown changes that are similar to muscle tissues that have not been used very much. The experience of child abuse is associated with fibromyalgia symptom severity and may shape the biological development of interoception in ways that predispose to pain and polysymptomatic distress.[9] Fibromyalgia and chronic pain have previously associated with HIV infection.[10]

A patient may have either an increase or a decrease in blood flow to muscle tissues. This may be the direct result of an abnormal nervous system. As a result of either an increased blood flow or a decreased blood flow, blood vessels can become a filter for blood to leak into muscle tissues. The blood or plasma that is leaking into muscles is the reason why individual tissues, such as the hands or feet swell up on the body.

In comparison to healthy controls, patients with fibromyalgia revealed significantly decreased levels of serotonin, somatomedin C, calcitonin, prostaglandin E2 and a significantly increased level of prolactin. No significant differences were found in the levels of ACTH, substance P and TSH.[11] These results suggest that the diagnosis of fibromyalgia can be confirmed by various biochemical parameters, hormones and other chemicals released by the body also affect symptoms of pain. Serotonin and norepinephrine are two chemicals in the central nervous system (brain and spinal cord) that calm down pain signals traveling to the brain.

Fibromyalgia also affects levels of norepinephrine, which is a chemical in the central nervous system that functions in response to short-term stress. Urine studies in people diagnosed with fibromyalgia have shown above normal urinary norepinephrine levels. These same high urinary norepinephrine levels also are seen in patients with anxiety. Just the opposite, people who don't have fibromyalgia, but who have a history of depression, do not show high urinary norepinepherine levels.

Another theory about the cause of fibromyalgia is related with the increase in substance P in the spinal fluid of people with fibromyalgia. An increase in substance P in the spinal fluid can cause the nerves that go to muscles to become excited. After these nerve endings are stimulated, muscles will become excited, and they will be tense and contract. Substance P is a neuropeptide which is widely distributed in the periphery and the central nervous system, where it is co-localized with other neurotransmitters such as serotonin or dopamine and where it acts as a neuromodulator.

SP has been proposed to play a role in the etiopathology of asthma, inflammatory bowel disease, emesis, psoriasis, as well as neuropsychiatric disorders including pain syndromes (e.g. migraine and fibromyalgia) and affective disorders, anxiety disorders, schizophrenia and Alzheimer's disease.[12]

Substance P is found basically in all neurons of the central nervous system as well as nerves that innervate to muscles. High substance P levels have been noted in the spinal fluid of people with fibromyalgia. Endorphins, substances produced by the body and deposited in the spinal cord to decrease pain transmission to the brain, slow down the pain-causing effects of substance P. low levels of endorphins in the brain and spinal cord may be another cause of pain associated with this condition.

A patient also may have symptoms similar to someone with low thyroid hormone production. This low blood level of thyroid hormone can cause one to have symptoms that include fatigue, weakness, and muscle aches. It is possible that the lower levels of serotonin in the central nervous system cause these symptoms.

Some researchers think that mental illness also could be a cause of fibromyalgia. Some doctors think that fibromyalgia is a made-up expression from people with depression or anxiety. The thought that fibromyalgia may be the result of a bipolar disorder is also being looked into. Researchers have discovered a higher lifetime rate of anxiety and depression among people suffering from fibromyalgia. In one study, 64 percent of patients suffering from fibromyalgia had depression for at least 12 months prior to its beginning. Comorbidity with fibromyalgia is associated with a high suicide risk in patients with migraines.[13]

However, in some people in chronic pain, depression and anxiety can be a result of their chronic pain symptoms. About 40 percent of people with fibromyalgia are depressed, whereas 10 percent of the healthy population suffers from depression as well. The common thinking among current researchers leans toward the assumption that depression does not cause fibromyalgia, but that it occurs after the fibromyalgia itself sets in.

Person-centered progressive resistance exercise improved physical fatigue in women with fibromyalgia when compared to an active control group.[14] Evidence of pathology and functional abnormalities of small nerve fibers exist as a potential correlate of pain in the fibromyalgia syndrome.[15]

Women with fibromyalgia have a decrease in body chemicals called endorphins. This is similar to morphine-like chemicals that reduce pain. Women suffering from fibromyalgia have a lower blood level of nociception than do normal women throughout the entire menstrual cycle. This could be a cause for their increase in pain sensitivity during that time. However, women suffering from fibromyalgia do not appear to have a decrease in their symptoms following menopause when their hormone levels are decreasing.

There is increased evidence that fibromyalgia can be genetically inherited. The exact gene that causes fibromyalgia has not been isolated, but several genes have been proposed as a possible explanation for the genetic inheritance of fibromyalgia, and they are being studied. Research into the causes of fibromyalgia must continue. Continued research may ultimately lead to the answer of why men and women respond to pain differently.

Low impact exercises can be a beneficial form of treatment for fibromyalgia syndrome in elderly patients. There is no agreement among doctors from different specialties as to the best treatment of fibromyalgia. Anesthesiologists will inject your muscles with a steroid mixed with a numbing medicine. Physical medicine and rehabilitation specialists will prescribe heat, cold, and other physical modalities for the treatment of your pain. Internists will prescribe various pills to control your pain. The combination of trigger point injections and acupuncture provides improved clinical outcomes.16 Physical exercise is one of the most efficient interventions to mitigate chronic pain symptoms in fibromyalgia.[17] Bone mass of women with FM may be more susceptible to changes in physical fitness than that of the women without fibromyalgia as well.[18]

Stress and depression cause the hormones and other chemicals in the body to become unbalanced and could lead to more symptoms of pain. It is important that a patient exercise or any type of low-impact aerobic activity. Aerobic exercise is extremely helpful in decreasing pain and improving sleep patterns. Swimming and water aerobics are excellent ways to accomplish this goal. They are some of the best exercise activities for patients with fibromyalgia.

These types of non-impact activities will help strengthen and condition muscles, unlike high-impact exercise that can actually do more damage to muscles. Exercise appears to stimulate brain regions involved in descending pain inhibition in fibromyalgia patients, decreasing their sensitivity to pain.[19]

Emerging evidence associates chronic pain syndrome, such as fibromyalgia, with endogenous pain modulatory system dysfunction, leading to an impaired descending pain inhibition.[20] Patients with fibromyalgia have an endogenous pain modulatory system dysfunction, possibly causing an impaired descending pain inhibition.

Massage and heat therapy are both good options. Acupuncture also has been shown to be of some benefit due to its effect on the release of the body's endorphins. Most doctors agree that medications, injections, and therapy alone will not be able to eliminate pain, but rather it will help one to manage y pain and cope with it better. Taking steroids to treat fibromyalgia will not improve symptoms of pain. People with other muscle or bone conditions such as rheumatoid arthritis do respond well to steroids. However, nonsteroidal anti-inflammatory medications such as ibuprofen may relieve or at least decrease muscle pain.

The major therapeutic approach for treating fibromyalgia, a chronic widespread pain syndrome, is pharmacotherapy-centered symptom management. Complexity of treatment often leads to multiple medication prescriptions.[21]

Tramadol (Ultram or Ultracet) may be extremely helpful to people suffering from fibromyalgia. It has two mechanisms of action that can effectively reduce pain. First, tramadol exerts its pain-relieving effects by stimulating receptors in the brain and spinal cord. Activation of these receptors can significantly block the amount of pain impulses that ultimately reach the pain center in the brain. Second, the added advantage of using this drug to treat pain is that it increases the levels of serotonin and norepinephrine in the spinal cord and brain.

The main goal in treating fibromyalgia is to attempt to break the pain cycle. One way of accomplishing this goal is to correct any disturbance in sleep patterns. Amitriptyline (Elavil) can be an important drug in restoring sleep. Numerous studies have shown that getting enough sleep can significantly reduce pain. Cyclobenzaprine (Flexeril) can be used.

In some people, nonsteroidal anti-inflammatory medications such as ibuprofen can be successfully used. Amantadine hydrochloride (Symmetrel) also may be used. This medication is an antiviral as well as an anti-Parkinson medication. Serotonin reuptake inhibitors (Paxil) may also have a positive effect on reducing pain.

Pregabalin was efficacious through 12 weeks for reducing pain and improving sleep quality in FM patients with baseline moderate or severe pain, with larger effects in the baseline severe pain subgroup.[22] Gabapentin may also reduce fibromyalgia pain.

A patient should avoid any narcotic types of pain-relieving medications. These narcotic medications could cause one to feel depressed. They also can reduce hormone production. A reduction in the levels of the hormone testosterone can occur in both men and women. In men, a large decrease of testosterone in the blood can cause depression and osteoporosis. In many cases, people with significant pain request narcotic therapy because he/she think it is the only thing that could possibly take care of relieving the pain. If they are prescribed to at all, only take them for three to five days.

Pain relieving creams that can be applied directly to the skin also are an effective ways to reduce pain symptoms. Capsaicin cream contains chemicals that are obtained from red peppers. These substances lessen the amount of substance P in the nerve endings around muscle tissue. Zostrix or a similar cream also may effective for you. This cream is expected to be more effective for managing pain than creams such as Ben-Gay that contain menthol. Ben-Gay is most useful in managing inflammatory pain such as arthritis. A patient may even find it helpful to have an injection of a local anesthetic and a steroid directly into the most sensitive areas of pain.

Psychological counseling can be another useful way to cope with the pain. A psychologist can help one deal with the suffering aspect of pain. The psychologist also may to teach biofeedback. This is a good way for one to learn relaxing techniques that can significantly reduce the pain. Aromatherapy also could be effective for helping manage pain. This method is more efficacious in women because their scent perception is better than men. A patient may also find that hypnosis can decrease pain intensity. The symptoms of fibromyalgia in men are generally fewer and milder than those of women. However, the conditions caused by this syndrome can be just as painful.

References

1. Ablin JN, Hauser W. Fibromyalgia syndrome: novel therapeutic targets. Pain Manag. 2016;6(4):371-381.
2. Burke NN, Finn DP, McGuire BE, Roche M. Psychological stress in early life as a predisposing factor for the development of chronic pain: Clinical and preclinical evidence and neurobiological mechanisms. J Neurosci Res. 2016.
3. Segura-Jimenez V, Soriano-Maldonado A, Alvarez-Gallardo IC, Estevez-Lopez F, Carbonell-Baeza A, Delgado-Fernandez M. Subgroups of fibromyalgia patients using the 1990 American College of Rheumatology criteria and the modified 2010 preliminary diagnostic criteria: the al-Andalus project. Clin Exp Rheumatol. 2016;34(2 Suppl 96):S26-33.
4. Hassett AL, Epel E, Clauw DJ, et al. Pain is associated with short leukocyte telomere length in women with fibromyalgia. J Pain. 2012;13(10):959-969.
5. Ghavidel-Parsa B, Bidari A, Maafi AA, et al. The impact of fibromyalgia on health status according to the types, demographic background and pain index. Clin Exp Rheumatol. 2016;34(2 Suppl 96):S134-139.
6. Li D, Yang L, Li J. [Fibromyalgia syndrome treated with acupuncture at the acupoints of the affected meridians and heavy moxibustion at painful points: a randomized controlled trial]. Zhongguo Zhen Jiu. 2016;36(2):147-151.
7. Baek SH, Seok HY, Koo YS, Kim BJ. Lengthened Cutaneous Silent Period in Fibromyalgia Suggesting Central Sensitization as a Pathogenesis. PLoS One. 2016;11(2):e0149248.
8. Brown D, Mulvey M, Cordingley L, et al. The relationship between psychological distress and multiple tender points across the adult lifespan. Arch Gerontol Geriatr. 2016;63:102-107.
9. Ortiz R, Ballard ED, Machado-Vieira R, Saligan LN, Walitt B. Quantifying the influence of child abuse history on the cardinal symptoms of fibromyalgia. Clin Exp Rheumatol. 2016;34(2 Suppl 96):S59-66.
10. Dotan I, Riesenberg K, Toledano R, et al. Prevalence and characteristics of fibromyalgia among HIV-positive patients in southern Israel. Clin Exp Rheumatol. 2016;34(2 Suppl 96):S34-39.
11. Samborski W, Stratz T, Schochat T, Mennet P, Muller W. [Biochemical changes in fibromyalgia]. Z Rheumatol. 1996;55(3):168-173.

12. Herpfer I, Lieb K. Substance P and Substance P receptor antagonists in the pathogenesis and treatment of affective disorders. World J Biol Psychiatry. 2003;4(2):56-63.

13. Liu HY, Fuh JL, Lin YY, Chen WT, Wang SJ. Suicide risk in patients with migraine and comorbid fibromyalgia. Neurology. 2015;85(12):1017-1023.

14. Ericsson A, Palstam A, Larsson A, et al. Resistance exercise improves physical fatigue in women with fibromyalgia: a randomized controlled trial. Arthritis Res Ther. 2016;18(1):176.

15. Doppler K, Rittner HL, Deckart M, Sommer C. Reduced dermal nerve fiber diameter in skin biopsies of patients with fibromyalgia. Pain. 2015;156(11):2319-2325.

16. Taw LB, Henry E. Acupuncture and Trigger Point Injections for Fibromyalgia: East-West Medicine Case Report. Altern Ther Health Med. 2016;22(1):58-61.

17. Flodin P, Martinsen S, Mannerkorpi K, et al. Normalization of aberrant resting state functional connectivity in fibromyalgia patients following a three month physical exercise therapy. Neuroimage Clin. 2015;9:134-139.

18. Gomez-Cabello A, Vicente-Rodriguez G, Navarro-Vera I, Martinez-Redondo D, Diez-Sanchez C, Casajus JA. Influences of physical fitness on bone mass in women with fibromyalgia. Adapt Phys Activ Q. 2015;32(2):125-136.

19. Ellingson LD, Stegner AJ, Schwabacher IJ, Koltyn KF, Cook DB. Exercise Strengthens Central Nervous System Modulation of Pain in Fibromyalgia. Brain Sci. 2016;6(1).

20. Truini A, Tinelli E, Gerardi MC, et al. Abnormal resting state functional connectivity of the periaqueductal grey in patients with fibromyalgia. Clin Exp Rheumatol. 2016;34(2 Suppl 96):S129-133.

21. Menzies V, Thacker LR, 2nd, Mayer SD, Young AM, Evans S, Barstow L. Polypharmacy, Opioid Use, and Fibromyalgia: A Secondary Analysis of Clinical Trial Data. Biol Res Nurs. 2016.

22. Clair A, Emir B. The safety and efficacy of pregabalin for treating subjects with fibromyalgia and moderate or severe baseline widespread pain. Curr Med Res Opin. 2016;32(3):601-609.

27. Reflex sympathetic dystrophy

Complex regional pain syndrome (CRPS) is a debilitating condition characterized by specific symptoms such as intense pain and loss of function. This syndrome can be so devastating that it affects quality of life. Complex regional pain syndrome (CRPS) is a chronic pain syndrome that causes intractable pain, disability, and poor quality of life for patients.

Reflex sympathetic dystrophy (RSD) can be a devastating entity if it is not diagnosed and treated within a timely fashion. Reflex sympathetic dystrophy usually affects one of the extremities but also can affect the face. Reflex sympathetic dystrophy is now called the complex regional pain syndrome (CRPS). It can occur in children as well. Reflex sympathetic dystrophy is serious, painful, and potentially disabling.

Pain associated with this entity is described as throbbing, burning, or aching. A patient can have pain just to touch. A patient can have swelling of the extremity as well as either warmth or coldness depending on the phase of your RSD and sweating.

A patient's hair may grow faster on the extremity with RSD at first, only to slow down as the disease progresses. The extremity will sweat. It can turn color. The nails in the affected limb can grow faster on the extremity that suffers from reflex sympathetic dystrophy.

Reflex sympathetic dystrophy usually occurs following an injury. However, a heart attack or stroke can cause you to have reflex sympathetic dystrophy. It can also be seen in the knee as well as in the shoulder. Simple bruises or sprains can trigger reflex sympathetic dystrophy.

Fractures account for 25 percent of reflex sympathetic dystrophy cases. Twenty percent of the RSD patients were postoperative on an arm or leg, whereas 12 percent occurred after a heart attack. Three percent occurred after a stroke. Approximately 37 percent of patients have emotional disturbances at the time of the onset of the reflex sympathetic dystrophy.

To determine the relationship, if any, between telomere length and pain, the researchers evaluated leukocyte telomere length in 66 women with central nervous system pain. There is a link between premature cellular aging and chronic pain as evidenced by telomere shortening. These preliminary data imply that chronic pain is a more serious condition than has typically been recognized in terms of bodily aging.

Complex regional pain syndrome (CRPS) is a progressive, chronic central nerve pain illness that is puzzling because the mechanisms for its pathogenesis have yet to be determined.[1] Certain injury mechanisms confer higher risk of CRPS. Injury increases CRPS nearly threefold.2 Open wounds, sprain and strains, superficial injuries, contusions, nerve and spinal cord injuries are main injury mechanisms.

Injury in the extremities confers a higher risk of CRPS as well. It's not well-understood why these injuries can trigger complex regional pain syndrome, but it may be due to a dysfunctional interaction between the central and peripheral nervous systems and inappropriate inflammatory responses.

The estimated overall incidence rate of CRPS is 26.2 per 100,000 person years. Females were affected at least three times more often than males. The highest incidence occurred in females in the age category of 61-70 years. The upper extremity was affected more frequently than the lower extremity and a fracture was the most common precipitating event.[3] The CRPS incidence is higher in patients with motor nerve injury and in patients with sensory nerve injury.[4] Genetic factors play a pronounced role in CRPS as well.[5] it is possible that the Herpes Simplex Virus contributes to CRPS.

A virus infection theory is an attractive hypothesis that accounts for many enigmas of CRPS.[6] A positive history for allergy/hypersensitivity reactions is a predisposing condition for CRPS I in this subset of orthopedic patients.[7]

It was once thought that reflex sympathetic dystrophy was a result of an emotional problem. However, many people do not suffer from emotional problems at the time of onset of reflex sympathetic dystrophy. To prevent a patient from having permanent disability, treatment needs to be started immediately when the diagnosis is suspected.

Treatment usually consists of oral medications as well as injection therapy by an anesthesiologist using local anesthetics. Steroids may also be used effectively to treat RSD. If your symptoms persist, sometimes you will need surgery to remove the offending nerves causing your pain.

Reflex sympathetic dystrophy can be potentially disabling. An early diagnosis and treatment can significantly improve your outcome. Further research in the exact cause of this disease and the appropriate treatment continues. If you have had reflex sympathetic dystrophy, it may have been called another condition.

Only recently have scientists throughout the world come together at an International Association for the Study of Pain meeting. These scientists devised a term to describe reflex sympathetic dystrophy that is now called complex regional pain syndrome (CRPS).

At one time it was called post-traumatic sympathetic dystrophy, algodystrophy, Sudeck's atrophy, transient osteoporosis, and post-traumatic vasomotor syndrome. The shoulder/hand syndrome was also used to describe reflex sympathetic dystrophy following a heart attack or a stroke. If a patient sustained actual nerve damage, the reflex sympathetic dystrophy was called causalgia.

A previous definition of causalgia was referred to the syndrome associated with known nerve injury, whereas reflex sympathetic dystrophy included those patients whose pain and associated symptoms were followed by a variety of causes. Injury associated with causalgia was more severe, whereas that associated with RSD was relatively minor. Now reflex sympathetic dystrophy is referred to as complex regional pain syndrome I, whereas causalgia is referred as complex regional pain syndrome II.

Causes of both of these syndromes include fractures as well as dislocations. Reflex sympathetic dystrophy and causalgia were originally described by Dr. Mitchell, a neurologist during the Civil War. He noted that some soldiers who had injuries to their hands or feet developed a syndrome that consisted of burning pain, pain to touch over the skin of the injured extremity, shiny skin, and skin that had different colors consisting of either redness or a blue cyanotic color. Blue or cyanotic discoloration usually occurs when skin or other tissues do not get enough blood and oxygen.

Dr. Mitchell also noted that the pain in the extremity was out of proportion to the injury. For example, if a patient sustained a sprain to the ankle, he/she would expect to have some pain. However, if a patient develops reflex sympathetic dystrophy, the pain is excruciating and unbearable. Mitchell noted the onset of reflex sympathetic dystrophy following gunshot wounds. The exact cause of reflex sympathetic dystrophy remains under investigation.

It was originally hypothesized that if the sympathetic nervous system became hyperactive, this hyperactivity was at least one of the causes of reflex sympathetic dystrophy. The sympathetic nervous system is one component of the autonomic nervous system. The other component of the autonomic nervous system is called the parasympathetic nervous system.

The autonomic nervous system regulates the circulation and breathing as well as stomach and bladder functions. A patient has no control over the autonomic nervous system. This distinguishes it from the peripheral nervous system which is usually under a patient's control.

When a patient has an injury to an extremity, for example, he/she will have pain impulses that go to the spinal cord as well as the brain. The impulses that are going to the spinal cord and brain are initiated by pain fibers in the tissue. These pain fibers are both enhanced and inhibited at all levels of the brain and spinal cord.

A patient's tissues produce pain-producing as well as pain-enhancing chemicals. This causes nerves to transmit pain impulses onto the spinal cord and ultimately to the brain. However, in the spinal cord a patient has chemicals that can stop or attenuate the pain impulses.

Chemical substances in tissues activate your fibers. These chemicals cause blood vessels to increase their diameter. When this happens, a patient will have warmth in the painful area as well as redness and increased temperature. As the blood vessels enlarge in diameter, a patient may also have swelling in the tissue. Chemicals such as acetychloline, potassium, and serotonin can stimulate pain in tissues.

Histamine in your tissues can also be a chemical that can cause you to have pain. However, histamine is being used in creams to decrease your pain in your skin and muscles. Further studies have shown that the release of histamine into your spinal cord can decrease your pain as well. The mechanisms by which histamine either cause pain or help relieve pain remain to be studied and elucidated.

Prostaglandins are also released if you have injury to your tissue. As mentioned previously, prostaglandins themselves do not produce pain; when they are around pain nerves, however, they sensitize these nerves to pain. Prostaglandins can intensify any inflammation that you may have and increase the action of bradykinin on your nerve endings. Substance P in your tissues can be a cause of significant pain. It is important for you to realize that there are many pain producing chemicals especially in reflex sympathetic dystrophy.

The reason for polypharmacy in the treatment of RSD is that many chemicals combine to cause your pain associated with the reflex sympathetic dystrophy. If a patient has increased sweating associated with reflex sympathetic dystrophy, this implies that the sympathetic nervous system has become overactive. However, if the reflex sympathetic dystrophy persists over time, the sweating in the hands or feet can significantly decrease. It is believed that with chronic reflex sympathetic dystrophy that the sympathetic reflexes do not remain active.

In 1916, a surgeon described that reflex sympathetic dystrophy pain could be relieved by surgically removing some of the sympathetic fibers that innervate the affected extremity. It was noted noted that patients who had his procedure had some pain relief and had decreased sweating and improvement in their skin color. This surgeon then thought that the sympathetic nervous system was involved in the etiology of reflex sympathetic dystrophy.

Over time the treatment of reflex sympathetic dystrophy included repetitive sympathetic blocks or removal of the sympathetic nerves, either surgically or by chemicals such as phenol. Sympathetic blocks involve placing a local anesthetic about the bundles of nerves which exist outside of the central nervous system. These nerve bundles which are called ganglia are in your neck as well as the lower back.

Early description of reflex sympathetic dystrophy included injuries without obvious nerve damage. Causalgia, on the other hand, was the description given to symptoms of reflex sympathetic dystrophy where a nerve had been actually injured, such as in a gunshot wound that was described by Dr. Mitchell during the Civil War. Sprains and strains can also be a cause of these syndromes as well as bursitis and tendonitis. Arthritis can also cause either reflex sympathetic dystrophy or causalgia. Head injuries and strokes can also cause reflex sympathetic dystrophy or causalgia.

A rare but devastating form of reflex sympathetic dystrophy can occur after a tooth extraction (facial RSD). Heart attacks can be associated with reflex sympathetic dystrophy of the upper arms. Painful reflex sympathetic dystrophy like symptoms can occur around the perineum (the area between the anus and urinary outlet) following surgery around this area. Sympathetic nerve fibers go to all parts of the body and, therefore, all parts of the body can be affected. The problem with reflex sympathetic dystrophy is that in many instances it is either over diagnosed or under diagnosed.

RSD is caused by an initiating traumatic event to the body, the onset of spontaneous pain as well as excruciating pain to touch as well as pain to a noxious stimulus that lasts longer than expected. The pain must be global. Evidence of swelling of the extremity, either an increase or a decrease in the skin blood flow as well as alterations in the color of the skin and sweating are noted.

The diagnosis of RSD must be excluded by the existence of other conditions that could account for the degree of the pain and dysfunction. For example, arthritis and inflammation can give a patient pain that is similar to that of reflex sympathetic dystrophy.

Causalgia also known as complex regional pain syndrome II, a patient will have the above mentioned symptoms but should also have a documented nerve injury. Furthermore, for the diagnosis of both of these entities, a patient should have documented temperature changes noted on the skin over the area of the reflex sympathetic dystrophy.

In the majority of cases most of the time the pain will be described as burning. The pain will develop after a traumatic event or after immobilization such as casting. The pain will be on one side. Only rarely can reflex sympathetic dystrophy spread to another extremity. The onset of the symptoms usually occurs within a month from the surgery or trauma.

Cold applications to the skin can worsen the pain. Movement of the joints can also cause pain. The skin should be shiny. The nails may grow faster on the side of the reflex sympathetic dystrophy. At first the hair will grow faster on the side of the reflex sympathetic dystrophy but eventually the hair pattern will decrease and a patient may lose hair in this area. Tremors or spasms maybe noted on the side of the reflex sympathetic dystrophy.

It was noted in 1946 that reflex sympathetic dystrophy needs to be diagnosed early because the treatment is more effective with an early diagnosis. In other words, early treatment positively affects the outcome. Blockade of the sympathetic nervous system is most effective for the treatment of the complex regional pain syndrome if it is performed within the first four to six weeks from the onset of the symptoms.

At one time, it was thought that a three-phase bone scan was useful for the diagnosis of complex regional pain syndrome. Studies were done as early as 1981. Individuals also used the three-phase bone scan for monitoring the progress of RSD. This imagery is related to the distribution of a radioactive isotope throughout the body, and a nuclear medicine doctor will note the distribution of this radioactive isotope in the affected extremity.

The distribution of the radioactive isotope is dependent upon blood flow as well as the activity of the bone. The problem with this test is that it has not been shown to be as good as previously assumed. Furthermore, if the three-phase bone scan is negative, this does not mean that a patient does not have reflex sympathetic dystrophy. A three-phase bone scan may be effective for staging the early or late forms of RSD.

Magnetic resonance imaging can aid in the diagnosis of RSD by identifying swelling in the center of the bone. This bone marrow edema is characteristic of complex regional pain syndrome. This study is more reliable than a three-phase bone scanning or plain x-ray exams. In 2002, it was reported in a pain medical journal that skin temperature differences in the arms and legs are extremely useful for the diagnosis of complex regional pain syndrome.

Contact and infrared thermography have both been recommended for the diagnosis of reflex sympathetic dystrophy, but the problem with thermography is that it can be influenced not only by skin blood flow but also by the temperature of the room environment as well as by muscle and deep tissue metabolism.

A newer method called laser Doppler imaging has been shown to be effective for the diagnosis of complex regional pain syndrome. This is a new entity and is not readily available in most medical centers or doctors' offices. It is a noninvasive procedure that takes no more than 10 minutes for the evaluation. It measures the skin blood flow. This laser Doppler is important because the results of this study are influenced by the superficial blood flow.

There are different phases of reflex sympathetic dystrophy. A test that measures all three of these phases is necessary. The only one to date that will detect all three phases is the laser Doppler device. After a patient has sustained an injury to the extremity, the blood vessels to the extremity become larger. This allows more blood flow to go to the extremity. The hand or foot will, therefore, feel warm and may appear to be red. This phase usually occurs within the first month of an injury. A three-phase bone scan at this time will demonstrate increased isotope activity in an extremity, which indicates phase I reflex sympathetic dystrophy.

As the RSD progresses, the blood vessels to an extremity will decrease in diameter. They go from the enlarged diameter to a normal appearing diameter. This is phase II. A three-phase bone scan will, therefore, appear normal at this time. A laser Doppler study, on the other hand, will reveal an abnormality of the sympathetic nervous system. A patient will have some swelling as well at this time and global pain about the extremity and sweating of the extremity as the sympathetic nervous system becomes overactive.

Phase II can progress on to phase III. During this phase, the blood vessels become extremely small and there is decreased blood flow to the hand, foot, or the affected extremity. This will cause the skin to become cold. By this time, the skin may become shiny and that the sweating in the hand or foot may have increased. A three-phase bone scan at this time can detect a significant decrease in the blood flow to the affected extremity.

After a patient has reached phase three of reflex sympathetic dystrophy, the disease is irreversible. The success rate for phase I is extremely high, which does decrease as a patient progresses to phase II. Symptoms and signs of complex regional pain syndrome may persist for a significant amount of time. Pain may be noted in 84 percent of individuals longer than 12 months. Ninety-one percent had temperature differences in their extremities after 12 months. Recurrence with exercise is noted in 97 percent of patients. Fifty-five percent continued to have swelling after 12 months. Muscle spasms are noted in 42 percent of individuals. Sweating is noted in 40 percent of patients. Nail growth continues in 52 percent of individuals, whereas hair patterns were present in only 35 percent of patients.

Be aware that on rare occasions RSD can spread into more than one extremity. This observation suggests that an individual may have a predisposition to develop RSD. If a patient has chronic RSD, he/she can have skin infections associated with persistent swelling of the skin as well as blood vessels that can spontaneously rupture. A patient may have a change in skin pigmentation and the fingernails or toenails on the affected extremity can become clubbed. The frequency of reflex sympathetic dystrophy shows a peak of the incidence of this entity around 50 years of age.

The distribution of RSD between men and women is almost equal for individuals younger than 50 years of age. However, for those over 50 years of age there is a predominance of reflex sympathetic dystrophy noted in women. Even though some investigators have questioned the existence of the sympathetic nervous system's influence on the pain associated with reflex sympathetic dystrophy, there is clinical evidence that this influence does actually exist. This led investigators to describe two types of pain. One is sympathetically maintained pain and is pain associated with chemicals released by the sympathetic nervous system.

The other type of RSD related pain is sympathetically independent pain, which is not associated with the chemicals liberated by the sympathetic nervous system into the bloodstream. This type of pain is not responsive to sympathetic blockade. Sympathetically maintained pain on the other hand, usually has a decrease in the pain component following a sympathetic block. Sympathetically maintained pain can be seen in other entities besides reflex sympathetic dystrophy. It may be seen in neuropathies, phantom limb pain, and shingles as well as neuralgias.

If a patient has had a nerve injury, the nerve will attempt to regrow and will sprout small sensory pain fibers. Sometimes as nerves attempt to grow together, the area where they come together can be extremely painful. Where the nerve endings come together can cause an extremely painful area called a neuroma. This neuroma is sensitive to the chemicals released by the sympathetic nervous system.

In 1995, it was proposed that inflammation with the release of prostaglandins function was the cause of pain in both RSD and causalgia. Furthermore, evidence indicates an inflammatory basis for the loss of bone mass that occurs in reflex sympathetic dystrophy. The COX-2 enzyme may be responsible for the pain associated with reflex sympathetic dystrophy. This is the reason why many doctors today treat reflex sympathetic dystrophy with the new COX-2-inhibiting drugs such as Celebrex. Furthermore, there may be an interaction between COX-2 enzyme and stimulation of the sympathetic nervous system.

Even though the injury usually occurs in the arms or legs, there can be distorted information processing within the spinal cord. In other words, changes in the spinal cord can occur secondary to the nerve injury in the arms or legs. Small inhibitory nerves in the spinal cord, called internuncial neurons, may be ineffective if a patient develops reflex sympathetic dystrophy. In addition to the central nervous system (composed of the brain and spinal cord) as well as the peripheral nervous system, which is composed of nerves outside of the brain and spinal cord, a patient also has a sympathetic nervous system.

Studies have shown that females are more vulnerable to sympathetically mediated pain than males. The chemicals that are involved that cause reflex sympathetic dystrophy are potentially affected by the sex hormones. It is believed that the hormone status at the time of the trauma is important for the development of the pain associated with reflex sympathetic dystrophy.

The effects of reflex sympathetic dystrophy on the central processing in your central nervous system may be the basis for the spread of reflex sympathetic dystrophy to your other extremities. Many recommendations for the treatment of reflex sympathetic dystrophy and causalgia exist. Because there are so many different treatments proposed, you should be aware that no single treatment is superior to the others. Remember that no treatment for complex regional pain syndrome is consistently successful. Complex regional pain syndrome (CRPS) is thought to have an auto-immune component.[8] There is a significant reduction in prevalence of CRPS however with the use of vitamin C.[9]

Early recognition and active treatment of the complex regional pain syndrome improves the outcome. For example, injections of local anesthetics about the sympathetic nervous system can alleviate the symptoms of reflex sympathetic dystrophy long term. These types of injections must be done early in the onset of the symptoms of reflex sympathetic dystrophy.

The injections can be done in the stellate ganglion, which provides sympathetic fibers to the arms, or the injections can be done in the lumbar sympathetic ganglion, which supplies sympathetic fibers to the legs. A virus infection theory is also an attractive hypothesis that accounts for many perplexities of CRPS.[6] Brachial plexopathy may be the direct cause of the reversible upper-limb paresis resulting from Herpes Zoster with CRPS-like symptoms.10

Steroids administered by mouth have been shown to be effective for the treatment of reflex sympathetic dystrophy. Steroids will decrease inflammation caused by prostaglandins. Anticonvulsive medications can be helpful in decreasing your pain. Gabapentin or pregabilin is frequently used now for the treatment of pain associated with the complex regional pain syndrome. Narcotic medications administered into the spinal fluid can also help decrease the pain. Sometimes a morphine pump, which sends a narcotic into the spinal fluid, needs to be implanted to control RSD pain.

Clonidine, which is frequently administered by a patch over the skin, can also be administered into the epidural space for the control of the pain as well. Antidepressant medication such as amitriptyline has also been shown to be effective in the management of pain associated with reflex sympathetic dystrophy and causalgia. Amitriptyline increases certain chemicals in the central nervous system that are helpful in decreasing the amount of pain that reaches the brain.

Implantation of a wire attached to a battery into your epidural space can also provide you with significant pain relief. This apparatus is called a dorsal column stimulator. Psychological intervention is also helpful. Because of the severity of the pain associated with reflex sympathetic dystrophy, a patient can develop fear, anxiety, and depression. Psychological intervention including the use of biofeedback and sometimes hypnosis can successfully be used to treat the pain.

Antidepressant medications can increase certain chemicals in the central nervous system that are helpful in reducing the amount of pain impulses that reach the brain. Some RSD patients may require psychological therapy, such as biofeedback, to help treat the fear, anxiety, and depression they may feel because of their pain condition.

Physical therapies remain the prerequisite of management but the roles of anti-inflammatory medication, sympathectomies and a team approach are emphasized as well.[11] Physical therapy is widely recommended as a first-line treatment. The efficacy of local anesthetic sympathetic blockade as treatment for CRPS I is questionable.[12] It may be concluded that RSD/CRPS can be a difficult entity to diagnose and treat. Remember that an early accurate diagnosis with the initiation of treatment in a timely fashion is essential for the successful treatment of this entity.

References

1. Aprile AE. Complex regional pain syndrome. AANA J. 1997;65(6):557-560.
2. Wang YC, Li HY, Lin FS, et al. Injury Location and Mechanism for Complex Regional Pain Syndrome: A Nationwide Population-Based Case-Control Study in Taiwan. Pain Pract. 2015;15(6):548-553.

3. de Mos M, de Bruijn AG, Huygen FJ, Dieleman JP, Stricker BH, Sturkenboom MC. The incidence of complex regional pain syndrome: a population-based study. Pain. 2007;129(1-2):12-20.

4. Demir SE, Ozaras N, Karamehmetoglu SS, Karacan I, Aytekin E. Risk factors for complex regional pain syndrome in patients with traumatic extremity injury. Ulus Travma Acil Cerrahi Derg. 2010;16(2):144-148.

5. de Rooij AM, de Mos M, van Hilten JJ, et al. Increased risk of complex regional pain syndrome in siblings of patients? J Pain. 2009;10(12):1250-1255.

6. Muneshige H, Toda K, Kimura H, Asou T. Does a viral infection cause complex regional pain syndrome? Acupunct Electrother Res. 2003;28(3-4):183-192.

7. Li X, Kenter K, Newman A, O'Brien S. Allergy/hypersensitivity reactions as a predisposing factor to complex regional pain syndrome I in orthopedic patients. Orthopedics. 2014;37(3):e286-291.

8. Reilly JM, Dharmalingam B, Marsh SJ, Thompson V, Goebel A, Brown DA. Effects of serum immunoglobulins from patients with complex regional pain syndrome (CRPS) on depolarisation-induced calcium transients in isolated dorsal root ganglion (DRG) neurons. Exp Neurol. 2016;277:96-102.

9. Meena S, Sharma P, Gangary SK, Chowdhury B. Role of vitamin C in prevention of complex regional pain syndrome after distal radius fractures: a meta-analysis. Eur J Orthop Surg Traumatol. 2015;25(4):637-641.

10. Eyigor S, Durmaz B, Karapolat H. Monoparesis with complex regional pain syndrome-like symptoms due to brachial plexopathy caused by the varicella zoster virus: a case report. Arch Phys Med Rehabil. 2006;87(12):1653-1655.

11. Bushnell TG, Cobo-Castro T. Complex regional pain syndrome: becoming more or less complex? Man Ther. 1999;4(4):221-228.

12. Bussa M, Guttilla D, Lucia M, Mascaro A, Rinaldi S. Complex regional pain syndrome type I: a comprehensive review. Acta Anaesthesiol Scand. 2015;59(6):685-697.

28. Shingles

Shingles is an infectious disease which is caused by a virus that causes herpes zoster and affects some of the nerves that go into the spinal cord. One or more nerves can be affected. Usually the shingles pain stays on one side of the body. The virus is called varicella zoster. Chicken pox is caused by the same virus that will cause shingles.

Anyone who previously had chickenpox may subsequently develop shingles. They can be male or female, young or old. In general, it is more common among older adults and certainly tends to be more severe in this group. Since shingles more commonly occurs in geriatric patients, it is important to recognize the effects that some medications and methods of treatment may have on older individuals. Leukocyte telomere length has gained attention as a marker of oxidative damage and age-related diseases.[1]

Individuals between the ages of 60 years and 80 years are most likely to come down with shingles. Shingles is actually a recurrence of the chicken pox virus. Shingles may occur spontaneously or may be induced by stress, fever, radiation therapy, tissue damage or immuno-suppression. This varicella zoster virus will remain within the area that connects the spinal nerve and the spinal cord. This area is called the dorsal root ganglia.

This virus typically reactivates when people are older than 50. This reactivation usually occurs after the immune system has been weakened, generally by another viral infection such as the flu or common cold. If a patient has cancer, he/she may be prone to develop shingles as well. The possibility exists that sporadic anti-cytokine autoantibodies in some subjects may cause an autoimmune immunodeficiency syndrome leading to uncontrolled VZV reactivation, nerve damage and subsequent PHN.[2]

When the virus is reactivated in the dorsal root ganglia, it goes along the nerves to the nerve endings. The virus at this time will cause the skin to develop lesions. A patient needs to be aware that any part of the central nervous system can be affected by this virus.

In rare cases, this virus can even affect the brain which causes encephalitis. The virus has been reported in some cases to affect the sympathetic ganglia as well, which can cause severe burning pain. This will cause a patient to have symptoms that mimic reflex sympathetic dystrophy.

If a patient has Hodgkin's disease, one risks developing shingles. If a patient has a history of cancer of the breasts, lungs, or gastrointestinal tract, a patient runs an increased risk of developing shingles. Early reports indicated that men and women were affected at the same rate. However, more recent studies have reported that men are affected more frequently than women. If a patient is debilitated, one also runs the risk of developing shingles.

Following chicken pox, antibodies are made in the body to fight the chicken pox virus. This is the reason why one usually does not get chicken pox again. If the immune system is compromised for any reason, however, the body's ability to combat the virus is greatly reduced. This is the reason why one may develop shingles.

If the immune system appears to be attacked, the body will immediately fight the shingles virus. If a patient is between the ages of 40 and 60, the chances of one developing post-herpetic neuralgia are 20 percent. If one is over 60 years of age, the chance of developing post-herpetic neuralgia will increase to 50 percent.

Post-herpetic neuralgia is a difficult entity to treat. Post-herpetic neuralgia can cause one to have agonizing pain as well as suffering. Some individuals have even committed suicide to escape this terrible pain. Sometimes one can develop burning pain associated with the herpes zoster virus.

However, it may be some time before the skin lesions appear. Before a patient develops a skin rash, the diagnosis of herpes zoster is difficult to make. After the skin lesions erupt, the diagnosis is easier to make. The post-herpetic neuralgia may be confused with other medical diseases. The problem with the post-herpetic neuralgia is that it can affect the central nervous system, which includes the spinal cord and brain.

Be aware that if a patient has severe burning pain that develops on one side of the body, one may or may not have a skin eruption, but one can have shingles. Sometimes the lack of a skin eruption confuses doctors as to whether one actually has of shingles, because skin lesions are so common.

If one does develop skin eruptions, the lesion will begin as redness. The redness over the skin will turn to blisters. These lesions on the skin breakdown. A crust then forms. If the skin, in addition to the nerves, is affected by the virus, one may develop scars as well as loss of skin pigment about the infected site.

Be aware that the virus can travel to the eyes. If one or anyone in the family has developed shingles and begins to complain of eye pain, this is a medical emergency. One must contact an ophthalmologist immediately. If left untreated, one may be blinded by the virus. The incidence of shingles is approximately 4 to 5 cases per 1,000 people. The chance of one developing shingles increases with the age. Usually when one has a viral infection; a patient will build up antibodies in the body that will help fight the virus.

As mentioned previously, shingles may be preceded by other events. Psychological stress can also trigger the onset of shingles. If one has a history of a prolonged use of steroids, one may also be prone to develop shingles. For reasons yet unknown, the Caucasian race appears to have a higher incidence of shingles than other races. The chest will be the most affected body part by shingles. A nerve coming off of the brain that distributes branches to the face called the trigeminal nerve is the next most common nerve affected.

Different types of laboratory tests are available to diagnose acute herpes zoster. As noted previously, virus recovery from the tissue and blood can provide a rapid diagnostic tool for early diagnosis. Occasionally, the virus can be recovered from the back of the throat. Different types of diagnostic tests that use various stains are available. After these scrapings are stained, they may show diagnostic material in the cells.

Many doctors advocate taking a small amount of the tissue (called a punch biopsy) so that they can do an examination under a specialized, high-powered microscope called an electron microscope. This is an extremely reliable test, and it can provide a diagnosis of whether one has the herpes zoster virus before one develop blisters on the skin.

Be aware that not every patient who develops shingles has severe, incapacitating pain. One may only complain of itching. On the other hand, one may complain of the most horrible pain that one could ever imagine. The pain can be either constant, or it can be intermittent. After one has been diagnosed with shingles, acyclovir, famciclovir, and valacyclovir can be used in the treatment of the viral infection. Antiviral medications are used to decrease the intensity and duration of the shingles and are used to prevent the chronic pain associated with post-herpetic neuralgia.

If one develops shingles and if the pain lasts longer than six weeks after the skin lesions have disappeared, one has developed post-herpetic neuralgia. A certain proportion of individuals who develop post-herpetic neuralgia will improve over time with no treatment. Approximately, 30 percent of individuals who develop post-herpetic neuralgia still complain of pain after one year. Two percent of individuals who suffer from post-herpetic neuralgia will have pain longer than five years.

Anxiety and depression are psychological factors that can affect the shingles as well as the post-herpetic neuralgia. As mentioned previously, stress can play an important role for the development of both shingles and post-herpetic neuralgia. Psychological stress in some instances can decrease the immune system, making one prone to develop shingles.

Two types of nerves conduct pain. One nerve is a larger nerve (Alpha delta) that conducts sharp, stabbing pain, whereas the other nerve is a small nerve (c fiber) that conducts burning pain. It appears that post-herpetic neuralgia affects the smaller nerves that cause one to have severe, burning pain. For some reason, on occasion the sympathetic nervous system can become overactive. This over activity of the sympathetic nervous system can cause blood vessels that are going to the tissue to decrease their diameter (constrict).

Some larger nerve fibers in the body transmit touch. Stimulation of these fibers can decrease the amount of pain impulses from pain fibers that reach the brain. Only so many impulses can be processed by the spinal cord. By stimulating the larger nerves by touch, theoretically one can decrease the number of pain impulses that reach the brain.

A significant problem associated with post-herpetic neuralgia is that these large nerves can be damaged and actually disappear. When these nerves are gone, there are no impulses to fight the burning impulses transmitted by the small nerves called C fibers. Sometimes as the nerves are being damaged by the virus that causes post-herpetic neuralgia, these nerves can become hyperirritable, causing one to suffer significant pain.

A patient must understand that this virus can injure and destroy the nerves that it affects. When the nerves become injured, they can develop areas of sensitivity at the site of nerve destruction. These sites can become hyperirritable. Studies have shown that these nerves can conduct spontaneous pain impulses. This increase in nerve electrical activity can recruit other pain transmitting nerves around the lesion.

When a patient has the acute herpes zoster attack, the pain is usually localized to the affected nerves. One may have a fever as well as weakness and fatigue. At this time, the pain could be shooting, dull, or even burning. The skin eruptions usually occur approximately four days later. The herpes zoster virus can go not only to the sensory nerves but also the nerves that go to the muscles. As a result, the muscles that are in the chest can be weakened.

Usually the weak muscle symptoms are reversible. If one has the initial stage of the viral infection, one is suffering viral replication. This means that the virus in the system is replicating rapidly. The immune system is usually depressed. As the disease progresses, the immune system should be able to fight the virus. As one go into a third phase, the body will continue to fight the virus with the antibodies. However, it is at this time that one could have permanent nerve changes.

Shingles can recur in 8 percent of individuals. Usually the shingles will occur at the same site affected previously. After one has developed crusts, these lesions will fall off in five to six weeks. After they have fallen off, they will leave an irregular scar. One may not have any feeling about the scar. If one has suffered from post-herpetic neuralgia for six months, the chance of a complete cure is remote.

One needs to realize that the virus associated with herpes zoster can be extremely destructive. It can cause nerve as well as tissue damage and bleeding into tissues. The nerves where they join the spinal cord can become extremely swollen, and bleeding can occur within the nerves. Significant nerve damage can occur within two weeks.

Remember, the initial stage of the infection is a viral replication. The virus duplicates itself rapidly. This is the reason why an antiviral medication must be administered as early as possible after the diagnosis has been made to decrease the rate of this replication. Not only is the virus recovered from blisters; it can also be recovered from the bloodstream. Occasionally, the virus can get into the fluid that surrounds the spinal cord and ultimately cause one to have meningitis.

A patient may be treated by the primary-care doctor or a dermatologist. One may have to go to an emergency room because of severe pain. Psychologists are also valuable in the management of the pain. All of these health-care providers can significantly help one manage the pain. One may find that each of these providers uses a different modality for the treatment of the pain.

If the pain is moderate, a mild analgesic such as tramadol or Tylenol with codeine may suffice for the management of the pain. If the pain becomes excruciating, these medications will not provide one with any significant pain relief. At this time, one may require more potent opioid medication such as oxycodone or hydrocodone. If these stronger narcotic drugs do not provide one with relief, one may require the administration of a strong opioid medication such as morphine.

Pain management in elderly individuals is unique because a patient may present with multiple underlying medical problems in addition to the pain problem. This makes the management of the post-herpetic neuralgia challenging. The correct diagnosis must be made before any treatment is initiated. Elderly individuals in nursing homes may have difficulty communicating their pain. If one is a family member of an elderly individual, he/she should help the relative's doctor by providing that doctor with a detailed history of the onset, duration, and severity of the post-herpetic neuralgia.

Lotions, different types of patches, nonsteroidal anti-inflammatory drugs, antidepressants, and muscle relaxants may all be needed to control the pain. One may even need injections of numbing medicines into the nerves. Placement of local anesthetics around the sympathetic nerves may be of benefit in reducing the pain, especially if the injection is done soon after the onset of the pain.

Topical agents are frequently used to treat shingles pain. These agents accelerate the healing of the skin and can decrease the pain associated with the shingles virus. A patch has been developed for the treatment of shingles. This patch has proven to be extremely useful in the management of shingles and post-herpetic neuralgia pain. A local anesthetic called lidocaine is placed within a patch system.

The lidocaine is placed within an adhesive. The adhesive binds to the skin. The lidocaine that is in this patch is dispersed through the skin and travels to the painful, hyperirritable nerve endings. When this drug reaches the nerve endings, it calms the painful nerves. Note that this patch will not cause one to have numbness about the skin.

A patient may need to take pills by mouth. If one is elderly, he/she must be aware that changes exist in the body with respect to target organ sensitivity to drugs. This means that the receptors that sit on the cells of some of the organs may not be as responsive to certain drugs as they would be if one were much younger.

As one ages, the absorption of drugs through the gastrointestinal system decreases as the age increases. On the other hand, some drugs are passively absorbed through the gastrointestinal system. This means that there will be no change in the blood level. The blood level will be the same as that of a younger individual who takes the same drug.

Tricyclic antidepressants are frequently used in the management of pain associated with post-herpetic neuralgia. The exact mechanism by which these drugs decrease the pain is unknown. The pain-relieving effect of amitriptyline (Elavil) has been shown in rats to decrease pain caused by certain nerves.

The correct dose of amitriptyline needed by elderly patients suffering from post-herpetic neuralgia is currently unknown. Higher doses definitely produce a greater decrease in the pain. However, the problem with using higher doses is that one may develop a significant decrease in the blood pressure. This is similar to that caused by clonidine.

A patient may benefit from the administration of a nonsteroidal anti-inflammatory drug because one may have a portion of the pain caused by the prostaglandins. An example of this drug is ibuprofen. The new COX-2 inhibitors may be somewhat safer for one because their incidence of side effects is less than the older NSAIDs. Because the virus does cause inflammation in the nerves and surrounding tissues, one can benefit from the use of nonsteroidal anti-inflammatory drugs.

Some narcotics, such as Demerol and Talwin, are associated with psychiatric side effects. It is best to avoid these two drugs in the geriatric population. If narcotics are to be used, mild narcotics should be initiated, as previously stated. Morphine is commonly used for severe pain.

Be aware if a patient is over 65 years old that one can have decreased renal function and can be at risk for the breakdown product of morphine. The same holds true with other narcotic medications. However, morphine does have a breakdown product that is pharmacologically active, meaning that it can cause sedation just as the intact morphine can. The metabolic breakdown products of Demerol can cause seizures. Muscle relaxants are sometimes used in the management of post-herpetic neuralgia pain. These medications are also used in elderly individuals.

Baclofen, which does stimulate some receptors in the spinal cord, can decrease the pain associated with post-herpetic neuralgia. It can also relieve any muscle spasms that occur as a result of this painful entity. Amantadine is a drug that can furthermore provide some relief for the management of post-herpetic neuralgia. It is an anti-Parkinson's medication. However, it also has NMDA receptor antagonist activity. These receptors can cause one severe pain when they are activated.

Baclofen, Amantadine, and Elavil can decrease burning pain associated with post-herpetic neuralgia while anticonvulsant medications can lessen the sharp, shooting pain. Another topical drug that is sometimes used is capsaicin cream. It can be purchased over the counter and can also be purchased by prescription at a higher concentration. This substance is found in hot peppers. It depletes and prevents the re-accumulation of substance P (a pain impulse transmitter) in the nerves. However, this medication does cause burning.

The burning sensation caused by the capsaicin prevents some individuals from using this drug. However, it can provide excellent benefits. It however, takes several days to deplete the substance P in the nerve endings.

Occurrence of HZ and progression to PHN adds extra burden on top of pharmacological treatment and impaired quality of life, especially in older patients who already have health problems to cope with in everyday life.[3] Osteoporosis risk factors included female gender, age, advanced Charlson Comorbidity Index, depression, and postherpetic neuralgia.[4]

Water therapy can be helpful because the warm water can be soothing and may also desensitize the nerves that are causing the severe pain. If the activities of daily living are limited because of the pain, consult an occupational therapist to learn how to preserve the daily-living activities.

A somatic block is an injection of the nerve with a local anesthetic. If one have significant relief but the pain returns, the doctor could do a permanent nerve block using a cold-producing modality. This is called cryo analgesia. A stellate ganglion or a lumbar sympathetic block can be used to manage the pain of the chest, lower extremities, upper extremities, or even the face. If one experience central pain, one will have burning pain sometimes from just light touch.

Sometimes an epidural injection using local anesthetics can provide relief. Further research is being done to evaluate the effects of the administration of epidural ketamine for the treatment of the pain. For the acute lesions, just an injection under the skin with a local anesthetic can provide pain relief. The different type of nerves that can be injected with a local anesthetic include the trigeminal nerve, the brachial plexus, the nerves under the ribs (called intercostal nerves), as well as the sciatic nerve.

It has been shown that sympathetic nerve blocks, if done early, can relieve pain associated with shingles and can also decrease the incidence of developing post-herpetic neuralgia. To be effective, they should be performed within the first two months after the onset of the symptoms. Stellate ganglion blocks are used for pain in the head, neck, and arms.

Thoracic epidural blocks are used for pain in the mid back and chest wall, whereas lumbar sympathetic blocks are used for the management of post-herpetic neuralgia pain in the lower extremities. The purpose of nerve blocks is to interrupt the pain impulses and to facilitate therapy and to help one increase the daily-living activities. Nerve blocks should be used if the pain is becoming too severe and cannot be controlled by non-narcotic medications.

If one has sympathetic pain that does not respond to the previously mentioned modalities, more permanent blocks of the sympathetic nervous system can be done using a modality called radiofrequency thermos coagulation. This device provides some heat about the sympathetic nerves. This device does not burn the nerves, but the heat essentially knocks the nerves out of commission. The procedure is done on an out-patient basis with only minimal discomfort. Radiofrequency thermo coagulation can provide one with a long-term interruption of the pain fibers and pain impulses. Occasionally, a dorsal column stimulator can be placed in the epidural space.

The epidural space is the space that surrounds the fluid that surrounds the spinal cord. The dorsal column stimulator is essentially an epidural catheter that has electrodes on it. The number of electrodes that are used depends upon the pattern of the pain. The dorsal column stimulator is placed within the body on a trial basis. The catheter is placed on an outpatient basis with x-ray. The end of the catheter attaches to a battery pack. How the dorsal column stimulator works actually works is debated. It is believed that the electrical interference with ascending pathways may be the mechanism for decreasing the pain impulse transmission.

The use of this device has been demonstrated to be effective for the management of post-herpetic neuralgic pain that is refractory to all other modalities. The goal of the stimulation is to decrease the pain by at least 50 percent. If one does obtain adequate pain relief, the stimulator is implanted permanently surgically. For pain that persists in the arms or legs and is refractory to other treatments, a nerve stimulator can be placed in the extremity to provide one with pain relief. Chemical substances that disrupt nerves have been used since 1930, for the treatment of post-herpetic neuralgia.

If all the previous modalities fail to provide one with relief, a narcotic pump can be placed within the body. The pump consists of a reservoir about the size of a hockey puck. It is connected with a tube that runs into the fluid that surrounds the spinal cord. Essentially this pump gives one a drop of a narcotic drug every minute or so and is another way of controlling the pain. The drug-delivery system is refilled approximately every 45-90 days. Before placing this pump, the doctor will do a trial of morphine and compare it to a saline solution to see whether one actually obtain pain relief from this device.

If the pain persists, one may require surgery. There is no single standard surgical procedure that is effective for the treatment of the post-herpetic neuralgia. A procedure called a dorsal root entry zone (DREZ) lesion has been shown to be effective in the management of post-herpetic neuralgia in some patients. Sometimes a neurosurgeon can interrupt the pain pathways by doing a procedure in the spinal cord.

Aging of the immune system is a major factor responsible for the increased severity of infections, reduced responses to vaccines, and higher cancer incidence in the elderly. A major category of stressors that contribute to the alterations within the T lymphocyte compartment is the family of herpes viruses. These viruses, usually acquired early in life, persist for many decades and drive certain T cells to the end stage of replicative senescence, which is characterized by a variety of phenotypic and functional changes, including altered cytokine profile, resistance to apoptosis, and shortened telomeres.[5]

High proportions of senescent CD8 (cytotoxic) T lymphocytess are associated with latent cytomegalovirus (CMV) infection in the elderly, and are part of a cluster of immune biomarkers that are associated with early mortality. Similar cells accumulate at younger ages in persons chronically infected with HIV-1. In addition to persistent viral infection, psychological stress as well as oxidative stress can also contribute to the generation of senescent dysfunctional T lymphocytes.

Despite controversy and few uncertainties, the Shingles vaccine significantly reduces herpes zoster and its complication incidence.[6] Up to now, no group of people with particularly high risk of herpes zoster-related complication who will beneficiate the most of the vaccination has been identified yet and only an age criteria has been considered for the recommendation.

The Zoster vaccine reduces the incidence of HZ and PHN, thereby reducing the burden of illness associated with HZ; improved uptake of zoster vaccine is needed.[7] Herpes zoster (HZ) arises in older people due to age-related decline in immunity. An age-related immune decline does not play a major role in cancer development in older people, but it may be important for some lymphomas.[8]

The features of the conserved genes and their relative order suggested a general scheme for divergence among these herpesvirus lineages.[9] In addition to the "core" conserved genes, the genome contains four distinct gene families which may be involved in immune evasion and persistence in immune cells: two have similarity to the "chemokine" chemotactic/proinflammatory family of cytokines, one to their peptide G-protein-coupled receptors, and a fourth to the immunoglobulin superfamily.

The efficacy of vaccines recommended for older-aged adults is consistently greater for females than for males. Gender differences as well as biological sex differences can influence vaccine uptake, responses, and outcome in older-aged individuals, which should influence guidelines, formulations, and dosage recommendations for vaccines in the elderly.[10]

References

1. Risques RA, Vaughan TL, Li X, et al. Leukocyte telomere length predicts cancer risk in Barrett's esophagus. Cancer Epidemiol Biomarkers Prev. 2007;16(12):2649-2655.

2. Bayat A, Burbelo PD, Browne SK, et al. Anti-cytokine autoantibodies in postherpetic neuralgia. J Transl Med. 2015;13:333.

3. Pickering G, Gavazzi G, Gaillat J, Paccalin M, Bloch K, Bouhassira D. Is herpes zoster an additional complication in old age alongside comorbidity and multiple medications? Results of the post hoc analysis of the 12-month longitudinal prospective observational ARIZONA cohort study. BMJ Open. 2016;6(2):e009689.

4. Wu CH, Chai CY, Tung YC, et al. Herpes zoster as a risk factor for osteoporosis: A 15-year nationwide population-based study. Medicine (Baltimore). 2016;95(25):e3943.

5. Effros RB. Telomere/telomerase dynamics within the human immune system: effect of chronic infection and stress. Exp Gerontol. 2011;46(2-3):135-140.

6. Ferahta N, Achek I, Dubourg J, Lang PO. [Vaccines against Herpes zoster: Effectiveness, safety, and cost/benefit ratio]. Presse Med. 2016;45(2):162-176.

7. Keating GM. Shingles (Herpes Zoster) Vaccine (Zostavax((R))): A Review in the Prevention of Herpes Zoster and Postherpetic Neuralgia. BioDrugs. 2016;30(3):243-254.

8. Mahale P, Yanik EL, Engels EA. Herpes Zoster and Risk of Cancer in the Elderly U.S. Population. Cancer Epidemiol Biomarkers Prev. 2016;25(1):28-35.

9. Gompels UA, Nicholas J, Lawrence G, et al. The DNA sequence of human herpesvirus-6: structure, coding content, and genome evolution. Virology. 1995;209(1):29-51.

10. Fink AL, Klein SL. Sex and Gender Impact Immune Responses to Vaccines Among the Elderly. Physiology (Bethesda). 2015;30(6):408-416.

29. Peripheral neuropathy

An estimated 20 million people in the United States have some form of peripheral neuropathy, a condition that develops as a result of damage to the peripheral nervous system. Peripheral neuropathies can present in a variety of forms and follow different patterns. Symptoms may be experienced over a period of days, weeks, or years. A neuropathy by definition is any disease of the peripheral nerves. These are the nerves that exist outside of the brain and spinal cord. A neuropathy typically occurs in middle aged and elderly individuals.

Elderly patients with peripheral neuropathies have a fourfold higher incidence of falls than elderly individuals without neuropathies. A disease of the nerves can cause a weakness as well as numbness in the area where the nerve travels. If only one nerve is affected by a disease state, it is called a mononeuropathy. The symptoms will depend upon the distribution of that nerve in the tissue. A polyneuropathy involves many nerves.

With a polyneuropathy, the symptoms are more exaggerated as compared to a mononeuropathy. A polyneuropathy can involve more than one extremity and is usually related to a metabolic disease. A mononeuropathy is usually related to a nerve compression.

Approximately, one in five adults over age 60 is affected by peripheral neuropathy. Basically, the symptoms of the neuropathy can be divided into two groups, one of which occurs where the symptoms are spontaneous and another, which involves maneuvers that can cause you to experience pain. Like neuralgias, you can also have shock-like stabbing pain. Neuralgia is "nerve pain" by definition. Sometimes the pain can radiate through the entire arm or leg.

Basically, any neuropathy may cause a burning, gnawing pain. Extreme pain from just a light touch can occur in tissues over the nerve. The onset of the pain following an injury to the nerve can either be of an immediate onset or a delayed gradual onset. The pain intensity can be affected by both emotion and fatigue. Not all neuropathies cause pain. Some neuropathies cause only numbness.

Nerve conduction testing examines the nerve while the EMG examines any effects on the muscles with respect to muscle pathology. The needles used for these tests are attached to an oscilloscope and can measure the speed of the transmission of impulses in the nerves or muscles. A nerve biopsy is needed as well for the doctor to diagnose a neuropathy. Mononeuropathies occur more often in diabetic patients than in the normal population. Diabetes can affect the muscles around the eye. A diabetic mononeuropathy can affect the nerves in the arms as well as the legs. A nerve lesion is a traumatic event to a nerve such as compression, which can cause a neuropathy.

Entrapment neuropathies such as the carpal tunnel syndrome are characterized by abnormal sensations in the area of the nerve as well as pain. Usually if the nerve is compressed, the blood supply to the nerve is also compromised. Entrapment neuropathies occur when a nerve is compressed. For example, tissue at the wrist can compress a nerve going to the hand and fingers, which can result in weakness and pain in the hand.

The basic pathology of an entrapment neuropathy is that the compression over the nerve can destroy the larger fibers that have myelin around them. As these nerves are destroyed, it leaves only the C-fibers in the affected nerve. With the preservation of the C-fibers, a patient will have pain as well as tenderness at the location of the nerve entrapment.

If a patient destroys the large nerve fibers, he/she will have mainly the smaller C-fibers left in the diseased nerve. These C-fibers will cause one to have significant burning pain. The exact causes of many neuropathies remain unknown. The drug Isonizid used for the treatment of tuberculosis can cause a patient have pain in the nerves. If a patient has a neuropathy, he/she may have numbness and weakness. Other types of drugs can also cause a neuropathy. For example, arsenic has been implicated as a cause of neuropathy. In addition, people who suffer with the HIV or AIDS can have extremely debilitating neuropathies associated with their disease.

If the thyroid glands do not produce enough thyroid hormone, one may develop pain related to a hypothyroid neuropathy. A patient may have pain or decreased or abnormal sensations in both the hands and feet. Compression of the nerves in the arms or legs for whatever reason can cause pressure damage to nerves. The neuropathy caused by this compression is called a compression neuropathy. Pressure over the nerve or nerves can come from a brace or cast or can come from tumors or muscle or connective tissue thickening.

Compression of the nerves can occur at different points throughout the body. Nerve conduction studies are helpful in diagnosing neuropathies. Nerve conduction studies are done by inserting a needle into the tissue and studying the conduction of the nerve impulses. Electromyography (EMG) can also be used to evaluate a compression neuropathy. This task can furthermore determine if the neuropathy has affected the muscles.

The carpal tunnel syndrome starts gradually with aching in the wrist that can extend to the forearm. Diagnosis of the carpal tunnel syndrome can be done by arthroscopy, which consists of putting a scope into the carpal tunnel. People can have a wide variety of carpal tunnel syndrome symptoms, but the condition typically causes hand and wrist pain and weakness. An MRI of the wrist and hand can be beneficial as well.

The carpal tunnel is a narrow passage in the wrist about the diameter of the thumb. The purpose of this tunnel is to protect the median nerve as well as the tendons that go to the fingers. The problem is that excessive pressure on this nerve will cause one to have numbness and pain and can lead to hand weakness. With proper treatment, most people who develop carpal tunnel syndrome can have normal restoration of their hand and nerve function.

This entity affects women more than men. The average age of the onset of this ailment is between 40 and 60 years of age. The carpal tunnel is the space between the bones in the hand at the wrist and the connective tissue over the tendons. The carpal tunnel contains the tendons that flex the wrist (bend it downward) and the median nerve. The symptoms usually begin in the dominant hand. However, the other hand can also be affected as well.

If a doctor taps over the middle of the wrist on the palm side, a patient have the production of pins and needles that go from the wrist to the fingers. This is called a Tinel's sign. The Phalen test is another test to diagnose carpal tunnel syndrome. A blood pressure cuff is applied to the arm. If a patient has a carpal tunnel syndrome, he/she will develop pins and needles in the hand when the blood pressure cuff is inflated.

Repetitive motion has been downplayed as a cause of carpal tunnel syndrome. It is important to know that carpal tunnel syndrome can be idiopathic. This means that the cause of the carpal tunnel syndrome is unknown. If a patient has a carpal tunnel syndrome, he/she runs a 1 percent chance that he/she will develop permanent injury. A patient will be given an anti-inflammatory drug or an injection of cortisone into the carpal tunnel to decrease the swelling in the tendons and ligaments within the tunnel. If this method fails, one may require surgery.

Surgery to release the tissue that is compressing the median nerve has been shown to be effective for the treatment of carpal tunnel syndrome. Elderly patients have low postsurgical symptom scores and express high levels of satisfaction after surgery for carpal tunnel syndrome. There have even been cases of gout or arthritis causing carpal tunnel syndrome that have been successfully treated by surgery. Surgical treatment appears to have better results than splinting.

A patient may develop reflex sympathetic dystrophy (RSD) for an unknown reason following carpal tunnel surgery. Carpal tunnel syndrome is treated frequently in a primary care environment. Workplace task modification and wrist splints can defer a referral for surgical decompression. Nerve and tendon exercises can be of benefit. Steroid injections into the mouth of the carpal tunnel can be helpful in some patients, especially in women.

Only a small percentage of patients with carpel tunnel syndrome actually require surgery. The chances of recovering completely following treatment are excellent. Research continues that is aimed at the prevention and rehabilitation of carpal tunnel syndrome. The incidence of an occupational carpal tunnel syndrome is usually a combination of genetics, the physiology, and the lifestyle factors in addition to general biomechanics. Therefore, no general rule of thumb applies to occupations in general.

The symptoms of carpal tunnel syndrome can progress. A patient does not want the nerve compressed for a significant period of time, because a permanent injury could occur.

The carpal tunnel syndrome can be due to a congenital predisposition. This means that the carpal tunnel is smaller than in other people. This can cause one to develop a carpal tunnel syndrome, especially if doing repetitive-motion work or using vibrating hand tools. A smaller carpal tunnel noted in women may be the reason why they are three times more likely than men to develop carpal tunnel syndrome . The carpal tunnel syndrome can occur in elderly patients using walkers and canes improperly. Weight bearing on the wrist of the aged patient can exert pressure over the median nerve which can cause a carpal tunnel syndrome.

Another type of neuropathy is a diabetic neuropathy. The prevalence of diabetes mellitus increases markedly with age. This means that advancing age is a strong risk factor for diabetic neuropathy, independent of the duration of diabetes mellitus Diabetes can be associated with a polyneuropathy, which means that many nerves are involved in the disease process. Numbness and abnormal sensations are the most frequent complaints associated with this neuropathy.

A patient can have complaints of burning pain ranging from mild to severe in both legs. Because diabetes can cause a patient to have a decrease in blood flow to the feet, make sure that one wears proper fitting shoes. Poor fitting shoes can cause ulcers on the bottom of the feet. Clinical complications of diabetic neuropathy in the elderly are often severe.

Sometimes both of the upper extremities can be involved with the diabetic neuropathy. The nerves in the extremities that have a myelin sheath around them will lose the sheath with a diabetic neuropathy. If one is diabetic and have an elevated blood sugar, for some reason this increased blood sugar can lower the pain threshold. This means that a patient will be more responsive to a certain pain stimulus Furthermore, if a patient has a diabetic neuropathy with an increase in the blood sugar, the tolerance to pain will be decreased. It has moreover been published in animal studies that an elevated blood sugar will reduce the analgesic effects of morphine in the animal model. In other words, glucose can affect the morphine pain receptors.

The sympathetic nervous system can also be altered if one suffers from a diabetic neuropathy. In many instances, the sympathetic stimulation can be decreased. A patient can subsequently have high blood flow in both extremities. However, this blood flow can be decreased by an increase in the activity of the sympathetic nervous system. Blood flow to certain areas of the body can be decreased by sympathetic stimulation of the sympathetic nervous system. This reduction in blood flow usually results in an improvement of the pain if the pain was caused by swelling of the tissue related to an increased blood flow to the tissue. Blood flow effect in a non-painful diabetic neuropathy has just the opposite effect.

Be aware that diabetes can cause multiple nerve disorders in the nerves outside of the brain and spinal cord. However, some of the nerves coming off of the brain can transmit pain fibers, and the diabetes can also adversely affect these nerves. Not only can one develop pain in the legs; a patient can furthermore develop weakness in the legs as a result of the diabetic neuropathy.

Diabetic neuropathy can be potentially very disabling. Furthermore, diabetes decreases the body's ability to heal itself. For example, if a patient has ulcers of the foot and so forth, he/she can have an impaired healing process of the involved nerves.

On occasion, some individuals with a diabetic neuropathy can have constant pain. The type of diabetic neuropathy is the diabetic amyotrophy. This entity occurs on one side of the body. It occurs most often in the nerves that go to the muscles. The nerves that go to the muscles are called motor nerves. The diabetic amyotrophy is a motor neuropathy. The diabetic amyotrophy neuropathy, as well as other diabetic neuropathies, can be seen if a patient has poor control over the diabetes. Diabetic neuropathies are found in middle-aged as well as elderly patients who suffer with diabetes. Careful attention to control over blood sugar in the long-term is the best way to prevent diabetic neuropathy. The treatment of painful diabetic neuropathy has included anticonvulsive medications.

Approximately one-half of elderly patients with painful neuropathies receive inappropriate analgesics. Propoxyphene which is now off of the market was the most commonly prescribed inappropriate drug, followed by amitriptyline, temazepam, alprazolam, lorazepam, and diazepam. Propoxyphene is cardio toxic in the elderly and the tricyclic antidepressants like Elavil (amitriptyline) have side effects that are considered unsafe in elderly patients.

Neurontin and Lyrica have become more popular over the past several years for the treatment of neuropathic pain in elderly patients but these drugs can cause confusion and delirium. Tricyclic antidepressant drugs such as Elavil can help to relieve the pain but can cause sedation and can cause a patient to fall. This drug should be avoided in elderly patients. Drugs used to treat neuropathic pain, such as opioids, tricyclic antidepressants, gabapentin, and pregabalin, are among those associated with sedation, dizziness, and falls, particularly in frail or vulnerable elderly patients

A drug that has been used successfully for the treatment of a painful diabetic neuropathy is mexiletine. This drug is essentially a medication that is used if you have abnormal heartbeats. This drug has been shown to be effective for the treatment of the diabetic neuropathy. The problem with mexiletine is that you can get side effects such as nausea and vomiting. Tremors, dizziness, and blurred vision can also occur.

Another medication that can help a patient control the painful diabetic neuropathy is a topical capsaicin cream. Almost 75 percent of patients with diabetic neuropathy who used this cream reported significant pain relief. The problem with this cream is that one can have side effects that include a burning sensation at the sight of the cream on application.

Diabetic neuropathy patients can develop an autonomic diabetic neuropathy. Autonomic nerves are supposed to keep the body running as it should. There are many functions that happen in the body without you thinking about them: the heart pumps, one breathes, and the stomach digests food. Those actions are controlled by the autonomic nervous system. The autonomic nervous system should maintain the body's homeostasis, which is its normal state.

If the autonomic nerves are damaged by the effects of diabetes, the body may have trouble maintaining homeostasis. Autonomic neuropathy can seem daunting because it can affect so many of the body's systems, from the digestive tract to how well one can see. However, the symptoms depend on what specific nerves in the autonomic nervous system are damaged.

Alcoholic neuropathy is fairly common in the United States. Approximately 20 percent of chronic alcoholics develop peripheral neuropathy related to their alcoholism. Increased incidence of alcoholism occurs within the elderly population. The neuropathy affects not only sensation but can affect strength in the lower extremities. Alcoholics who develop this neuropathy complain of burning feet. As the neuropathy becomes more severe, the alcoholic will develop weakness in both legs. Occasionally the arms can be affected as well. One important treatment for this neuropathy is to stop drinking.

When alcohol consumption has been abolished, the neuropathy can recover, but the recovery is slow. The alcoholic neuropathy is believed to be due to a deficiency of thiamine as well as other B vitamins. Alcoholics usually have an inadequate food intake. The alcohol can affect the absorption of vitamins through their gastrointestinal systems.

Alcoholics have a greater need for thiamine but are not obtaining the thiamine in their diet. It is furthermore known that alcohol itself can exert a direct toxic effect on nerves in the arms and legs. Besides stopping alcohol consumption, alcoholics should take nutritional supplements containing both thiamine and a vitamin B complex. Because of the natural diminution of postural reflexes and the nerve cell degeneration that occurs with advanced age, these patients may be more at risk for the clinical problems associated with a peripheral neuropathy, such as frequent falls and loss of balance.

Cigarette smoking and vigorous physical activity have an impact on telomere length. Smoking was related to shorter telomere length while vigorous physical activity was related to longer telomeres. Lifestyle may play an important role in telomere dynamics and also suggest that engaging in healthy behaviors may mitigate the effect of harmful behaviors on telomere length.1 One published study reported that telomere length in old age does not have a significant association with age-related physical and cognitive decline or mortality.[2]

If a patient has kidney failure, a severe neuropathy can occur that is called a uremic neuropathy. This type of neuropathy is associated with chronic renal failure. Uremia is the presence of an excessive amount of urea as well as other nitrogen waste compounds that are in the bloodstream. Normally, these waste products are excreted by the kidneys into the urine. However, if one has kidney failure, the urea is not eliminated from the bloodstream. This will cause the urea to accumulate in the blood. This will cause drowsiness as well as nausea and vomiting and can progress to death.

With uremia, a patient has a 50 percent chance that he/she can develop a uremic neuropathy. This disease is becoming less prevalent because of the treatment of kidney failure with hemodialysis as well as kidney transplants. This disease progresses slowly. At first, it affects the sensory nerves. It can progress to cause weakness in the muscles about the feet. With dialysis, this disease will stabilize. It can even improve with dialysis. If this disorder worsens during dialysis, the frequency and duration of the dialysis will be increased until the symptoms improve. After a renal transplant, a patient can expect to have a significant improvement in the renal neuropathy. Elderly patients may improve with dialysis.

As previously mentioned, thiamine deficiency as seen in alcoholics can cause neuropathies. This is another class of neuropathy called nutritional neuropathy. This class of neuropathy is seen not only in alcoholics but in individuals who are on restrictive diets. Peripheral neuropathy may occur as a result of malnutrition, which occurs in some elderly patients because of an unbalanced diet. Thiamine deficiency can lead to heart failure.

With this nutritional neuropathy, a patient may have hand, feet, and calf pain. One may have some numbness and weakness in the extremities. The administration of thiamine can reduce the symptoms. Severe nutritional deficiency can cause a patient to develop significant pain related to the nutritional neuropathy. If one doesn't get enough thiamine, he/she can develop beriberi. This is a result of a deficiency of vitamin B1 (thiamine).

Beriberi is another nutritional neuropathy that is widespread in rice-eating countries. It is noted in individuals who eat polished rice from which the thiamine-rich seed coat is removed. Two types of beriberi exist. One form is called wet beriberi. In this type of beriberi, there is an accumulation of tissue fluid in the body. With dry beriberi, there are signs of starvation. The nervous system can degenerate if a patient is not obtaining a proper amount of thiamine. Furthermore, nutritional deficiencies in a woman at the time of conception can cause abnormalities in a fetus, which can cause significant harm.

Pellagra is another neuropathy caused by nutritional deficiency. It is characterized by weakness, tingling, and even pain. This neuropathy is caused by niacin deficiency. Niacin is also a B vitamin. Pellagra is a result of a poor diet that does not have enough niacin or doesn't have sufficient tryptophane. Tryptophane is an amino acid from which niacin can be synthesized in the body. Pellagra is more common in corn-eating communities.

Chemicals also can a neuropathy. Cisplatin is an agent used in chemotherapy to treat tumors. This chemical can cause a painful peripheral neuropathy as well. The neuropathy associated with this drug can severe pain in the extremities. However, this neuropathy is reversible at the end of the chemotherapy.

Arsenic is another chemical associated with a painful neuropathy. It can also cause renal failure. Arsenic can be toxic to the heart and can cause the heart to stop. It takes one to two weeks for a patient to develop a neuropathy associated with arsenic ingestion. A patient will have burning pain as well as tingling and numbness in the extremities associated with this neuropathy.

Thallium is an insecticide as well as a rodentcide (kills rats and mice). It can also be used to image the heart by the cardiologist when examining for heart disease. The symptoms can progress through a stoppage of the heart. A patient can develop a psychosis as well as confusion, which can lead to a coma. This chemical can affect the nerves that are involved in the breathing. If one recovers from this poisoning, the recovery may never be complete. One of the hallmarks of this disease is the loss of hair.

A large number of older adults are at risk of neuropathic pain because many diseases that cause neuropathic pain increase in incidence with age, such as diabetes mellitus, herpes zoster, low back pain, cancers, limb amputation, and stroke. Each type of neuropathy requires a distinctive type of treatment. In the majority of instances, there is no cure.

References

1. Latifovic L, Peacock SD, Massey TE, King WD. The Influence of Alcohol Consumption, Cigarette Smoking, and Physical Activity on Leukocyte Telomere Length. Cancer Epidemiol Biomarkers Prev. 2016;25(2):374-380.

2. Harris SE, Deary IJ, MacIntyre A, et al. The association between telomere length, physical health, cognitive ageing, and mortality in non-demented older people. Neurosci Lett. 2006;406(3):260-264.

30. Cancer pain

High telomerase activity is detected in nearly all human cancers but most human cells are devoid of telomerase activity.[1] Aging, cancer, and chronic disease have remained at the forefront of basic biological research for decades. Telomere shortening is associated with cancer development, primarily through the induction of genomic instability. The majority of studies have indicated that individuals with shorter blood telomeres may be at a higher risk of developing various types of cancer.[2]

Within this context, significant attention has been paid to the role of telomerase, the enzyme responsible for lengthening telomeres, the nucleotide sequences located at the end of chromosomes found in the nucleus.[3] Alterations in telomere length and telomerase activity are a common denominator to the underlying pathology of these diseases. Telomere shortening occurs in many organs and tissues and is accelerated by oxidative injury and rapid cell turnover.

Short telomeres initiate chromosomal instability and may eventually contribute to tumorigenesis.[4] Telomere shortening is associated with cancer development, primarily through the induction of genomic instability. The majority of studies have indicated that individuals with shorter blood telomeres may be at a higher risk of developing various types of cancer.[2] The simultaneous evaluation of two biomarkers-telomere length and telomerase activity-could be useful for the assessment of the invasive capacity and aggressiveness of tumor cells from breast cancer patients.[5]

Telomerase-positive activity was identified as a marker that confers a trend toward a poor prognosis. In CRC, results support the use of telomere status as an independent prognostic factor.[6]

Cancer pain is usually not evident until the cancer growth has become far advanced. Most non-solid tumors cause minimal pain while solid tumors like prostate cancer can cause significant pain. If a patient has myeloma, he/she will have a malignant formation of plasma cells.

Plasma cells are antibody-producing cells found in bone forming tissue as well as in the lungs and abdomen. This increase in plasma cells can affect organs and cause painful symptoms. Usually bone pain is the most common pain noted involving multiple myelomas. The bone pain associated with this entity involves primarily the back. This disease can destroy bone. With significant destruction of bone, the bone can collapse. If the bones in the Vertebral column collapse, the collapsed bone can injure the spinal cord.

Multiple myeloma can be an extremely painful entity affecting bone and is usually treated by an oncologist. Lung cancer is common in the United States. Lung Cancer is a disease that begins in the tissue of the lungs. The lungs are sponge-like organs that are part of the respiratory system.

During breathing, air enters the mouth or nasal passage and travels down the trachea. The trachea splits into two sets of bronchial tubes that lead to the left and right lung. The bronchi branch off into smaller and smaller tubes that eventually end in small balloon-like sacs known as alveoli. The alveoli are where oxygen is taken up by the body, and carbon dioxide is removed.

The vast majority of lung cancer cases fall into one of two different categories: Non-Small Cell Lung Cancer is the most common type of lung cancer, making up nearly 80% of all cases. This type of lung cancer grows and spreads more slowly than small cell lung cancer. Small Cell Lung Cancer makes up nearly 20% of all lung cancer cases. It is associated with cancer cells smaller than most other cancer cells. These cells may be small, but they can rapidly reproduce to form large tumors. Their size and quick rate of reproduction allow them to spread to the lymph nodes and to other organs throughout the body. Cigarette smoking causes this type of cancer.

Symptoms of lung cancer include the following: coughing, short-ness of breath, wheezing, pain in your chest, shoulder, upper back, or arm, coughing up blood, frequent pneumonia, generalized pain and hoarse-ness. Lung cancer can spread to your brain liver or bone. As a result, you may experience headaches, seizures, abdominal pain or bone pain. Non-small cell lung cancer can be treated with surgery while small cell cancer is treated with chemotherapy. Sometimes, a small segment of the lung can be removed while in other cases, the whole lobe must be removed.

Colon cancer is another common cancer. The colon is the part of the body where the waste material is stored. The rectum is the end of the colon adjacent to the anus. Together, they form a long, muscular tube called the large intestine.

Tumors of the colon and rectum are growths arising from the inner wall of the large intestine. Benign tumors of the large intestine are called polyps. Malignant tumors of the large intestine are called cancers. Cancer of the colon and rectum can invade and damage adjacent tissues and organs. Cancer cells can also break away and spread into other parts of the body.

Factors that increase a person's risk of colorectal cancer include high fat intake, a family history of colorectal cancer and polyps, the presence of polyps in the large intestine, and chronic ulcerative colitis. If colon cancer is suspected, a barium enema x-ray or a colonoscopy will be indicated. Surgery is the most common treatment for cancer of the rectum and colon. If the cancer has spread a patient may also require chemotherapy. If the cancer is limited to the rectum, a patient may be treated with radiation therapy.

High incidences of small cell carcinoma and adenocarcinoma of the lung, astrocytoma and glioblastoma multiforme of the brain and mesothelioma of the lung were found in those who had a high accumulation of Asbestos in the eyes and upper respiratory system (nose, larynx, trachea, etc.).

When measured non-invasively using the Bi-Digital O-Ring Test (BDORT), brain tumors had the highest concentration of Asbestos. Relatively high levels of Asbestos were found in: squamous cell Carcinoma of the lungs & esophagus, adenocarcinoma of the larynx & breast, myelogenic leukemia, arteries of these cancers, left ventricle of failing heart, myocardial infarction, some of the narrowed arteries, varicose veins, cataracts, balding heads, hot flashes, Alzheimer's disease and autism. A small, round or ellipsoidal area, with diameter of 5 mm or less, was found near the center of every cancer tissue

Some cancers can be gender specific. For example, a female can develop cancer of your breasts, cervix, uterus, or ovary. If a patient is male, one can develop cancer of the testicles, prostate gland or breast. Cancer-related pain can be excruciating in some cases. Breast cancer is the most common malignancy in women in the United States. Approximately, 182,000 women develop breast cancer and more than 46,000 die with it. It occurs in one in eight women. Approximately, two-thirds of cases occur after menopause. Fifteen percent of cases occur before the age of 40.

Some breast cancers can affect the ducts of the breasts, whereas other types affect the lobules of the breasts. Cancer of the ducts usually occurs on one side of the body, whereas lobular cancer is bilateral. Mammography is recommended every 1 to 2 years if you are older than 40 years of age.

A pathologist will stage the cancer. Staging determines the severity of the cancer. A 0 stage cancer is confined to an area of the organ. A cancer stage greater than III usually means that the cancer has spread beyond the affected organ. The survival rate depends upon the stage of the cancer.

The stages are based upon the severity of the cancer. The higher stage correlates with a lower survival rate. If a patient has cancer in the breast that has not spread to the bones or other organs, the 5-year survival rate is greater than 95 percent. However, if the cancer has spread into other areas of the body, the 5-year survival rate is only 10 percent.

If the cancer is only in the tissue, a patient may only need removal of that part of the tissue from the breast. Despite a reduction in the number of deaths from cancers made possible by the development of early detection tests, improvements in treatment, changes in the age distribution of the population, and changes of personal behaviors as a result of awareness, breast cancer remains a major health problem worldwide.[8] Breast cancer is the most common cancer and second leading cause of cancer death in women.

Breast cancer can also occur in males. Males can have an enlargement of their breast tissue. Estrogens stimulate breast development. Androgens such as testosterone inhibit breast development. Male breast cancer is usually on one side and presents as a firm mass that appears to be fixed to the male's underlying muscle. There may even be a nipple discharge. There may also be retraction of the skin around the male breast.

With respect to female cancer, cervical cancer accounts for approximately 2 to 3 percent of all cancers involving women in the United States. More than 15,000 cases of cervical cancer are diagnosed each year, and approximately 5,000 women die from this disease.

Risk factors for developing carcinoma from the cervix include suppression of the immune system, a history of genital herpes or genital warts, multiple sexual partners, partners with penile warts or cancer, low economic status, intercourse before age 17, and cigarette smoking.

Usually cancer of the cervix is painless. A Pap smear detects many cases of cervical cancer. Cancer from the cervix can spread and can cause one to experience lower-back pain, leg pain, weight loss, or swelling in the legs. If a patient has an abnormal Pap smear, a biopsy of the cervix is necessary. If the biopsy is unable to determine whether a suspicious-looking tissue is cancerous, a patient will have a greater portion of the cervix removed, which is called a cervical conization.

As with most cancers, a pathologist will assign a numeric stage to the cancer. A high number means that the cancer has spread beyond the organ where it began. If the cancer is only confined to the cervix, the 5-year survival rate is 100 percent. If the cancer has spread throughout the pelvis and involved the bladder or rectum, the 5-year survival rate is 20 percent.

Approximately, 34,000 cases of cancer of the uterus occur each year in the United States. The incidence of this uterine tumor decreases yearly. The death rate has decreased each year since 1950. Usually this cancer will occur if a patient is a postmenopausal woman. Women who undergo menopause after age 52 are more prone to develop uterine cancer.

Obesity contributes to an increase in this type of cancer. If a patient is taking estrogen replacement and is over age 52, she has an increased risk of developing uterine cancer. As with the other cancers mentioned throughout this chapter, there are stages. Stage 0, which is the cancer in the uterus, has a 100 percent success rate. If the cancer involves the bladder or the rectum, the survival rate decreases to 20 percent.

Standard therapy for uterine cancer is an abdominal hysterectomy with removal of both ovaries. Ovarian cancer develops in 1 in every 70 women. Approximately, 1 percent of women die from this cancer. Approximately, 24,000 cases of ovarian cancer are diagnosed in the United States each year. More than 13,000 women will die with ovarian cancer each year. The incidence of cancer of the ovary is increased in women who have never been pregnant and is more prevalent in women who have had late onset of menopause or have been on a high-fat diet.

Males suffer from gender-specific tumors as well. The testes secrete testosterone and estradiol, which are two hormones. Testicular cancer represents approximately 2 percent of all cancers in men. It is the second most common cancer in men between the ages of 20 and 34 years of age. These tumors usually manifest as an enlargement of the testicle. A male with a testicular tumor can have breast enlargement. Approximately, 10 percent of these tumors will have distant spread of the cancer at the time of the diagnosis.

These tumors are staged through measurement of certain chemical markers in the bloodstream as well as imaging studies or surgery. Some of these cancers are quite sensitive to radiation therapy. Other tumors that are confined to the testes are cured through removal of the testicle followed by radiation therapy. If a cancer is localized to the testicle, the 5-year survival rate approximates 100 percent. If the cancer has spread throughout the body, the survival rate drops to 20 percent.

Most men over 55 years of age may have an enlargement of their prostate gland. Almost two thirds of these men will have symptoms of prostatism. They will have decreased force of their urine stream and retention of their urine in their bladder after they urinate. They wake up frequently at night to urinate. Over time, they may not be able to hold their urine. Prostatism is a benign entity. However, prostatism can be a symptom of cancer. Cancer symptoms may be without significant symptoms initially but as the cancer advances can become severe.

Prostate cancer is the second most common tumor in men. Lung cancer is the most common. Approximately, 200,000 new cases are diagnosed each year in the United States. Prostate cancer is more common among African Americans and men who have a family history of prostate cancer. The problem with prostate cancer is that it is usually painless and has no other symptoms that are seen with prostatism. Prostate cancer can be detected by routine digital examination or elevation of the prostate-specific antigen (PSA).

In many instances, an MRI will be done to see whether the tumor has spread to other organs. Other chemical body markers can be measured as well if cancer is suspected to be present in another organ. A bone scan may be necessary to detect a cancer that has gone to the bones. If a patient has prostate cancer, the surgeon may do a prostatectomy, radiation therapy, hormone therapy, or chemotherapy. If the tumor is confined to the prostate gland, a prostatectomy, radiation therapy and/or hormone therapy may be necessary.

If the prostate cancer has spread beyond the prostate, radiation therapy is usually the treatment of choice. If the prostate cancer has disseminated throughout the body, a patient will be treated with hormone therapy. The prostate cancer is usually testosterone sensitive. The doctor will prescribe hormone therapy that will lower the testosterone in the bloodstream. This can be done through castration.

An important association has been described between chronic obstructive pulmonary disease (COPD) and lung cancer, where different mechanisms have been proposed. There is no unique cause for this association, as COPD is by itself a heterogeneous disease, in which their classical phenotypes (i.e., emphysema and chronic bronchitis) each play an important role in lung cancer development.[9]

Clinical and molecular studies have found that lung cancers that develop in patients with COPD and/or emphysema appear to be more aggressive and have a distinct molecular profile when compared with tumors from patients without an underlying lung disease.

Chronic inflammation and oxidative damage caused by obesity, cigarette smoking, and chronic gastroesophageal reflux disease (GERD) are major risk factors associated with Barrett's esophagus and esophageal adenocarcinoma.[10] Chronic lymphocytic leukemia (CLL) is the most common leukemia in the Western world.

Shorter mean telomere length in leukemic cells has been associated with more aggressive disease. Germline polymorphisms in telomere maintenance genes affect telomere length and may contribute to CLL susceptibility.[11] A genetic predisposition to longer telomere length is associated with an increased risk of CLL, suggesting that the role of telomere length in CLL etiology may be distinct from its role in disease progression.

Several pieces of evidence indicate that a complex relationship exists between constitutional telomere length and the risk of cutaneous melanoma.[12] Although the general perception is that longer telomeres increase melanoma risk, some studies do not support this association.

The role of telomeres and telomerase in colorectal cancer is well established as the major driving force in generating chromosomal instability.[6] However, their potential as prognostic markers remains unclear. Telomerase-positive activity was identified as a marker that confers a trend toward a poor prognosis.

A shortened telomere in peripheral blood and tumor tissue might indicate poor survival for cancer patients. However, by calculating the telomere length ratios of tumor tissue to adjacent normal mucosa, the lower ratio might indicate better survival.[13]

There is no reason why cancer pain cannot be controlled. There are multiple modalities now available to adequately control cancer pain. One of the most feared consequences of cancer is pain. To treat the pain appropriately, a multidisciplinary approach may be necessary. Almost 90 percent of psychiatric disorders noted in cancer patients are a reaction against the disease itself or treatments used to cure the cancer. An extremely painful disease is the most feared effect associated with cancer. Approximately 15 percent of cancer patients whose cancer has not spread develop significant pain. If the disease is advanced, 60 to 90 percent of patients report significant pain. Unfortunately, 25 percent of all cancer patients die while still experiencing considerable pain.

As a tumor grows it can compress nerves in areas of the body, which can cause pain. Most of the pain can respond to narcotic drugs. If the pain is in the central nervous system, or if it affects some of the nerves outside of the brain and spinal cord, a patient has neuropathic pain. Neuropathic pain causes symptoms that are sharp and electrical shock like. This type of pain can be controlled by anti-seizure medications such as Neurontin or Lyrica. A patient can have pain that is severe and excessive for the extent of tissue damage that has occurred. This type of pain is called idiopathic and usually has a psychological pathology associated with it.

Anticonvulsant medications can relieve severe lancinating pain when the tumor affects a nerve. In the United States, about 5 percent of all anticonvulsant medications are prescribed for pain management. Nerve injury caused by cancer, chemotherapy, or radiation therapy is controlled with anticonvulsant medications. Nonsteroidal anti-inflammatory medications may relieve bone pain related to a cancer.

Narcotics can relieve cancer pain. Morphine is the standard of comparison for the rest of the narcotic analgesics. A sustained-release preparation is available called MS Contin releases the drug over 8 to 12 hours.

OxyContin also provides a release of oxycodone over 8-12 hours. There is also a drug that a patient can take once a day that will give a sustained release over 24 hours called Kadian.

Dilaudid is stronger than morphine, but it has a shorter duration of action than morphine. Methadone is another drug that can be prescribed for cancer pain. It is very effective when given in a pill form. Another drug more potent than morphine is Levo-Dromoran. It is stronger than morphine and can last up to 16 hours per dose.

Opana, a long-acting oxymorphone is also available. Fentanyl is a potent drug that is more potent than the drugs mentioned. A transdermal fentanyl patch gives a patient a continuous dose of morphine. There is also an oral fentanyl lozenge that is available for treatment of breakthrough pain. Breakthrough pain means additional pain, which can occur when your activities increase.

Demerol (meperidine) is another drug that is available for pain management. It is not recommended for chronic pain because the break-down products of this drug can cause seizures and also because of its relatively short duration of pain-relieving action, one and a half to two hours, as compared to other opioid preparations.

Another drug called Ultram (tramadol) is a weak narcotic-binding receptor drug that can decrease the pain. It also inhibits the reuptake of norepinephrine and serotonin, which are two chemicals that exist in the central nervous system that can also decrease the pain.

Clonidine (Catapress) may help control some cancer pains. The FDA has approved clonidine for epidural use. The epidural space is the spinal fluid that surrounds the spinal cord. Clonidine administered into the epidural space can control some pains that are caused by the cancer. Narcotic medications can be placed into the epidural space or actually even placed into the fluid that surrounds the spinal cord through an implanted pump.

A snail toxin called Prialt can also be placed in a spinal pump to control the pain. This pump deposits the drug in the spinal fluid. Other routes of drug administration are the oral routes, but you do not have to swallow a pill.

Sublingual (under the tongue) morphine when it is in a high concentration (Roxanol 20 mg/ml) can provide pain relief. Actiq is a fentanyl preparation on a stick that resembles a lollipop. Actiq works quickly to provide pain relief. An adhesive oral fentanyl disc is available which can control pain as well. Rectal suppositories are another way of providing a patient with narcotic medications. Rectal suppositories are available for hydromorphone, oxymorphone, and morphine. The rectal administration of morphine, for example, can provide pain relief within 10 minutes.

Cancer cannot always be successfully treated. Remember however, that cancer pain can be successfully treated. In order to do so, a timely and accurate diagnosis must be done. This is one of many reasons why an individual should have a routine yearly physical examination.

References

1. Kumar M, Lechel A, Gunes C. Telomerase: The Devil Inside. Genes (Basel). 2016;7(8).
2. Barczak W, Rozwadowska N, Romaniuk A, et al. Telomere length assessment in leukocytes presents potential diagnostic value in patients with breast cancer. Oncol Lett. 2016;11(3):2305-2309.
3. Ait-Aissa K, Ebben JD, Kadlec AO, Beyer AM. Friend or foe? Telomerase as a pharmacological target in cancer and cardiovascular disease. Pharmacol Res. 2016;111:422-433.
4. Tahara T, Shibata T, Kawamura T, et al. Telomere length shortening in gastric mucosa is a field effect associated with increased risk of gastric cancer. Virchows Arch. 2016;469(1):19-24.
5. Ceja-Rangel HA, Sanchez-Suarez P, Castellanos-Juarez E, et al. Shorter telomeres and high telomerase activity correlate with a highly aggressive phenotype in breast cancer cell lines. Tumour Biol. 2016.
6. Fernandez-Marcelo T, Sanchez-Pernaute A, Pascua I, et al. Clinical Relevance of Telomere Status and Telomerase Activity in Colorectal Cancer. PLoS One. 2016;11(2):e0149626.
7. Omura Y. Asbestos as a possible major cause of malignant lung tumors (including small cell carcinoma, adenocarcinoma & mesothelioma), brain tumors (i.e. astrocytoma & glioblastoma multiforme), many other malignant tumors, intractable pain including fibromyalgia, & some cardiovascular pathology: Safe & effective methods of reducing asbestos from normal & pathological areas. Acupunct Electrother Res. 2006;31(1-2):61-125.
8. Oztas E, Kara H, Kara ZP, Aydogan MU, Uras C, Ozhan G. Association Between Human Telomerase Reverse Transcriptase Gene Variations and Risk of Developing Breast Cancer. Genet Test Mol Biomarkers. 2016.
9. Sanchez-Salcedo P, Zulueta JJ. Lung cancer in chronic obstructive pulmonary disease patients, it is not just the cigarette smoke. Curr Opin Pulm Med. 2016;22(4):344-349.

10. Wennerstrom EC, Risques RA, Prunkard D, et al. Leukocyte telomere length in relation to the risk of Barrett's esophagus and esophageal adenocarcinoma. Cancer Med. 2016.

11. Ojha J, Codd V, Nelson CP, et al. Genetic Variation Associated with Longer Telomere Length Increases Risk of Chronic Lymphocytic Leukemia. Cancer Epidemiol Biomarkers Prev. 2016;25(7):1043-1049.

12. Menin C, Bojnik E, Del Bianco P, et al. Differences in telomere length between sporadic and familial cutaneous melanoma. Br J Dermatol. 2016.

13. Xu Y, Goldkorn A. Telomere and Telomerase Therapeutics in Cancer. Genes (Basel). 2016;7(6).

31. Chest pain

Aging is commonly defined as the accumulation of diverse deleterious changes occurring in cells and tissues with advancing age that are responsible for the increased risk of disease and death. Chest pain in both elderly men and women can be serious. Even though minor medical conditions can cause chest pain, a heart attack, it can be potentially fatal. Cardiovascular disease is the primary cause of chest pain in the elderly population. Epidemiology and genetic studies indicate that patients with telomere length shorter than average are at higher risk of dying from heart disease or stroke.[1]

Around 12 percent of women and 20 percent of men over 65 years of age suffer from ischemic heart disease. Chest pain may also be caused by the following factors: reflux esophagitis, pulmonary embolism, cancer, pleurisy, fractured ribs, or shingles. In addition, telomere shortening has been demonstrated in patients with coronary heart disease, premature myocardial infarction, hypertension and diabetes mellitus.[2] Telomere shortening is a feature of cellular ageing common to a range of human tissues. Shorter telomeres are associated with an increased likelihood of mortality.

The chest houses several organs, such as the lungs, heart, and esophagus, and any pain left in the chest should never be taken lightly in elderly patients. Right sided chest pain usually does not have a cardiac reason associated with it, but it should not be neglected. Many common viral infections, like the cold or flu, can result in pain on the right side of the chest. Gallbladder problems and inflammation of the liver can also cause right sided chest pain. Telomerase reverse transcriptase maintains telomere ends during DNA replication by catalyzing the addition of short telomere repeats.

The expression of telomerase is normally repressed in somatic cells leading to a gradual shortening of telomeres and cellular senescence with aging.3 Telomeres are noncoding functional DNA repeat sequences at the ends of chromosomes that decrease in length by a predictable amount at each cell division. When the telomeres become critically short, the cell is no longer able to replicate and enters cellular senescence.

The chest region comprises of the ribs, the cartilages, the chest muscles, lungs, pleura or the covering membranes of the lung, heart as well as the covering of the heart or the pericardium. Any one of these structures can give rise to pain. This is apparently a painful condition pertaining to the joint between the ribs and the relevant cartilage. The condition can arise suddenly and will be an intensely painful event which can be misinterpreted as a heart-related condition. Lung inflammation (pleuritic pain) which originates from the pleura of the lungs may cause intense pain that can be felt in taking a deep breath.

If the heart muscles do not obtain enough oxygen, some of the heart muscle can become injured, and even some of the muscle can die. This can lead to some dysfunction in the remainder of the muscle that is trying to pump blood out of the heart to the rest of the body. The injured muscle can't pump blood efficiently if at all. The patient can subsequently develop angina or a myocardial infarction.

Angina is common in people over the age of 60. Angina pectoris occurs when myocardial oxygen demand exceeds myocardial oxygen supply. Usually angina is relieved by rest. Ageing is associated with changes at the molecular and cellular level that can alter cardiovascular function and ultimately lead to disease.[4]

Angina chest pain in men may spread to the jaws and arms. Numbness and pain radiating from the chest into the left arm is especially characteristic of angina pain in men. In women with a decrease in oxygen to the heart muscle for some reason, symptoms of angina pain include pressure in the center of the chest accompanied by pain in the neck or arms. Angina or heart pain occurs when the demand for blood by the heart exceeds the supply of the arteries. Biological age may be distinct from chronological age and contribute to the pathogenesis of age-related diseases.

Mean telomeres lengths provide an assessment of biological age with shorter telomeres, indicating increased biological age. Biological age may play a role in the etiology of coronary heart disease and have potentially important implications for our understanding of its genetic etiology, pathogenesis, and variable age of onset.[5]

A myocardial infarction (heart attack) or death of a segment of the heart muscle occurs following an interruption of the blood supply to the heart muscle. A heart attack can cause sudden severe chest pain. There is a danger that the heart could go into an irregular heartbeat called an arrhythmia. If one has a severe arrhythmia, the heart can stop, which is referred to as a cardiac arrest. If a patient has an interruption of the blood flow going to the heart, he/she can have an irreversible injury to the heart muscle. This injury usually begins within 20 minutes from the time of the loss of blood flow to the heart muscle.

The extent of the heart muscle injury is related to the amount of obstruction that the arteries have in the heart vessels. It is also related to the length of time that the heart muscle is without blood flow. The will probably have other vessels in the heart that supply the heart muscle. This is collateral circulation. This collateral circulation can get some blood flow to the muscle that is without blood flow. When the heart muscle is without oxygen and when the heart muscle dies, the electrical conduction of impulses through the muscle is decreased or stopped. This is the mechanism by which the heart develops abnormal heart beats. Telomerase activation could be a therapeutic strategy to prevent heart failure after a heart attack.[6]

Together, the limited capacity for regenerative growth in cardiac muscle after injury and the prevalence of ongoing sporadic cell death due to apoptosis in chronic heart failure states pose one of the paramount challenges in heart failure therapeutics. In adults, the unique self-renewal potential of progenitor/stem cells is associated with telomerase reverse transcriptase, an RNA-dependent DNA polymerase that maintains the lariat-like loop capping chromosome ends. Researchers have identified telomere uncapping, mediated by down-regulation of telomere repeat-binding factor 2 (TRF2) as a novel trigger of cell death in human dilated cardiomyopathy.[7]

Angina pectoris is chest pain that results from decreased oxygen from the heart muscle. Angina pectoris is usually pain under the breastbone. The may perceive discomfort instead of pain or pressure. The pain, if it is present or the pressure sensation can radiate to the neck or arm, which is usually the left arm. Shortness of breath may also be reported. Angina pectoris is usually elicited by physical exertion. Occasionally psychological stress can cause the patient to have angina pectoris. The stress can cause the heart rate to increase, which increases the oxygen demand. The importance of cardiorespiratory fitness and exercise training in the prevention of biological aging is important.[8] Moderate amounts of exercise training protects against biological aging, while higher amounts may not elicit additional benefits.

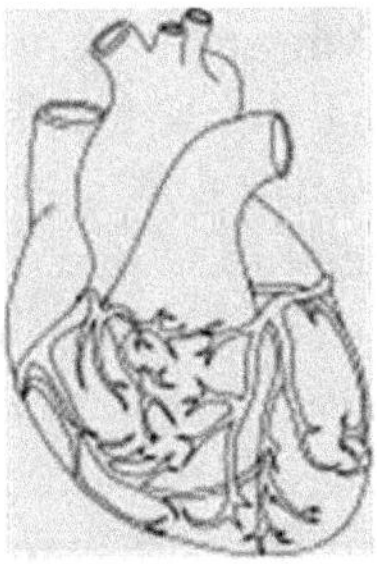

Figure 1. If an artery that supplies blood and oxygen to the heart muscle becomes occluded, the patient may experience chest (anginal) pain and/or have a heart attack (myocardial infarction).

Coronary heart disease is usually related to atherosclerosis, which can occur in the heart arteries as well as other arteries throughout the body. Atherosclerosis is a build-up of fat and other materials in the walls of arteries that cause them to become narrowed. This entity is caused by many factors. If he is hypertensive and has an elevated cholesterol and smoke, he is at a higher risk for developing atherosclerosis. If he is obese and has a sedentary lifestyle, the risk for atherosclerosis is increased. If a patient is over 60, is a male, and has a family history of coronary artery disease, he is prone to develop this disease.

At first, a patient will develop a buildup of a type of "bad" cholesterol called low-density lipoproteins (LDL) in the walls of the blood vessels about the heart. These low-density lipoproteins eventually can calcify. This calcification will narrow the lumen, or diameter of the blood vessels, causing a decrease in the amount of blood that can pass through them. This is similar to calcium building up in the plumbing in the residence.

If the repetitively deposit calcium in the pipes, eventually the pipes will close off. The same analogy is true for the blood vessels in the heart. When tone has a deposit of calcium in the blood vessels, the heart will still pump blood through these vessels. It takes a decrease in the diameter of the blood vessels by approximately 70 percent to decrease the blood flow.

Many diverse factors lead to the progression of atherosclerosis. Increasing age and a family history of coronary artery disease may predispose a patient to develop this entity. The male sex is an important risk factor for developing coronary artery disease and for having a heart attack, but coronary heart disease is also the leading cause of death in women over 50 years of age.

Women will generally have their symptoms approximately 10 years later than men. The risk of coronary artery disease increases with the use of birth control pills and with the onset of menopause. However, the risk of coronary artery disease could be increased with hormone therapy following the onset of menopause.

If a patient has an elevated blood pressure, a patient is also at risk for developing coronary artery disease. In fact, hypertension is a major risk factor for developing this disease. If a patient has a family history of hypertension or if a patient is beginning to have an increase in the blood pressure, a patient may need to change his/her lifestyle. A patient will need to stop smoking.

If a patient is obese, he/she will need to decrease his/her weight. Sodium restriction is important for a patient control of a patient hypertension, which can ultimately decrease coronary artery disease. Aerobic exercise is also necessary to decrease a patient risk for developing coronary heart disease. Exercise is extremely important if a patient have risk factors for developing coronary artery disease.

Smoking is another patient factor that can cause one to be at a high risk for developing coronary artery disease.

A patient should be aware that the cholesterol level must not be alowed to become elevated because it can increase the risk of developing coronary artery disease. If a patient has a high level of low-density lipoprotein cholesterol, the have an elevated chance of developing coronary heart disease. Plaques (deposits of fat and calcium in the blood vessels) are usually the most common causes of obstruction to blood flow in the arteries about the heart, but other factors can also cause obstruction of blood flow in the heart. Vegetations, small growths that can develop on the valves in the heart from infections, can extend up to the coronary arteries and cause them to become blocked.

Diseases such as rheumatoid arthritis can affect the caliber of the coronary arteries as well. A patient must be aware that if he/she has had or needs radiation therapy for cancer treatment, that radiation therapy can cause one to have coronary artery disease. Cocaine use has become more and more prevalent in the United States. However, cocaine use can make the arteries in the heart to go into spasm. Cocaine can accelerate the deposition of fat and calcium in the blood vessels, which can cause a patient to have angina as well as a heart attack.

Sometimes a decrease in the blood flow in the arteries about the heart can lead to decreased blood flow to the heart muscle tissue, and a decrease in oxygen to the heart will cause a possible injury to the heart muscle. The heart muscle is dependent upon a balance of oxygen supply as well as demand. At rest, the heart should receive adequate oxygen, or a patient may complain of chest pain. However, if a patient runs a mile or runs up steps, the oxygen demand to the heart muscle is increased. The blood vessels that deliver the blood carrying oxygen to the heart must provide the heart muscle with an adequate blood flow.

If the blood vessels are narrowed, the heart cannot get enough blood carrying oxygen to the heart muscle. As a result, some of the heart muscle could become injured and die. This is what happens to the heart muscle when a patient suffers a myocardial infarction.

A patient will usually develop chest pain when the heart oxygen demand exceeds the supply of oxygen that the blood vessels are supplying to the heart. Usually if the heart begins beating faster, the increase in oxygen demand is met by an increased blood flow in the arteries about the heart.

The small arteries around the heart muscle will increase their diameter to provide the heart with more oxygenated blood. If the vessels cannot dilate, the heart will not receive enough oxygen, and the will experience pain in the chest. Fat and calcium within the heart vessels will restrict the amount of blood that goes to the heart.

Men may have chest pain with radiation of pain to their left arms. A recent study of women finds that fatigue, and sleeplessness are accurate predictors of an impending heart attack. Exhaustion, sleep deprivation, and nausea were frequently seen in women who were having impending heart attacks. Fatigue and sleeplessness are warning signs for heart attacks in women.

It is thought that this research will alter the way doctors diagnose and treat women who are likely to suffer heart attacks. The appearance of fatigue and sleeplessness in addition to nausea and vomiting in addition to women's heart-attack risk factors should alert the doctor that a woman needs to be thoroughly examined for the possibility of a heart attack. Furthermore, women should not ignore these warnings.

Think Symptoms is a National Institute of Nursing Research funded study investigating symptoms suggestive of acute coronary syndrome (heart attack or unstable angina) in women and men. Many women who had heart attacks did not have any chest pain during their heart attacks. However, more than 70 percent of the women who had heart attacks reported feeling unusual fatigue. These new findings differ from the previous findings that chest pain was the most important symptom for identifying heart attacks in both men and women. Other, previously discounted symptoms such as fatigue, sleeplessness, nausea, anxiety, and shortness of breath are important signs of heart disease as well.

Forty eight percent of women report sleeplessness, whereas 42 percent reported shortness of breath. Thirty-five percent of women in the study complained of anxiety. These symptoms interfered with the daily activities of the women in the study. The study was sponsored by the National Institute of Nursing Research. It involved 515 women. The women in the study were mostly Caucasian. These women were diagnosed with a heart attack within the previous six months prior to entering the study.

Women, however, should look beyond the results of this study and look at other risk factors such as whether they smoke, are overweight, or have high-cholesterol levels. Furthermore, diabetes and a family history of heart disease can make them prone to heart attacks as well. The results of this study are important because numerous studies have shown that men, on the other hand, experience chest pains before a heart attack. There are physiologic differences between men and women who may account for these differences in symptoms associated with a heart attack.

Hormones are different for men and women, and women have smaller arteries that supply their heart muscles. These physiologic differences may account for the differences in heart attack symptoms. The need to realize that heart disease is the number-one killer of women as well as men in the United States. When a woman has a heart attack, she is more likely to die than men. They are also more probable to have a repeat heart attack within a year as opposed to men. According to the American Heart Association, approximately 6.3 million men and 6.6 million women have histories of heart attacks. In the year 2000, more than 500,000 people died from heart disease.

Different types of angina have been described that can occur in both men and women. Stable angina is angina that is chronic and is usually caused by physical activity or emotional stress. Stable angina is usually heart-related pain relieved by rest or nitroglycerin. Unstable angina, on the other hand, can increase with rest.

Other types of unstable angina can occur at low activity levels. Unstable angina may not be responsive to nitroglycerin. Sometimes the can develop spasms of the arteries that supply the heart muscle. This type of spasm is called Pinzmetal's angina and can be relieved frequently with nitroglycerin.

Stable angina is a term used to describe pain that is predictably caused by narrowing of coronary arteries and a given stress to the heart. On the other hand, unstable angina describes a new pattern of pain not previously experienced, for example, pain previously felt after a flight of stairs is now suddenly experienced at rest. Unstable angina is a medical emergency that should be immediately evaluated by a doctor.

Pain that remains in one area and is not referred to other areas and is stabbing and fleeting is usually not angina pectoris. The heart rate and blood pressure can be normal, although heart pain will often cause an increase in heart rate and blood pressure. A striking variability exists in the susceptibility, age of onset and pace of progression of cardiovascular diseases. This is inadequately explained by the presence or absence of conventional risk factors. Differences in biological aging might provide an additional component of the observed variability.[9] Telomere length provides a potential marker of an individual's biological age; shorter telomeres reflect a more advanced biological age.

Telomere length at birth is mainly determined by genetic factors. Telomere attrition occurs as a consequence of cellular replication and can be accelerated by harmful environmental factors such as oxidative stress. When telomeres reach a critical threshold the cell will enter senescence and becomes dysfunctional.

Telomeres are remarkably shorter in patients with aging associated diseases, including coronary artery disease and chronic heart failure. In addition, numerous conventional cardiovascular risk factors are associated with shorter telomere length. The rate of progression of cellular ageing in late midlife relates to vascular damage, independently from contribution of cardiovascular risk factor exposure.[10]

If the patient has heart muscle damage, the injured tissue will release chemicals. If these heart isoenzymes are increased, this may be a sign that the patient is having a heart attack. If the patient has a history of risk factors for coronary artery disease and if the symptoms are stable, the doctor may do a pharmacologic stress test.

A dobutamine echocardiogram study may be done. The patient will be given a drug that will increase the heart rate. The will be monitored with a continuous EKG to see if there are any changes on the EKG that suggest decreased perfusion to the heart muscles. Occasionally, the cardiologist may want to do a coronary angiogram, which is a test that uses a dye to assess the extent of the coronary artery disease.

A chest pain syndrome that may be more prevalent in women is an entity called syndrome X. this syndrome, the may be an exaggerated response of the small arteries that go to the heart muscles. This excessive response is constriction of the diameter of the arteries. When this happens, there is decreased blood flow going to the heart.

Painless myocardial infarctions can occur in both sexes. These painless myocardial infarctions are usually discovered on routine EKGs. Women have significantly greater back and jaw pain as well as nausea and vomiting than men when they present with symptoms of an acute coronary syndromes. If they have these symptoms, the may be having a heart attack, and the must seek medical attention immediately. Men have more chest pain as well as sweating when they are having a heart attack. Essentially men and women can experience the same symptoms, but the proportions of the symptoms are more prevalent in women than men.

The prevalence of the cardiac syndrome X is higher in women when compared to men. Estrogen deficiency has been shown to play a major role in the origin of cardiac syndrome X. Estrogen has properties on blood vessels that can increase the diameter of the blood vessels. The results of this study demonstrate that the blood vessels in the heart can be modified by sex hormones. A further study reveals that an estrogen deficiency contributes to the development of angina and that in women, this angina can be treated with estrogen supplements.

Men are more likely to be hospitalized for unstable angina than women. In the year 2000, one study by cardiologists in one area reported thee were approximately 30,000 hospitalizations for men and approximately 16,000 hospitalizations for women of a similar age. The reason for this data is being examined. Research has demonstrated a smaller proportion of women who suffer from angina have coronary artery disease than men who have angina.

Research continues to demonstrate that heart disease, which has not always been considered a serious problem for women, is now a serious problem for women. With more women smoking today, the incidence of heart disease has risen. Approximately, 240,000 women in the United States die from heart disease each year. Heart disease is the second-leading killer of women under age 55. Cancer is the primary reason why women die. However, by age 55 heart disease causes more deaths in women than cancer.

Studies have shown that if women control their weight and work with their doctor to control their blood pressure and modify their lifestyles, they can minimize the risk of heart disease and minimize the risk of having a heart attack. The problem in this country is that obesity is increasing and is near epidemic. Almost 50 percent of adults in the United States are overweight. These findings suggest that more individuals will develop high blood pressure, and eventually more individuals will develop coronary artery disease, and one can expect that there will be more deaths related to myocardial infarction.

Women have not been included in research studies done on the heart until recently. The reason for this was that most premature heart attacks occurred in men before age 55. Women who develop heart disease at older ages were not included in the studies. Furthermore, researchers eliminated women in their earlier studies because it was thought that women's hormones could alter the results of the studies on the incidence of heart attacks and deaths. The good news is that there have been inclusions of women in studies of coronary artery disease following the institution of the Women's Health Initiative about 10 years ago.

Hormone-replacement therapy may be useful for the prevention of heart disease. It is known that estrogen does affect the caliber of the arteries that go to the heart and also affects the muscles in the walls of the arteries. If the blood clots too readily, the can have a stoppage of the blood flow in the coronary arteries.

The estrogen hormone may have an effect on the body's ability to form clots. Estrogen therapy can be associated with a stroke, and the risks of this therapy must be discussed with the physician. Aspirin can affect the body's ability to clot and if a patient is having angina, or if the patient suspects he/she is having a heart attack, aspirin can be lifesaving. Current studies are being done examining the effects of nutrients for the prevention of heart disease.

Angina is treated by controlling the risk factors. This includes decreasing the blood pressure if the patients are hypertensive. It also means that the patients should stop smoking cigarettes. If the cholesterol is elevated, he/she should reduce the cholesterol and take any cholesterol-lowering drugs that a doctor may prescribe and strive to exercise and reduce the fat in the diet.

All treatments for coronary heart disease have the same goals: to improve quality of life and relieve symptoms, particularly angina. The medicines used to treat coronary heart disease and angina reduces the risk of dying for many people with these conditions. Nitroglycerin is a commonly prescribed drug for the treatment of angina. Nitroglycerin will relieve the angina pain by making the blood vessels going to the heart wider. The increased blood flow will permit more oxygen to go to the heart. This increased oxygen will keep up with the demand of the heart.

If medication fails to control the angina, coronary artery bypass surgery is sometimes necessary. A blood vessel is grafted onto the blocked artery. This allows the blood flow to bypass the blockage so that blood can go to the heart muscle to provide the heart muscle with needed oxygen. The surgeon can use an artery inside the chest or take a vein from the leg.

Another treatment that can be used to increase the artery size is called balloon angioplasty. This involves insertion of a catheter that has a tiny balloon on the end of it into an artery either in the arm or the leg. The balloon is inflated briefly to widen the vessel in places where the arteries are narrow. Additionally, a coronary stent can be used. Stents are implanted through the veins with a catheter. A coronary stent is a stainless tube with slots. It is mounted on a balloon catheter in a collapsed state. When the balloon is inflated, the stent expands or opens up and pushes itself against the inner wall of the coronary artery. This holds the artery open when the balloon is deflated and removed. Elderly patients who undergo coronary artery stenting have significantly higher rates of procedural complications and worse six-month outcomes than younger patients.

Over 1 million new and repeat cases of heart attack occur each year. Approximately, 44 percent of these patients die. Almost 13 million individuals who have angina or a heart attack are still living. The number of men and women living are nearly equal. Since 1990, the death rate from coronary artery disease has actually decreased.

More than 6 million people in the United States suffer from angina. Another study revealed that 400,000 new cases of stable angina occur each year. The incidence of angina is greater in women than men. Furthermore, the incidence of angina in women over age 20 was highest in African-American women followed by Mexican American followed by Caucasian women. The same is true for racial differences in men.

Smoking increases the risk of coronary artery disease. If a patient is obese, he/she should make dietary changes to decrease the cholesterol and weight. Nitroglycerin and other vasodilator medications will make the blood vessels going to the heart larger, therefore, increasing the amount of oxygen that the heart receives. If the heart rate is too fast, beta blockers, such as propranolol, may slow the heart rate and decrease the contraction of the heart muscle to help conserve oxygen.

Calcium-channel blockers, such as Verapamil, may be necessary to decrease the incidence of having angina or heart attack. Exercise regimens may be necessary to strengthen the heart muscles. Surgical interventions such as coronary artery bypass surgery, balloon angioplasty and stent placement may be needed to improve blood flow to the heart if medications are not successfully treating the condition.

The understanding of cardiovascular aging and telomere biology may open up new avenues for interventions, such as stem cell therapy or agents that could retard this aging process over and beyond conventional risk factor control.[11] Together, the limited capacity for regenerative growth in cardiac muscle after injury and the prevalence of ongoing sporadic cell death due to apoptosis in chronic heart failure states pose one of the paramount challenges in heart failure therapeutics.[7] Cell DNA research may eventually change this process. Telomere shortening in peripheral blood leukocytes is a promising index of ischemic heart disease risk in older people and deserves further investigation as a potential mechanism.[12]

References

1. Zhang B, Chen L, Swartz KR, et al. Deficiency of telomerase activity aggravates the blood-brain barrier disruption and neuroinflammatory responses in a model of experimental stroke. J Neurosci Res. 2010;88(13):2859-2868.

2. Balasubramanyam M, Adaikalakoteswari A, Monickaraj SF, Mohan V. Telomere shortening & metabolic/vascular diseases. Indian J Med Res. 2007;125(3):441-450.

3. Bressler J, Franceschini N, Demerath EW, Mosley TH, Folsom AR, Boerwinkle E. Sequence variation in telomerase reverse transcriptase (TERT) as a determinant of risk of cardiovascular disease: the Atherosclerosis Risk in Communities (ARIC) study. BMC Med Genet. 2015;16:52.

4. Yeung KR, Chiu CL, Pears S, et al. A Cross-Sectional Study of Ageing and Cardiovascular Function over the Baboon Lifespan. PLoS One. 2016;11(7):e0159576.

5. Brouilette S, Singh RK, Thompson JR, Goodall AH, Samani NJ. White cell telomere length and risk of premature myocardial infarction. Arterioscler Thromb Vasc Biol. 2003;23(5):842-846.

6. Bar C, Bernardes de Jesus B, Serrano R, et al. Telomerase expression confers cardioprotection in the adult mouse heart after acute myocardial infarction. Nat Commun. 2014;5:5863.

7. Schneider MD. Dual roles of telomerase in cardiac protection and repair. Novartis Found Symp. 2006;274:260-267; discussion 267-276.

8. Denham J, O'Brien BJ, Prestes PR, Brown NJ, Charchar FJ. Increased expression of telomere-regulating genes in endurance athletes with long leukocyte telomeres. J Appl Physiol (1985). 2016;120(2):148-158.

9. Huzen J, de Boer RA, van Veldhuisen DJ, van Gilst WH, van der Harst P. The emerging role of telomere biology in cardiovascular disease. Front Biosci (Landmark Ed). 2010;15:35-45.

10. Masi S, D'Aiuto F, Martin-Ruiz C, et al. Rate of telomere shortening and cardiovascular damage: a longitudinal study in the 1946 British Birth Cohort. Eur Heart J. 2014;35(46):3296-3303.

11. Nilsson PM, Tufvesson H, Leosdottir M, Melander O. Telomeres and cardiovascular disease risk: an update 2013. Transl Res. 2013;162(6):371-380.

12. Starr JM, McGurn B, Harris SE, Whalley LJ, Deary IJ, Shiels PG. Association between telomere length and heart disease in a narrow age cohort of older people. Exp Gerontol. 2007;42(6):571-573.

32. Facial neuropathy and neuralgia

Facial neuropathy and neuralgias or pathology and pain of the nerves of the face have been recognized for centuries. These types of pain, especially trigeminal neuralgia, can be severe. The pain associated with trigeminal neuralgia has been well defined. A common type of pain syndrome is pain related to temporal mandibular-lar joint disorders. This usually involves the joint between the mandible, and the maxilla. When these two bones meet, they form a joint called the temporomandibular joint.

The trigeminal nerve, which has three branches: ophthalmic, maxillary, and mandibular. Other nerves also can cause facial pain. The facial nerves, glossopharyngeal nerve, the vagus nerve, and some cervical nerves go to various parts of the mouth areas and facial areas and can cause pain. Trigeminal neuralgia affects mainly adults, especially the elderly. If the pain is coming from a nerve, typically the pain is sharp and stabbing. On the other hand, if the pain is coming from the muscles, it is generally continuous and dull. Pain from the blood vessels is usually of a throbbing nature.

Trigeminal neuralgia is also called tic douloureux. Tic douloureux is defined as a sudden stabbing pain felt in the face. It usually occurs on one side of the face. One of the nerves that supplies sensation to the face is the trigeminal nerve. This is the nerve that comes off of the brain stem. This trigeminal nerve is the cause of the trigeminal neuralgia. If the exit of the trigeminal nerve from the brain stem is depressed by a blood vessel or other tissue, this can be the cause of the pain. Compression of the trigeminal nerve with blood vessels occurs in approximately 80 percent of trigeminal neuralgia.

The trigeminal nerve provides sensation to the face, teeth, mouth and nose. Symptoms can be triggered by touching the face, brushing the teeth, feeling a breeze of air, putting on makeup, shaving, or merely touching certain parts of the face. The trigeminal nerve, has three branches:1. Ophthalmic (around the eye); 2. Maxillary (around the upper jaw); and 3. Mandibular (around the lower jaw). The pain may be limited to one or more of these branches.

Trigeminal neuralgia is one of the most common causes of facial pain with the highest incidence in individuals greater than 60 years old. 1Trigeminal neuralgia (TN) refers to sharp, lancinating pain in the areas supplied by trigeminal nerve. Both pharmacological and surgical lines of treatments are available for the treatment of TN.

Trigeminal neuralgia is a severe neuropathic pain in the distribution of one or more branches of the trigeminal nerve, which occurs in recurrent episodes, causing deterioration in quality of life, affecting everyday habits and inducing severe disability. The pain of trigeminal neuralgia comes from the trigeminal nerve. This nerve carries the feelings of touch and pain from the face, eyes, sinuses, and mouth to the brain. Trigeminal neuralgia may be part of the normal aging process. Trigeminal neuralgia may be caused by: Multiple sclerosis or pressure on the trigeminal nerve from a swollen blood vessel or tumor. Often, no cause is found.

One of the most common neuralgic pains affecting the face is the pain of TN. Although numerous lines of treatment options are available for its treatment, all these have one or the other drawbacks.[2] Trigeminal neuralgia is a serious health problem, causing brief, recurrent episodes of stabbing or burning facial pain, which patients describe as feeling like an electric shock. The consequences of living with the condition are severe.[3]

Infratentorial arteriovenous malformations (AVM) associated with the trigeminal nerve root entry zone are a known cause of secondary trigeminal neuralgia.[4] Although microvascular decompression (MVD) has become the best surgical treatment for trigeminal neuralgia, it does not achieve 100% cure rate.[5] Repeat Gamma Knife radiosurgery (GKRS) is an established option for patients whose pain has recurred after the initial procedure, with reported success rates varying from 68% to 95%.[6]

Tests that are done to look for the cause of the problem include: Blood tests MRI of the head and Trigeminal nerve reflex testing.

Local subcutaneous injection of botulinum toxin-A for TN treatment has considerable therapeutic effects lasting several months and is safe for this indication. At least one-quarter of patients in one study maintained complete analgesia.[7] The first-line treatment for the management of in adults is an antiepileptic-carbamazepine or oxcarbazepine. There is a lack of research on the use of antiepileptics in the elderly however. The use of antiepileptics raises a number of problems due to the polypharmacy therapy common in older patients. Other medicines include: gabapentin, lamotrigine, phenytoin, valproate, and pregabalin. Muscle relaxants including baclofen, or clonazepam may be beneficial. Tricyclic antidepressants (amitriptyline, nortriptyline, or carbamazepine) may also be beneficial.

The three primary surgical options for the treatment of trigeminal neuralgia are: Trigeminal Glycerol Rhizolysis (TGR). Microvascular Decompression (MVD) and Gamma Knife (GK) treatment. With Trigeminal Glycerol Rhizolysis, a needle is advanced under X ray until it reaches a small pocket of fluid surrounding the trigeminal nerve. Glycerol will destroy the nerve which will eliminate or decrease the pain. TGR is the preferred surgical approach for elderly patients with some medical issues who are in such extreme distress that they need urgent and immediate relief.

With microvascular decompression, a small incision will be made behind the ear on the same side as the trigeminal neuralgia pain. The surgeon will expose the trigeminal nerve. Once the nerve is exposed a careful inspection is done for vascular compression of the nerve (the nerve is compressed by the blood vessel). After detecting the vascular compression, the surgeon will elevate the blood vessel off of the nerve and place pledgelets of Teflon under the nerve. Gamma Knife treatment itself is silent, completely painless and lasts roughly 30 minutes. In the majority of patients take six to eight weeks to notice major improvement in the trigeminal neuralgia pain.

Micro vascular decompression continues to be the procedure of choice for the treatment of trigeminal neuralgia in patients reluctant to medical treatment, including elderly patients because age is not a contraindication.[1] The incidence of trigeminal neuralgia in elderly patients is high. However, for those with poor fitness, the optimal surgical treatment for those refractory to medical treatment is controversial. CT-guided percutaneous radiofrequency thermocoagulation is safe and effective for classic TN patients 70 years or older, including poor-fitness patients.[8]

Trigeminal neuralgia related to multiple sclerosis (MS) is more difficult to manage pharmacologically and surgically. Gamma Knife surgery has been proved safe and effective in this special group of patients.[9] A high percentage of patients that are surgically treated for trigeminal neuralgia consult their dentist first and receive possibly unjustified dental treatment. Differential diagnoses include odontogenic pain syndromes as well as atypical orofacial pain.[10]

TN is one of the most common causes of facial pain. A higher prevalence of psychiatric co-morbidities, especially depressive disorder, has been proven in patients with TN might increase the risk of subsequent newly diagnosed depressive disorder, anxiety disorder, and sleep disorder, but not schizophrenia or bipolar disorder.[11]

Carotidynia is a form of vascular neck and face pain in which the vascular change occurs in the carotid artery in the neck. The disorder is not uncommon, and most patients have a prior history of migraine. They present with pain in the neck and face, and are often thought to have a disorder such as chronic sinusitis or trigeminal neuralgia. The diagnosis can be made from the type and location of the pain and the finding of a tender and swollen carotid artery on the same side.[12]

If a patient has a history of arthritis, he/she can have joint problems within the temporal mandibular joint (TMJ). This pain is caused by dislocations of the small discs within the TMJ. This can result in inflammation as well as dysfunction of the joint and cause persistent and chronic inflammation, which in turn will cause chronic pain.

TMJ not only manifests itself as pain and discomfort but defines the conditions that have developed in seniors that leads up to being dizzy or having vertigo. Aging causes a lack of normal motion in the bones of the skull. The bones in the skull are not rigid.

Two of the bones, the temporals, affect balance. When these bones lose motion ability, it can affect the balance. This happens as one ages and wears the teeth down. The lower jaw shifts due to this wear and many seniors end up with this as a contributing factor to some component of dizziness.

Muscles involved in chewing can refer pain to the sides of the head. Sometimes heat and muscle relaxants can relieve some of the pain. The TMJ muscle pain can originate from psychological causes. Stress, which can cause a patient to grind the teeth, leading to dental irritation, can cause the muscles to become overactive. This can cause the muscles about the jaw to become spasmodic and can fatigue easily.

Temporomandibular joint disease (TMJ), is a complex health condition that affects the mandible, or jaw bone, of anyone at any age. For older adults, especially those who are at-risk for developing arthritis, the onset of TMJ is a risk that can often lead to secondary health complications. TMJ disorders occur in 12 percent of individuals in the United States. The actual cause of TMJ remains unknown. One's facial pain may have led to changes, which may affect an older patient's nutrition.

Unlike traditional types of arthritis, where physical therapy and medications are effective, TMJ often does not respond to medications and, instead, requires more aggressive forms of treatment. For many elderly adults who have TMJ, there is a need for facial massages, home warm compresses, and even the use of steroid blocks in the neck and face to alleviate facial pain. Without proper treatment of the TMJ arthritis, older adults have a greater tendency to fall into a process of not eating and, ultimately, this can lead to malnutrition.

If a patient has an abnormal mouth bite, a patient can develop pain in the TMJ joint. When the teeth are properly aligned, especially during chewing, the muscles will be of a normal tone. If a patient has an abnormal bite, the muscles around the jaw can develop areas of spasm. Sometimes the muscles that are involved in chewing fail to relax. This muscle behavior causes a patient to have myofascial trigger points in the muscles involved with chewing. Not only will a patient have pain in the muscles and the TMJ; a patient also will eventually have TMJ dysfunction. The dental specialist can make a special orthotic device for a patient that can be placed intermittently, which will allow the jaw muscles to relax. This modality will ultimately decrease the myofascial trigger points.

If a patient has TMJ, a patient can have ringing in the ears and hearing loss as well as pain around the ear. Heat and massage as well as analgesic medications can reduce the TMJ pain. The nervous habits can result in TMJ pain as well. There have been reports of TMJ pain related to individuals holding their telephone on their shoulder for hours at a time. These maneuvers compress some of the muscles, leading to myofascial pain and trigger points. It has been shown that women are more prone to TMJ than men.

The discs in the joints can displace or wear out and cause a patient TMJ pain. This is called intra-articular TMJ pain. If the disc is displaced forward, a patient may develop clicking, popping noises when a patient open and close the mouth. A patient can also have pain as well as the limitation of the jaw movement. Over time, a patient will develop wear-and-tear changes, leading to osteoarthritis of the joint. The capsule around the TMJ can become inflamed as well as deranged.

In the central nervous system, there are areas that exist in the spinal cord and the brain that inhibit painful impulses from reaching the pain center in the brain. It is possible that TMJ may be associated with impairment in the inhibitory system. This allows pain impulses from the jaw to reach the brain without being filtered or decreased in intensity.

If a patient has a decrease in the inhibition in the spinal cord, a patient will have exaggerated responses to both painful stimuli and psychological stimuli. For some reason, increased pain sensitivity throughout the body is more prevalent in patients with TMJ. The enhanced pain sensitivity noted among patients with TMJ was done in a clinical laboratory setting.

TMJ patients in general have a lower pain threshold than normal subjects for an unknown reason. TMJ patients in general can have more physical and psychological symptoms of stress. TMJ individuals report greater stress than healthy individuals. This finding is important because stress can cause a patient to clench the teeth. This clenching of teeth can affect the muscles for chewing as well as the TMJ joint.

Both fatigue as well as psychological distress can increase the pain. As time progresses, the pain will become constant. X-rays can identify changes in the TMJ space. Traumatic injuries can also cause a patient to experience TMJ pain as well. If a patient has rheumatoid arthritis, he/she can develop TMJ pain. Rheumatoid arthritis is usually on both sides of the body, whereas osteoarthritis is usually confined to one side.

If a patient has rheumatoid arthritis, this disease can progress to the TMJs on both sides of the head. In addition to x-rays, a patient may need a magnetic resonance image (MRI). A CT can also be used to examine the TMJ. At present, MRIs are the most effective tool for diagnosing TMJ problems. The TMJ specialist can also inject to dye into the joint. This injection of dye, called an arthrography, can help diagnose the disc displacement.

If a patient has a displacement of the TMJ disc, the mouth will deviate to one side as a patient open the mouth. If a patient has a popping or clicking in the jaw, a patient may have disc pathology. If an injection into the TMJ provides a patient with significant relief, the pain is intra-articular or coming from within the TMJ itself. However, if injection into the muscle provides a patient with pain relief, this tells the health-care provider that the pain is coming from outside the joint. Furthermore, by injecting around the nerve that goes to the TMJ, this maneuver can provide information as to whether the TMJ is the source of the chronic pain.

These injections are safe. Since most TMJ sufferers are missing pieces of their actual jaw bone or cartilage that helps keep the jaw in place, the muscles actually have to work harder to chew. When these muscles get fatigued, the jaw pops out of place, the TMJ joints get inflamed, and the headaches and jaw pain occurs. A patient should avoid chewy foods as well as crunchy foods.

Surgery is sometimes indicated for the management of a TMJ problem. When less-invasive procedures fail to alleviate TMJ pain, oral surgery procedures can be done. These include using a scope to reposition the discs. The oral surgeon can also remove the discs. Implantations can be done into the TMJ. Using a scope is less invasive than opening the TMJ joint. A patient needs to remember that the most conservative therapies are usually the best therapies.

TMJ prevalence peaks between the ages of 25 and 44. After age 44, the chance of a patient developing TMJ decreases with increasing age. For some reason, female patients who develop TMJ were more likely than males to have chronic pain. Studies have shown that sex is a definite risk for the development of TMJ.

TMJ is most noted in women during their reproductive years. The reason for this finding is not known. The problem with doing gender-specific studies on TMJ patients is that only a small number of males actually seek treatment for TMJ. A study in 1994 demonstrated that women have more physical and psychological symptoms with TMJ than males. However, in the study, males had greater psychological-related symptoms.

Studies have also been done to determine whether TMJ psychosocial symptoms were different from women when compared to men. Higher levels of stress, depression, and anxiety have been reported in the TMJ population in general when compared to healthy individuals who do not suffer from TMJ.

It was previously reported that if a patient suffers from TMJ that the patient has a higher rate of psychopathology than normal control individuals. A patient must be aware that psychopathology is strongly associated with generalized muscle pain throughout the body. The psychological disorders reported in TMJ patients are higher in females than males. If a patient has a history of sexual abuse or trauma, a patient has a higher risk of developing TMJ.

Close to 50 percent of TMJ patients have a history of sexual or physical abuse. An abuse history makes a patient more prone for depression and anxiety. An abuse history in general is associated with increased physical as well as psychological symptoms if a patient suffers from chronic pain. An abuse history is related to the increased pain complaints as well as the psychological disturbances.

Sexual abuse has been noted to be associated with an increased risk of generalized muscle pain in females but not in males. Be aware that females are more often the victims of sexual and physical abuse. As a result, the effect of abuse on pain response is more likely to be noted by females than by males.

Pain in the mouth and face can come from the teeth, jaws, the temporal mandibular joints, the muscles involved in chewing, and from the salivary glands. The nose and sinuses can also be a source of pain.

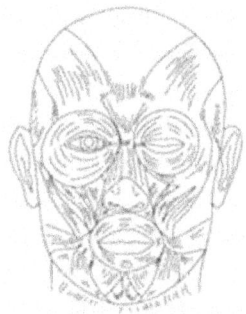

Figure 1. Facial pain can be caused by pathology in the facial bones, teeth, nerves, muscles, TMJ joint, etc.

If a patient develops an abscess and if the abscess becomes severe, a patient may need surgical drainage of this abscess and antibiotic therapy. An infection from the tooth could spread to other tissues in the mouth and to the neck. If the situation causes a patient to have significant swelling about the throat, especially about the airway, a patient may have trouble breathing. The airway can be compromised so severely that a patient could die. A dry socket is actually a localized inflammation of the bone where a tooth was removed. This pain can start two or three days after the tooth was removed and can last approximately two weeks.

A patient can also develop pain that comes from the salivary glands. The parotid gland as well as other salivary glands can be a site of infection. Furthermore, a small stone can block the parotid duct. The gland toward the bottom of the face and upper neck can swell. The pain will increase at the sight or smell of food. Sometimes the swelling and pain can decrease after a patient eat but can recur following another meal. If the stone remains in the duct, it may have to be removed surgically.

A patient can experience pain that is called atypical facial and oral pain. This type of pain may be related to psychiatric problems. An example of atypical facial pain is phantom tooth pain in which a tooth has been pulled, but the individual still reports complaints of pain in the area of the extracted tooth. If a patient has phantom tooth pain, the dentist may provide a patient with fillings or different treatments, none of which will provide a patient with significant relief in most instances.

The dentist may even extract neighboring teeth. If a patient have diabetes or have some vitamin deficiencies, a patient can develop a syndrome that causes a patient to have a burning mouth as well as a burning tongue. Sometimes psycho-genic factors can give one a pain syndrome of this type. The doctor and dentist will do a thorough physical examination, including x-rays. In many stances, a psychiatric consultation is indicated. Usually the tricyclic antidepressants such as Elavil will decrease the pain if a patient has these symptoms.

Schizophrenia and hypochondriasis or other emotional problems can also cause a patient to suffer facial pain for unknown reasons. As with many of the other pain syndromes in this book, there is no one definable treatment for facial pain, especially atypical facial pain. The health-care provided will obtain a complete history and do a thorough physical examination with the possibility of doing other tests before initiating definitive treatment. With this information in mind, a patient can be an extreme help to the health-care provider by keeping an accurate diary of the pain symptoms.

A stroke can also cause a patient to have pain in the facial area. Be aware that coronary artery disease can also cause a patient to have facial pain. If a patient suffers from this type of pain, nitroglycerin can sometimes relieve it. Remember that the pain from a heart attack can go into the jaw. If a patient has had a whiplash injury, one of the nerves off of the cervical spine can send nerve branches to the skin over the angle of the lower jawbone. This type of pain can cause a patient to have significant sharp pain.

On occasion local anesthetics and steroids can be used to decrease this pain. A patient can have facial pain that has been called atypical facial pain or facial pain of a psychological origin. This type of pain is usually associated with psychiatric symptoms. It can be seen in malingers as well as drug abusers.

Jaw pain in the elderly patient may have other causes. Dentists' diagnoses are complicated by patients' underlying medical conditions, age-associated physical changes, and the increased rate of some jaw diseases in the elderly. Facial pain may result from brain tumors or from a bone infection. Chest pain caused by insufficient blood flow to the heart radiates to the jaw in 9% to 18% of cases.

Symptoms of gastroesophageal reflux may mimic chest pain and can affect the jaw. Diseases that involve the nerves and jaw fractures can cause facial pain. Cranial arteritis is an inflammation of the blood vessels in the head that may produce pain in the chewing muscles. Arthritis may develop in the temporomandibular joint, producing pain. Changes in dentition and oral habits developed to support ill-fitting dentures may produce jaw pain.

A diagnosis of oral pain can be difficult. Pain in the mouth and face is common. It is fortunate that in most cases, the cause of the pain can be easily determined. However, the anatomy of the area about the face and throat is complex. Another type of pain is glossopharyngeal neuralgia. This type of pain has trigger areas around the tonsils or the back of the throat or even at the base of the tongue.

The injection of local anesthetics and steroids will not usually provide long-term pain relief. These types of neuralgias ordinarily require the use of anticonvulsant medications. Carbamazepine has been used for years for the treatment of trigeminal neuralgia, but now a newer anticonvulsant medication; pregabilin (Lyrica) can be helpful in alleviating the pain.

Leukocyte telomere length shortening occurred at the same rate among adults with and without severe chronic periodontitis. This suggests that LTL shortening may have occurred earlier in the life course. [13]

The diagnoses of bone marrow associated malignancies such as Acute and Chronic Lymphocytic Leukemia, Acute and Chronic Myelogenous, leukemia, Hodgkin's Lymphoma, Non-Hodgkin's Lymphoma, and Multiple Myeloma are often missed without a blood test. Increasing normal cell telomere and a longevity gene product can often improve both pathology and the prognosis.[14]

References

1. Martinez-Anda JJ, Barges-Coll J, Ponce-Gomez JA, Perez-Pena N, Revuelta-Gutierrez R. Surgical management of trigeminal neuralgia in elderly patients using a small retrosigmoidal approach: analysis of efficacy and safety. J Neurol Surg A Cent Eur Neurosurg. 2015;76(1):39-45.
2. Yadav S, Sonone RM, Jaiswara C, Bansal S, Singh D, Rathi VC. Long-term Follow-up of Trigeminal Neuralgia Patients treated with Percutaneous Balloon Compression Technique: A Retrospective Analysis. J Contemp Dent Pract. 2016;17(3):263-266.
3. Allsop MJ, Twiddy M, Grant H, et al. Diagnosis, medication, and surgical management for patients with trigeminal neuralgia: a qualitative study. Acta Neurochir (Wien). 2015;157(11):1925-1933.
4. Choudhri O, Heit JJ, Feroze AH, Chang SD, Dodd RL, Steinberg GK. Persistent trigeminal artery supply to an intrinsic trigeminal nerve arteriovenous malformation: a rare cause of trigeminal neuralgia. J Clin Neurosci. 2015;22(2):409-412.
5. Du Y, Yang D, Dong X, Du Q, Wang H, Yu W. Percutaneous balloon compression (PBC) of trigeminal ganglion for recurrent trigeminal neuralgia after microvascular decompression (MVD). Ir J Med Sci. 2015;184(4):745-751.
6. Helis CA, Lucas JT, Jr., Bourland JD, Chan MD, Tatter SB, Laxton AW. Repeat Radiosurgery for Trigeminal Neuralgia. Neurosurgery. 2015;77(5):755-761; discussion 761.
7. Li S, Lian YJ, Chen Y, et al. Therapeutic effect of Botulinum toxin-A in 88 patients with trigeminal neuralgia with 14-month follow-up. J Headache Pain. 2014;15:43.
8. Tang YZ, Jin D, Bian JJ, Li XY, Lai GH, Ni JX. Long-term outcome of computed tomography-guided percutaneous radiofrequency thermocoagulation for classic trigeminal neuralgia patients older than 70 years. J Craniofac Surg. 2014;25(4):1292-1295.
9. Tuleasca C, Carron R, Resseguier N, et al. Multiple sclerosis-related trigeminal neuralgia: a prospective series of 43 patients treated with gamma knife surgery with more than one year of follow-up. Stereotact Funct Neurosurg. 2014;92(4):203-210.

10. von Eckardstein KL, Keil M, Rohde V. Unnecessary dental procedures as a consequence of trigeminal neuralgia. Neurosurg Rev. 2015;38(2):355-360; discussion 360.

11. Wu TH, Hu LY, Lu T, et al. Risk of psychiatric disorders following trigeminal neuralgia: a nationwide population-based retrospective cohort study. J Headache Pain. 2015;16:64.

12. Murray TJ. Carotidynia: a cause of neck and face pain. Can Med Assoc J. 1979;120(4):441-443.

13. Sanders AE, Divaris K, Naorungroj S, Heiss G, Risques RA. Telomere length attrition and chronic periodontitis: an ARIC Study nested case-control study. J Clin Periodontol. 2015;42(1):12-20.

14. Omura Y, O'Young B, Jones M, et al. Newly discovered quick, non-invasive screening method of bone marrow malignancies including various leukemias, Hodgkin's lymphoma, non-Hodgkin's lymphoma, & multiple myeloma by abnormality of small rectangular area within bone marrow organ representation areas of the face. Acupunct Electrother Res. 2012;37(1):13-47.

33. Osteoporosis

The Body Mass Index (BMI), bone mineral density (BMD), and telomere length are phenotypes that modulate the course of aging. Over 40% of their phenotypic variance is determined by genetics.[1]

Osteoporosis affects 20 million Americans and results in more than 1.3 million bone fractures in the United States every year. In a lifetime, women lose more than half of their spongy bone, which comprises the center of bones, and approximately 30 percent of the non-spongy (compact) bone, which composes the outer aspect of bones. Osteoporosis can be a significant bone disease because it is potentially disabling.

Approximately, 30 percent of all postmenopausal Caucasian women will suffer from fractures related to osteoporosis. More than one-third of all women and one-sixth of all men over 65 years of age will sustain a hip fracture. This is a frightening statistic because hip fracture Osteoporosis is the most common type of bone disease that is related to the breakdown of substances that exist in a patient's bones and is common in elderly individuals. If a patient suffers from osteoporosis, a patient will have a progressive reduction in bone minerals as well as the structural components of bones, but the normal composition of bone is preserved.

Osteoporosis is a metabolic disease of bone, which leads to a reduction in bone density. The affected bones become thinner, and are more likely to (fracture which may result in pain and other complications, including loss of independence. Body mass complications can be fatal. It is estimated that the annual cost of health care for those with osteoporosis in lost national productivity as well as medical costs exceed $10 billion in the United States alone.

In recent decades the population of both elderly men and women has grown substantially worldwide. Aging is associated with a number of pathologies involving various organs including the skeleton. Age-related bone loss and resultant osteoporosis put the elderly population at an increased risk for fractures and morbidity.2   Body mass index (BMI), bone mineral density (BMD), and telomere length are phenotypes that modulate the course of aging. Over 40% of their phenotypic variance is determined by genetics.1

During a lifetime, bone is constantly being made and is constantly being lost. In normal circumstances, the production and reduction of a patient's bone are balanced. Osteoporosis can result if a patient do not make enough bone, or if a patient have an accelerated decrease in a bone minerals and the matrix structure (the components of bone, which make bones hard) of a patient's bone or both.

Bone density increases significantly during puberty. This increase in bone density is the result of a response to sex steroids. If a patient has had a delay in the onset of puberty, a patient may have a decrease in bone density. Factors that can affect bone mass include exercise or lack of exercise, calcium intake, growth hormones, sex hormones, genetics, race, and gender.

Genetics play an important role in the development of osteoporosis. Studies have demonstrated that bone density is lower in the daughters of women who have osteoporosis than in those women who do not have osteoporosis. Bone density tests in identical twins have been done indicating that genetics is an important factor in the development of osteoporosis. These studies have suggested that most of the genetic differences in bone density are the result of a gene that is linked to a vitamin D receptor gene.

Further study has revealed that variations of the vitamin D receptor gene result in differences in bone density changes of 10 percent to 12 percent in osteoporosis-prone individuals. Additional study is being done on the effect of the vitamin D receptor gene and the severity of osteoporosis in both men and women.

Men in general have been shown to have higher bone densities than women. Furthermore, African American men have higher bone density than Caucasian men. The same is true with African-American and Caucasian women. Even though osteoporosis is a disease that mostly affects women, osteoporosis can be seen in a small percentage of men.

A woman's first menstruation occurs when her reproductive organs become active and can take place at any time between the ages of 10 and 18. Studies have revealed that calcium supplementation can enhance prepuberty bone accumulation. An increase in physical activity can also increase bone density at the time of puberty.

When a patient approaches 40, the bone density can begin to decline. Bone density decreases are noted in women before menopause. In men, a decrease in their bone density occurs somewhere between 20 to 40 years of age. In women, after menopause has occurred, the rate of bone loss accelerates. During the first 10 years of menopause, the women's spongy bone is lost faster than the outer bone. Osteoporosis is normally without symptoms until a fracture occurs. Usually the fracture is in one of the bones of the back. However, the wrists, hips, ribs, pelvic bone, and legs can sustain fractures. The bones in the spine can have a loss of height, which is called a compression fracture.

A patient will also lose height as the bones in the back compress. Hip fractures are dangerous for elderly patients. Usually a hip fracture will cause a patient to need hospitalization. On occasion, a hip has to be replaced surgically. Medical complications, such as a pulmonary embolus, that can be associated with hip surgery in elderly patients can be fatal. With osteoporosis all of the bones can be affected, and each of the bones can be at an increased risk for a fracture. If a patient has a low calcium intake and is not physically active, the patient is at risk of developing osteoporosis.

There is a type of osteoporosis that is called idiopathic osteoporosis. The cause of this type of osteoporosis is unknown, but it does affect middle-aged men and premenopausal women. Being weightless in space can contribute to the onset of osteoporosis. Individuals who suffer from anorexia nervosa also develop osteoporosis. There are other causes of osteoporosis besides the ones just mentioned. Hyperthyroidism and hyperparathyroidism in addition to a body's overproduction of cortisone (a steroid) are causes of osteoporosis. If a patient has a decrease in growth hormone, one may be prone to develop osteoporosis.

It is important for a body to absorb calcium through the system. If a patient has a history of a gastrectomy (removal of a portion of the stomach), cirrhosis of the liver, or any other gastrointestinal malabsorption syndrome, the patient is more prone to develop osteoporosis. If a patient has a history of multiple myeloma or leukemia, a patient may develop osteoporosis. The exact cause of this finding is presently unknown.

If a patient has been immobilized for any reason, a patient may also develop osteoporosis. If a patient is unable to walk or exercise for whatever reason due to immobilization, a patient may develop osteoporosis. Alcohol can contribute to the development of osteoporosis. Chemotherapy can also cause osteoporosis. Steroid use has been implicated in the development of osteoporosis as well.

Other diseases have a link to osteoporosis. An autoimmune disease is a disorder in which the body attacks its own tissue. The joints can become damaged by antibodies. Systemic lupus erythematous is an autoimmune disease commonly known as lupus. If a patient has lupus, he/she will become fatigued and have painful joints in addition to developing skin rashes. Ninety percent of individuals diagnosed with lupus are women. If a patient has lupus, he/she are at an increased risk for developing osteoporosis.

Steroids are prescribed for the treatment of lupus. The fatigue caused by lupus results in a decrease in exercise and activity. These factors increase the risk of developing osteoporosis. Furthermore, the disease itself can decrease the bone mass. Individuals, who are HIV positive, can also develop osteoporosis. The reason for the increase in osteoporosis in patients with HIV infection is not known.

It is possible that the virus may infect the cells that produce bone. In addition to Caucasian women being more prone to developing osteoporosis, Asian American women are also at a high risk for developing osteoporosis. African-American and Hispanic women are at a lower risk for developing osteoporosis. The reason for the effect of race on the development of osteoporosis remains to be seen.

A diagnosis of osteoporosis can be made by a plain X-ray. If a patient has a vertebral bone compression in the mid back, for example, there will usually be a decrease in the height of the affected (compressed) bone that can be seen on X-ray. Sometimes a bone scan is needed to diagnosis-sis osteoporosis. If a patient has a bone scan, a doctor will inject a radioactive material into the vein.

A patient will have a picture of the body taken by a special camera. Compression fractures, which were not diagnosed by other means, can be detected on a bone scan. Osteoporosis can also be diagnosed by measuring theb one mineral density. The bone density value will be compared to a normal value that is noted for a patient's of the same sex. A bone-density test can predict the probability of a patient developing a fracture related to the bone density value.

Quantitative computed tomography can also be used and is effective for diagnosing osteoporosis because it will not only measure the bone mineral density, this test can also measure the density of the spongy bone within the back and hip bones. However, this test is expensive and will expose a patient to radiation. Different types of tests are being used and being developed to diagnosis osteoporosis. Bone scanning can be useful for the diagnosis of compression fractures. If a patient has a decreased bone density, the doctor should attempt to determine the cause of the osteoporosis.

Not all fractures associated with osteoporosis are painful. A patient may have a fracture and not know it. The doctor will probably measure the level of the parathyroid hormone in the blood if a patient develops non painful bone fractures, which are not associated with bone trauma such as a fall. This is important because an elevation of parathyroid hormone can decrease the bone mass.

Because a decrease in testosterone may be associated with osteoporosis in men, male patients should have their testosterone blood levels measured when they have their yearly physical examinations. Bone density testing is important early in the development of osteoporosis because there is no cure for osteoporosis. In other words, there is no way to reverse osteoporosis after it has become established. However, early treatment can prevent the progression of osteoporosis.

If it has been determined that alcohol is a cause of the osteoporosis, a patient must stop consuming alcohol. If the thyroid levels are elevated, this disease should be treated early to decrease the progression of the osteoporosis. Physical therapy and mild aerobic exercise may be important in retarding the timely development of osteoporosis. If a patient has a compression fracture of one of the bones in the spine, a back brace can provide a patient with pain relief. The physical therapist may want to strengthen the stomach muscles as well as the muscles in the back.

Not only should a patient be educated in the diagnosis and treatment of osteoporosis, the doctor may also need education in the diagnosis and treatment of this disease. A study published in an orthopedic surgeon journal reported that orthopedic surgeons are frequently the first health-care providers to evaluate patients with fractures. This study reported that orthopedic surgeons, however, have been slow to develop awareness for identifying individuals who have osteoporosis who could benefit from drug therapies. Only 50 percent of patients who have a history of a hip fracture were referred for bone density testing.

Furthermore, a Canadian survey done in 1998 revealed that orthopedic surgeons had little interest in evaluating and treating osteoporosis in patients who had fractures. Doctors need to realize that a patient who sustained a hip fracture is identified as an individual who has a high probability of developing osteoporosis. This individual is at a high risk for having a future bone fracture.

If a patient has had a hip fracture, a patient is a probable candidate for bone density testing. Communication between a patient's orthopedic surgeon and primary-care doctor is essential. This communication could facilitate the diagnosis of decreased bone density in individuals who have suffered hip fractures.

Cortical bone is a compact form of bone that makes up the outer shell of the bones. It consists of a hard, solid mass made up of bony tissue that is arranged in concentric layers. This is similar to the layers noted in a tree. The compact bone will surround the spongy bone. Bone is composed of collagen fibers that contain bone salts, which are mainly calcium carbonate salts as well as calcium phosphate salts. As previously stated, during the first 5 to 10 years of menopause, women can lose 10 to 15 percent of their compact bone and 25 percent of the spongy bone. It is important for a patient to know that this bone loss can be prevented by estrogen-replacement therapy. However, estrogen therapy can be associated with an increased risk of a stroke and heart disease.

The amount of bone loss varies among women, which has led medical investigators to derive a classification of osteoporosis. If the osteoporosis is more severe than is expected for the age, a patient have type I postmenopausal osteoporosis. If a patient have type I osteoporosis, a patient are at a higher risk to have compression or crush fractures of the bones in the spine.

A patient may also be prone to a fracture at the bone above the wrist on the side of the thumb. This type of fracture is called a Colles fracture. If the bones are weak and fragile, a patient can easily sustain a bone fracture. These types of fractures are related to bone density loss. If a patient have a decrease in the estrogen, a patient may have the production of chemicals that may decrease the bone mass.

An initially rapid rate of bone loss in the post-menopausal period is followed by a slower loss of bone throughout the rest of life. The loss of bone mass does result from normal aging and occurs in both men and women. This type of bone loss is called type II osteoporosis.

Fractures can occur in type II osteoporosis as well as in type I osteoporosis. Fractures can occur in the hip, pelvis, wrist, the bones in the legs, and the bones in the back. Sometimes type II osteoporosis is associated with a defect in the absorption of calcium through the gastrointestinal system. As a patient age, the calcium absorption through the stomach and intestine can decrease.

A decreased absorption of this important substance will decrease the amount of calcium in the blood stream. Studies do not support the notion of the occurrence of a generalized premature cellular aging in osteoporotic patients.[3] Adipose tissue may represent a promising autologous cell source for the development of novel bone regenerative therapeutic strategies in the treatment of age-related osteoporosis.[4]

In the body, a patient has various chemicals stimulated by a growth factor. Growth factor tells the body to make new cells and to maintain the cells that are already present in the body. These chemicals sit on the outer surface of the cells. Growth factor is needed in wound healing if a patient has had an injury to one of the tissues (bone, muscle, nerve).

Estrogen, a female sex hormone, increases the production of this growth factor. Be aware that growth factor stimulates bone formation. If a patient has a decrease in estrogen, a patient can diminish the formation of bone. As a result, a decrease in estrogen will decrease the ability to form bone.

In the body a patient have two parathyroid glands. These glands are around the thyroid gland at the base of the neck above the breastbone (the sternum). The parathyroid glands stimulate the production of parathyroid hormone, which is produced if a patient has a decrease in calcium in the bloodstream. Parathyroid glands produce parathyroid hormone. This hormone produced by the parathyroid gland is released into the bloodstream. The parathyroid hormone controls the distribution of both calcium and phosphate throughout the body. A high level of parathyroid hormone will cause the transfer of calcium from the bones to the bloodstream.

If the parathyroid hormone level decreases in the bloodstream, it will lower the blood calcium level. If a patient has a decrease in the estrogen hormone, a patient will have a decrease in the blood calcium levels as well. If the estrogen goes down, the bone sensitivity to the transfer of calcium from the bones to the bloodstream is increased. Therefore, a patient will lose the bone density as the blood level of estrogen decreases.

If the calcium in the bloodstream increases, a patient will decrease parathyroid hormone secretion. Estrogen deficiency can decrease bone matrix formation in a body. A patient should now be aware that sex hormones play an important role in the maintenance of the bone structure. A patient should now realize that when the sex hormones decrease as the patient ages and that this decreased hormone level could adversely affect the skeletal system. Age corrected mean telomere restriction fragment length was associated with longitudinal bone loss for different distal forearm sites.[5]

Osteoporosis occurs more often in women than in men. However, it is also seen in men. It is estimated that more than 2 million men in the United States suffer from osteoporosis. Approximately, 20 percent of all hip fractures in the United States occur in men. Compression fractures in the bones of the spine can occur in men as well. Bone fractures related to osteoporosis accounted for $2.7 billion, which is one fifth of the total cost of osteoporotic fractures, in the United States in 1994.

This observation demonstrated that osteoporosis is not solely a "woman's disease." Osteoporosis develops less often in men than in women because men have more bone mass and larger skeletons. Therefore, the bone loss in men starts later and progresses more slowly. Telomeres progressively shorten with repeated somatic tissue cell division, their length being an indicator of cellular ageing. Telomeric dysfunction may be implicated in a variety of diseases.[6]

The development of osteoporosis in men has been recently recognized as an important public health issue. Men suffering from osteoporosis are a long-neglected group of individuals. The National Institutes of Health are currently studying osteoporosis in men. The results of this study should help doctors understand how to prevent and treat osteoporosis in men. Remember that when bone is lost, it cannot be replaced. Middle-aged and elderly men should have their testosterone levels measured periodically.

It has been documented that telomere-associated cellular senescence may contribute to certain age-related disorders, including an increase in cancer incidence, wrinkling and diminished skin elasticity, atherosclerosis, osteoporosis, weight loss, age-related cataract, glaucoma and others. Shorter telomere length in leukocytes is associated cross sectionally with cardiovascular disorders and their risk factors, including pulse pressure and vascular aging, obesity, vascular dementia, diabetes, coronary artery disease, myocardial infarction (although not in all studies), cellular turnover and exposure to oxidative and inflammatory damage in chronic obstructive pulmonary disease.[7]

As previously stated, a reduced level of testosterone in men can cause osteoporosis. Thirty percent of men with osteoporotic fractures of the bones in their spine have low testosterone levels. Testosterone therapy may retard the development of osteoporosis-is in men. The research has shown that a decrease in estrogen in men can be a cause of osteoporosis. Be aware of the fact that men also have estrogen secreted in their bodies.

The prevention and treatment of osteoporosis include synthetic estrogen or progesterone therapy if a patient is postmenopausal. However, a patient must take calcium in addition to the hormone therapy. A synthetic estrogen called raloxifene has been approved for the treatment of osteoporosis. This drug will increase the bone density. It has fewer side effects than other types of estrogen drugs.

Postmenopausal women who exercise for 60 minutes 3 times a week and take calcium supplements can stop bone loss. It is recommended that individuals over 50 use calcium supplements. If a patient does not want to use a calcium supplement, calcium-rich foods such as milk, yogurt, and cooked dry beans will provide a patient with calcium. Furthermore, some cheeses can increase the calcium in the bloodstream.

Most individuals have trouble getting enough calcium in their diet and end up needing calcium supplements. Remember that vitamin D is also an important vitamin that is necessary for strong bones. If a patient is not out in the sun at all, a patient should drink vitamin D-fortified milk or eat vitamin D-fortified foods. Remember that vitamin D is important because it helps the body to absorb calcium. Vitamin D can help a patient increase the calcium absorption through the gastrointestinal tract by up to 65 percent.

One must be aware that drugs used to treat asthma can increase the risk of fractures if patients are prone to osteoporosis. Inhaled steroids can be used for the treatment of asthma. This drug increases the risk of sustaining a bone fracture. Steroids are used not only for the treatment of asthma but also for the treatment of rheumatoid arthritis and some bowel disease.

If a patient are taking steroids for longer than three months, a patient may need to discuss this with the doctor and a patient and the doctor should consider a prescription for Fosamax, which is used to treat osteoporosis. Smoking also increases bone loss. Hip and spinal bone fractures are higher in men and women who smoke. Research is being done to determine how nicotine damages bone. Preliminary investigations reveal that nicotine can inhibit absorption of calcium that is needed for bone health.

Just like women, men need to take calcium. Men can inherit osteoporosis from their fathers. Caucasian men are at a higher risk of developing osteoporosis than other races. Osteoporosis in men can be diagnosed by a bone mass measurement. This is a special type of x-ray that emits a trace amount of radiation. Middle-aged men who have complaints of back or hip pain may be candidates for a bone mass measurement as well as a measurement of the testosterone in their bloodstream.

Research has demonstrated that there is gender bias with respect to men who have suffered hip fractures. Doctors in the past have felt osteoporosis was a woman's disease. We now realize that osteoporosis affects both women and men. Medications to prevent bone loss are, for the most part, ignored for middle-aged and older men who have sustained hip fractures. Hip fracture complications are a cause of death in approximately 17 percent of women and 6 percent of men in the United States. By the age of 70, bone loss is equal in both men and women.

The absorption of calcium from the gastro intestinal system decreases with age. The United Stated recommended dietary allowance of calcium is up to 1,000 milligrams per day. Calcium can retard the osteoporosis but cannot completely stop it. An increase in calcium in the bloodstream may not protect a patient from compression fractures of the bones in the spine. Calcium therapy can help a patient if a patient are a woman and postmenopausal. Some endocrinologists have recommended that if a patient is postmenopausal that a patient should consume 1,500 milligrams per day of calcium.

As stated earlier in this chapter, sex steroids are important for the maintenance of proper bone density. Oral estrogen as well as estrogen in the form of a patch worn on the skin can prevent bone loss if a patient is estrogen deficient. Bone loss is rapid in the first years of menopause, so estrogen therapy is of great benefit if it is administered before a patient begin to lose a significant amount of bone mass. Studies have demonstrated that estrogen therapy decreases the risk of bone fractures in postmenopausal women.

It is recommended that if a patient is taking estrogen supplements that a patient also take calcium supplements. Estrogen supplements are not without side effects. If estrogen is not administered along with progestin, a patient runs the risk of cancer. Estrogen replacement can be related to breast cancer as well as heart disease. These studies with respect to cancer are controversial, however. Other studies have noted that estrogen therapy can decrease the chance of a patient having a heart attack by up to 50 percent.

Calcitonin is another drug that a patient could take to prevent bone loss in the vertebral bodies throughout the spine. Calcitonin is most effective in early and late menopause. Calcitonin is available for intranasal use. Calcitonin has been shown to produce pain-relieving effects. Calcitonin is most useful if a patient has a history of osteoporosis and has chronic pain related to fractures related to the osteoporosis. Elderly individuals appear to be prone to vitamin D deficiency. Decreased vitamin D and decreased calcium in elderly patients' bloodstreams can lead to accelerated bone loss. It has been shown that vitamin D plus calcium can reduce the incidence of fractures in elderly women.

Studies have been done that suggest that eating foods rich in soy protein helps protect older women from bone loss. Women in their 20s who ate diets that were high in soy protein did not demonstrate any improvement in their bone density. Some compounds found in soy are chemically similar to human estrogens.

Some studies suggest that eating a soy diet can slow bone loss in postmenopausal women. A new form of vitamin D supplements can help women regain some bone mass loss due to osteoporosis. The new vitamin D supplement is more potent than previous vitamin D supplements. This new compound is called 2MD. It promotes the growth of cells that are responsible for making bone. Current studies that are being done in animals are prominent. This new form of vitamin D may become an important alternative to hormone therapy. This new drug has not been tested in humans.

Falls can cause significant injury to the hips or the bones in the legs if a patient has osteoporosis. A recent study has demonstrated that vibrating shoe insoles can help elderly individuals improve their balance and prevent falls because the soles increase awareness as to where the feet are positioned. The rationale for this device is that the nervous system in elderly individuals, women and men, decreases touch and position sense.

Touch and position sense are needed to maintain balance. It is thought that if a patient can stimulate the nervous system in the soles of the feet, improvement will be seen in the balance and posture control of elderly individuals. Improvement in the balance of aging individuals is extremely important because bone fractures can be potentially lethal for them.

Recent research has revealed that one in five elderly individuals who have suffered a hip or wrist fracture because of osteoporosis received the treatment that they need to prevent future fractures of their bones. Only 22 percent of elderly women and elderly men received a prescription drug for one of the drugs used to treat osteoporosis. It is important that elderly individuals who have sustained a fracture receive osteoporosis treatment medications because they are five times more likely to suffer another fracture.

Telomere length is emerging as a biomarker for aging and survival is paternally inherited and associated with parental lifespan. Telomere-associated cellular senescence may contribute to certain age-related disorders, including an increase in cancer incidence, wrinkling and diminished skin elasticity, atherosclerosis, osteoporosis, weight loss, age-related cataract, glaucoma and others.[8]

Shorter telomere length in leukocytes was associated cross-sectionally with cardiovascular disorders and its risk factors, including pulse pressure and vascular aging, obesity, vascular dementia, diabetes, coronary artery disease, myocardial infarction (although not in all studies), cellular turnover and exposure to oxidative and inflammatory damage in chronic obstructive pulmonary disease.

By using osteoporosis drugs, they can reduce the risk of a future fracture by as much as 60 percent. Be aware that more than 550,000 hip and wrist fractures occur in elderly individuals suffering from osteoporosis every year. An initial fracture in an elderly individual should signal a red flag to a doctor that this individual probably has osteoporosis and needs prescription medications.

Telomere length is emerging as a biomarker for aging and survival is paternally inherited and associated with parental lifespan. Telomere-associated cellular senescence may contribute to certain age-related disorders, including an increase in cancer incidence, wrinkling and diminished skin elasticity, atherosclerosis, osteoporosis, weight loss, age-related cataract, glaucoma and others.

Shorter telomere length in leukocytes was associated cross-sectionally with cardiovascular disorders and its risk factors, including pulse pressure and vascular aging, obesity, vascular dementia, diabetes, coronary artery disease, myocardial infarction (although not in all studies), cellular turnover and exposure to oxidative and inflammatory damage in chronic obstructive pulmonary disease. Osteoporosis can decrease the calcium in the spine and hips.

If a patient has had a fracture of one of the bones in the spine, treatment that puts bone cement into the bone can be used to treat any compression fracture that a patient may have. Be aware that leakage of this bone cement, called polymethylmethacrylate, can be associated with an embolus to thelungs, heart and lung failure, and death. The techniques that use this cement are called vertebroplasty and kyphoplasty.

The value and safety of these procedures continue to be studied. Vertebroplasty involves the injection of the bone cement into the vertebral bones. Kyphyplasty introduces a surgical instrument into one of the bones in the spine with intent to elevate the compressed bone. When this instrument is withdrawn, the space left is filled with bone cement. Each of these procedures remains to be studied.

If a patient has decreased bone density, he/she must take the medicines prescribed. Studies have shown that compliance is sometimes as low as 66 percent. This means that only 66 percent of individuals in a study actually took the medications prescribed for them. Women who did not take their osteoporosis medications developed significant further decrease in their bone densities.

On the other hand, a study of postmenopausal women who had a history of fractures related to osteoporosis did not receive drug treatment for the osteoporosis within a year following their fracture. Improved adherence to osteoporosis treatment can be done if women are educated regarding their bone densities and the effects of drugs on their bone density.

Bisphosphonates are an important class of drug for osteoporosis. These drugs can increase the minerals in the bones in the back. Furthermore, the chance of a patient having a vertebral fracture is decreased if a patient is in late menopause. These drugs can also prevent bone loss in early menopause. Bisphosphonates can inhibit bone breakdown, preserve bone mass, and even increase bone density in thespine and hip, reducing the risk of fractures. Examples of these medications include alendronate (Fosamax), ibandronate (Boniva), risedronate (Actonel) and zoledronic acid (Reclast).

Bisphosphonates may be especially beneficial for men, and people with steroid-induced osteoporosis. They're also used to prevent osteoporosis in people who require long-term steroid treatment for a disease such as asthma or arthritis. Side effects, which can be severe, include nausea, abdominal pain, difficulty swallowing and the risk of an inflamed esophagus or esophageal ulcers.

that can be taken once a week or once a month may cause fewer stomach problems. If a patient can't tolerate oral bisphosphonates, the doctor may recommend periodic intravenous infusions of bisphosphonate preparations. There have also been reports of serious side effects with bisphosphonates, such as osteonecrosis of the jaw, a rare type of thigh fracture, irregular heartbeats and visual disturbances.

The longer telomeres revealed in people more heavily exposed to ionizing radiation probably indicate activation of telomerase as a chromosome healing mechanism following damage, and reflect defects in telomerase regulation that could potentiate carcinogenesis.[9] Walking speed may be an objective indicator of successful aging. Frailty and successful aging may be considered two sides of the same entity, and fast walking speed may be used as an objective indicator of successful aging.[10]

Raloxifene (Evista) is a drug that belongs to a class of drugs called selective estrogen receptor modulators (SERMs). Raloxifene mimics estrogen's beneficial effects on bone density in postmenopausal women, without some of the risks associated with estrogen, such as increased risk of uterine cancer and, possibly, breast cancer. Hot flashes are a common side effect of raloxifene. A patient should not use this drug if a patient has a history of blood clots.

Teriparatide (Forteo) is an analog of parathyroid hormone and is used to treat osteoporosis in postmenopausal women and men who are at high risk of fractures. It works by stimulating new bone growth, while other medications prevent further bone loss. Teriparatide is given once a day by injection under the skin on the thigh or abdomen. Long-term effects are still being studied.

During the acute stage of osteoporotic fractures, attention is directed toward relieving the pain with pain pills, including narcotics and muscle relaxants for spasm that occurs related to the fracture. Heat, massage, and rest can also be of benefit to a patient.

Physical therapy in many instances can help a patient with the pain. If a patient has a fracture of one of the vertebral bodies in the spine, a corset or a back brace can decrease the pain. Exercise can be useful if it strengthens the abdominal and back muscles. Prevention is the best treatment. A calcium supplement that contains Vitamin D, such as OsCal-D, will strengthen the bones and help prevent osteoporosis.

Protein intake is also important because protein intake far below Recommended Daily Allowance could be particularly detrimental for both the acquirement of bone mass and the preservation of bone integrity with aging. Prescription medications such as Fosamax will keep a patient from losing more bone mass. A patient should do light weight-bearing exercises to help maintain and build the bone mass. Adequate dietary calcium intake and maintaining a physically active lifestyle in late decades of life could potentially translate into a reduction in the risk of osteoporosis and hence improve the quality and perhaps quantity of life in the elderly population.

References

1. Lill CM, Liu T, Norman K, et al. Genetic Burden Analyses of Phenotypes Relevant to Aging in the Berlin Aging Study II (BASE-II). Gerontology. 2016;62(3):316-322.

2. Syed FA, Ng AC. The pathophysiology of the aging skeleton. Curr Osteoporos Rep. 2010;8(4):235-240.

3. Kveiborg M, Kassem M, Langdahl B, Eriksen EF, Clark BF, Rattan SI. Telomere shortening during aging of human osteoblasts in vitro and leukocytes in vivo: lack of excessive telomere loss in osteoporotic patients. Mech Ageing Dev. 1999;106(3):261-271.

4. Mirsaidi A, Kleinhans KN, Rimann M, et al. Telomere length, telomerase activity and osteogenic differentiation are maintained in adipose-derived stromal cells from senile osteoporotic SAMP6 mice. J Tissue Eng Regen Med. 2012;6(5):378-390.

5. Bekaert S, Van Pottelbergh I, De Meyer T, et al. Telomere length versus hormonal and bone mineral status in healthy elderly men. Mech Ageing Dev. 2005;126(10):1115-1122.

6. Tamayo M, Mosquera A, Rego JI, Fernandez-Sueiro JL, Blanco FJ, Fernandez JL. Differing patterns of peripheral blood leukocyte telomere length in rheumatologic diseases. Mutat Res. 2010;683(1-2):68-73.

7. Babizhayev MA, Vishnyakova KS, Yegorov YE. Oxidative damage impact on aging and age-related diseases: drug targeting of telomere attrition and dynamic telomerase activity flirting with imidazole-containing dipeptides. Recent Pat Drug Deliv Formul. 2014;8(3):163-192.

8. Babizhayev MA, Kasus-Jacobi A, Vishnyakova KS, Yegorov YE. Novel neuroendocrine and metabolic mechanism provides the patented platform for important rejuvenation therapies: targeted therapy of telomere attrition and lifestyle changes of telomerase activity with the timing of neuron-specific imidazole-containing dipeptide-dominant pharmaconutrition provision. Recent Pat Endocr Metab Immune Drug Discov. 2014;8(3):153-179.

9. Reste J, Zvigule G, Zvagule T, et al. Telomere length in Chernobyl accident recovery workers in the late period after the disaster. J Radiat Res. 2014;55(6):1089-1100.

10. Woo J, Leung J, Zhang T. Successful Aging and Frailty: Opposite Sides of the Same Coin? J Am Med Dir Assoc. 2016.

34. HIV/AIDS

Older people are at increasing risk for HIV/AIDS and other sexually transmitted diseases (STDs). A growing number of older people now have HIV/AIDS. Greater than 10% of persons with AIDS in the United States are over 50 years of age, and the number of elderly persons in their 60s and 70s living with HIV/AIDS is increasing. About 19 percent of all people with HIV/AIDS in this country are age 50 and older. Accelerated telomere shortening in lymphocytes has been associated with a variety of human pathologies, including HIV disease, Down syndrome, and cardiovascular disease.[1]

Aging of the immune system is a major factor responsible for the increased severity of infections, reduced responses to vaccines, and higher cancer incidence in the elderly.[2] A major category of stressors that contribute to the alterations within the T lymphocyte compartment is the family of herpes viruses.

These viruses, usually acquired early in life, persist for many decades and drive certain T cells to the end stage of replicative senescence, which is characterized by a variety of phenotypic and functional changes, including altered cytokine profile, resistance to apoptosis, and shortened telomeres.

HIV infection induces changes to monocyte phenotype and function in young HIV-positive males that mimic those observed in elderly uninfected individuals, suggesting HIV may accelerate age-related changes to monocytes. Importantly, these defects persist in virologically suppressed HIV-positive individuals.[3]

High proportions of senescent CD8 (cytotoxic) T lymphocytes are associated with latent cytomegalovirus infection in the elderly, and are part of a cluster of immune biomarkers that are associated with early mortality. Similar cells accumulate at younger ages in persons chronically infected with HIV-1. In addition to persistent viral infection, psychological stress as well as oxidative stress can also contribute to the generation of senescent dysfunctional T lymphocytes.

Because older people don't get tested for HIV/AIDS regularly, there may are even more cases than currently known. Many factors contribute to the increasing risk of infection in older people. In general, older Americans know less about HIV/AIDS and STDs than younger age groups because the elderly have been neglected by those responsible for education and prevention messages. Late presentation to HIV care leads to increased morbidity and mortality.[4]

With the increased use of agents for erectile dysfunction, there have been increases in sexual activity among older adults. With this increase in sexual activity, the number of HIV and AIDS cases has increased drastically. The problem that has arisen in the United States is that many adults over age 65 are not protecting themselves against AIDS. Some of these individuals do not think that they are at risk for HIV infection. The incidence of AIDS in individuals over 50 continues to increase in the United States. In women over 50, the number of new AIDS cases more than doubled between 1991 and 1996. In older men, the increase was similar.

Aids is caused by a virus. A virus is a biological particle that is composed of a genetic material called DNA or RNA and a protein. A virus is not considered to be a living organism. Viruses are organisms that are essentially between living and nonliving things. Viruses can take over the genetic machinery of a cell or cells that they infect. By taking over the whole cell that they infect, they ultimately control the genetic machinery of the cell. The genetic machinery directs the cell's fate.

A virus can replicate itself within a host cell or do nothing once it infects the host cell. When a virus replicates itself in a host cell, thousands or even millions of copies of itself can be released from the cell and then go on to infect other cells. HIV, for example, can enter a body from unsafe sex practices or contaminated blood, enter cells, and make millions, billions, and even trillions of copies of itself that go on to infect other cells in a body.

The decline of the immune system appears to be an intractable consequence of aging, leading to increased susceptibility to infections, reduced effectiveness of vaccination and higher incidences of many diseases including osteoporosis and cancer in the elderly.[5] Senescent T cells have also been identified in patients with certain cancers, autoimmune diseases and chronic infections such as HIV.

A virus, therefore, is a highly effective means of causing one to develop and have an infection. A virus will consist of either RNA or DNA that is encased in a protein outer coat, which is called a capsid. If the virus gets into a body, it can cause a disease unless it is attacked by antibodies. A virus that causes a disease is called virulent. If the virus gains entrance into a body but does not cause a disease, it is called a temperate virus. It is not clearly understood why a virus will be temperate or virulent.

Viruses are not considered living organisms. The cells in a body reproduce naturally. A virus, on the other hand, can reproduce only by invading one of a patient's cells. The virus then uses chemicals and other structures within cells, referred to as genetic material, to make more viruses. A virus cannot reproduce unless the virus can invade a cell. A virus is a lifeless particle that has no control of its movement. It is spread randomly through the wind, in water, food, by blood, or by body secretions.

With respect to HIV, blood and body secretions are important mechanisms by which this virus spreads from one person's body into someone else's body. The science of virology is relatively new. A virus was first isolated in 1935.

Electrophoresis is now used to examine different properties of a virus. Electrophoresis is a process that separates molecules based on their electrical charges. Different types of viruses exist depending upon the genetic material that it contains. HIV, which is the causative virus of AIDS, is very complex. HIV has two strands of RNA inside of it.

These two RNA strands are surrounded by two layers of a protein. A layer of fatty substances surround the inner proteins. The protein sugar complex on the fatty layer forms the outer coat of the virus. HIV is a virus that infects and destroys CD4 cells. CD4 cells are part of the body's immune system. The immune system protects the body from invaders. When the immune system loses too many CD4 cells, it becomes weak and is unable to fight off germs. At this point, you are at risk of getting AIDS-related that can cause serious illness or death.

Viruses in general are classified as DNA viruses or RNA viruses, depending on whether RNA or DNA is within the viral structure. In other words, a virus contains either RNA or DNA, but never both. The difference between an RNA virus and a DNA virus is the fashion in which they change the genetic machinery of the cell that they infect. When the virus is inside of a cell, a DNA virus usually produces new RNA, which in turn makes more viral proteins.

On the other hand, the DNA from the virus that has infected your cell may join the DNA of a cell and then direct the synthesis (creation) of newer viruses. An RNA virus works in a different fashion. An RNA virus can enter a cell and make new proteins directly. The polio virus is an RNA virus.

The HIV virus is a different type of virus, called a retrovirus. In a retrovirus, RNA makes DNA with the help of an enzyme. This new DNA then makes new RNA. The RNA then makes the proteins that become part of new viruses. In 1881, Louis Pasteur grew a weakened form of the rabies virus. He knew that if he could inject a weakened form of the virus, he could help the body to use its mechanisms to fight the rabies virus and prevent it from replicating.

If a patient is given a weak form of a virus, he/she will not have the symptoms normally associated with a virus such as fever and chills. Louis Pasteur showed that a single injection of a weak virus could provide one with future immunity from a normal infectious virus. Following injection of a weak form of a virus into a body, the body will construct antibodies to destroy not only the weakened virus (vaccine) but also the strong infectious form (virulent form) of the virus.

Louis Pasteur's original experiment is the basis of the development of vaccines to combat viral infections. When a virus, such as HIV or any other virulent virus attacks one of a patient's cells, first the virus attaches to the cell. The virus will attach itself to the outer membrane of the cell at an area called a receptor site.

When the virus attaches to a receptor site, the virus will release an enzyme that weakens a spot on the wall of the cell membrane. After the virus has weakened the outer wall of the cell, it will then inject the RNA from itself into the cell through the hole in the cell wall.

Sometimes the whole virus can go right through the hole in the cell wall without just injecting its RNA. When the virus is inside of the cell, the HIV complex can make RNA, which in turns makes DNA. The DNA can then take complete control of the cell. The DNA can tell the cell to make new DNA, which is an RNA that is needed to make new viruses.

When the new viruses are made, an enzyme is released that destroys the outer wall of the cell. When this wall is destroyed, the new viruses that have been made within the cell are now released into the body. These viruses will go to infect different cells of different tissues within the body at this time.

A temperate virus does not cause a disease immediately. Therefore, even though a virus is within the cell or cells, it may take time for it to do any damage to a cell. This example is the reason why HIV can be present in the body for some time before causing symptoms. The majority of the other viruses that commonly cause people to become sick are either DNA or RNA viruses. A retrovirus more commonly infects animals.

Most viral infections are contracted from particles in the air or from touching infected individuals. The retrovirus that can cause AIDS can be transmitted by one of three means: Exposure to infected blood products, sexual contact with infected people, and an infection from a mother to her baby. The infection with this virus appears within two to six weeks following infection.

Early symptoms of infection with HIV are much like flu symptoms and include muscle pain, joint pain, headaches, as well as a sore throat and fever. Antibodies to the HIV virus develop in a body within three to six months of an infection. Later symptoms, which take up to 10 years to develop, as those of AIDS, result from the destructive effects of HIV on the immune system and are characterized by unusual types of pneumonia, cancer, central nervous system infections, and other problems.

After the HIV virus enters a cell, the virus can set up a chronic infection in which new virus particles are constantly produced. A patient may develop some antibodies to the virus. When the level of the body's antibodies decreases, a patient can develop AIDS. Progression to AIDS, which is a syndrome following infection with the virus, can begin with a low red blood cell count. Other factors can be necessary for a patient to contract the HIV infection and for the development of progression to AIDS.

There are four high-risk groups for developing AIDS, as follows: homosexual and bisexual men, hemophiliacs and transfusion recipients, intravenous drug abusers, children born to infected mothers. Homosexual and bisexual men account for approximately 37-40 percent of the reported cases of AIDS in the United States. However, this number is increasing. The majority of women with AIDS in the United States are in childbearing years.

Though Black and Hispanic men who have sex with men (MSM) are at an increased risk for HIV, few HIV risk reduction interventions that target HIV-positive MSM, and even fewer that use technology, have been designed to target these groups.

Despite similar rates of social media and technology use across racial/ethnic groups, online engagement of minority MSM for HIV prevention efforts is low. Efficacy trials of technology-based HIV prevention interventions targeting high-risk minority HIV-positive MSM are warranted.6

Disparities in HIV prevalence between black and white MSM continue to increase. Black MSM may be infected with HIV at younger ages than other MSM and may benefit from prevention efforts that address the needs of younger men.[7] Early linkage to care and antiretroviral (ARV) treatment are associated with reduced HIV transmission.

Male-to-male sexual contact represents the largest HIV transmission category in the United States; men who have sex with men (MSM) are an important focus of care and treatment efforts.[8] Mobile populations are at increased risk for HIV infection. Exposure to HIV prevention messages at all phases of the migration process may help decrease im/migrants' HIV risk.[9]

The number of individuals with AIDS does not take into account the high number of HIV-infected asymptomatic women. Remember that an HIV infection takes time to develop AIDS. The risks for a woman to expose herself to the HIV virus are through unsafe sex practices, intravenous drug use, and transfusions. A significant number of HIV-infected women have given birth to HIV-infected babies.

There is speculation that pregnancy can accelerate the disease progression of HIV. This rate of AIDS development is faster than for homosexual men or intravenous drug users; approximately 40 percent of asymptomatic carriers of the virus in these categories will develop AIDS.

The AIDS virus will decrease the lymphocytes, which are cells that normally exist in the bloodstream. Lymphocytes are important mediators of the immune system. These cells help fight the development of various diseases. The average time of onset of your viral infection to development of AIDS varies months to years with a mean time of approximately 10 years.

Health-care providers cannot test an individual for HIV without permission. To check a patient for an HIV infection, a doctor must obtain an informed consent from the patient. Informed consent is a legal requirement and means that a doctor must inform a patient that he/she will be tested for HIV.

A patient must sign an agreement that gives a doctor the right to do this test. Without informed consent, a doctor is violating a patient's rights. Informed consent is required in most states before a patient can be tested for HIV.

If a patient received blood products between 1987 and 1995, he/she is at an increased risk of developing AIDS. If a patient has active tuberculosis, he/she runs a higher risk of contracting the HIV virus. Furthermore, if an individual is a health-care provider and have had a needle stick, he/she runs the risk of exposure to the virus.

The name for the initial viral test performed is ELISA (enzyme-linked immunosorbent assay). If /a patient has a positive screening test using ELISA, the infection with the HIV complex is confirmed by a repeat ELISA test as well as another test called a Western blot test.

If a patient is pregnant and has been infected with the HIV virus, the incidence of a premature birth is increased as well as mental retardation of the baby. Otherwise, there is no evidence that the HIV virus affects the outcome of a pregnancy if a patient has no symptoms. If a patient has the HIV virus, he/sheu should be immunized with some vaccines for other diseases.

When AIDS becomes manifest, a patient can develop significant pain with multiple causes. A HIV virus infection is characterized by a deterioration of the body's immune system. This deterioration in the immune system will cause a patient to develop AIDS. A patient has important immune cells in the body called CD4+T. During the HIV infection; the number of these cells progressively declines. When these cells fall to a critical level, a patient is vulnerable to infections as well as cancers.

The HIV virus induces AIDS by causing the death of the CD4+T cells in the body. These cells are important for the normal function of the immune system. The AIDS virus also interferes with their normal function. When this happens, a patient's ability to fight other infections is diminished. The HIV virus is called a slow virus. This means that the course of infection with the HIV virus has a long interval between the initial infection and the onset of the AIDS symptoms.

The HIV virus is unique in that it escapes the body's immune responses. Once infected, a patient can progress to AIDS in an average of 10 years. Combinations of three or more anti-HIV drugs called highly active antiretroviral therapy can delay the progression of the HIV disease for prolonged periods.

As the body's immune system is overwhelmed, increased quantities of the virus enter the bloodstream from cells that were infected. With the increased use of agents for erectile dysfunction, there have been increases in sexual activity among older adults. With this increase in sexual activity, the number of HIV and AIDS cases in elderly patients has increased drastically.

This virus can cause a patient to have a neuropathy. A neuropathy is a lesion in the nerves that are outside of the spinal cord and brain. AIDS can cause one to have a painful neuropathy. A neuropathy associated with AIDS can be intermittent or constant. The pain can vary in severity from mild to severe. The pain can be burning, shooting, aching, or stabbing. It is believed that the HIV virus can cause nerve damage, which is the cause of the neuropathy. A patient can develop headaches from the HIV virus meningitis. Also one can have abdominal pain related to gastrointestinal disease and chest pain related to pneumonia.

The use of receiving an influenza vaccine is if a patient has AIDS is controversial. There is a chance that this vaccine could promote HIV replication for up to three months following a vaccination. If a patient has the HIV virus, he/she runs the risk of being infected with the varicella zoster virus. If one is exposed to chicken pox or shingles, he/she may need an antiviral medication.

A patient should have a tuberculosis test in addition to the other recommended tests. This test is called a PPD test, which is a protein extract from cultures of tuberculin bacteria. This test will tell if a patient has been in contact with tuberculosis. It takes 48 to 72 hours for this test to become positive. If one has a positive test, he/she should receive tuberculosis treatment, which consists of treatment with an antituberculin drug or drugs.

If a patient has been infected with the HIV virus, he/she runs the risk of other bacterial infections. One can also develop gastrointestinal infections as well as pulmonary infections. One can develop a salmonella infection as well as a bacterial pneumonia. Bacterial pneumonias occur frequently in HIV-infected patients. These bacterial pneumonias can be a result of streptococcus pneumonia or H. influenza pneumonia.

A common fungal infection is candidiasis. This fungus can affect the mouth, esophagus, and vagina. These fungal infections are common in HIV-infected individuals. The severity of a fungal infection as well as the other diseases mentioned depends on the degree of suppression of the immune system.

Oral and vaginal fungal infections usually respond to topical therapies. A patient can also develop a fungal infection of the central nervous system. The cryptococcus neoformans fungal infection is the most common cause of central nervous system fungal infections in patients who have developed AIDS.

Some fungal infections are more prevalent in certain areas of the United States. A patient can also develop a histoplasmosis fungal infection if he/she lives around the Ohio Valley, although this type of infection is not limited to this area. A patient can develop a fever, weight loss, and an enlargement of the liver and possibly the spleen. This fungus can affect the bone marrow and decrease some of the blood cells.

Another fungal infection that is prevalent in the southwestern United States that can cause patient problems is the coccidioides immitis. This fungal frequently affects the lungs. Aspergillosis is another fungus that can infect a patient. When these different organisms affect the body, a patient can have generalized pain, including muscle pain, joint pain, and headaches. One of the leading causes of death in individuals with AIDS is the pneumocystis carinii pneumonia. This is the most common infection in AIDS patients and is the leading cause of death in this patient population. Not only does this disease affect the lungs; it can affect other parts of the body as well.

If one has have AIDS, a patient can also develop tumors associated with AIDS. These tumors include Kaposi's sarcoma as well as Hodgkin and non-Hodgkin lymphoma. Another type of infection that a patient can develop is a protozoan infection. A protozoa infection example is toxoplasma gondii, which can cause a serious infection of the central nervous system.

Cryptosporidium is an infection that can give a patient chronic diarrhea. Usually this parasite can be observed in the stool. Other protozoal infections can cause a patient to have chronic diarrhea as well. Another protozoon that can cause generalized infections in the body is the strongyloides protozoa.

Gender differences between men and women are noted. With respect to AIDS, women's bodies differ from men's bodies. Drug companies are doing studies to see whether there is any evidence that women respond differently to the AIDS drugs. A study at Johns Hopkins revealed that women were progressing to AIDS at the same rate as men, but it only took half the viral infection that it took to infect men.

It is now known that there are gender differences in HIV. A study in Kenya revealed that women were often infected by multiple virus variants as opposed to men. In other words, the HIV infecting the men appeared to be of one type of HIV virus, whereas women have several different variants of the virus. It was speculated that the virus was mutating faster in women than in men. Women naturally have more cells in their bodies that recognize and attack the HIV virus.

It is thought that women's stronger immune response than men to the virus could force the virus to mutate or it is possible that women have a greater infection of the virus than men. In other words, women probably get a larger dose of the virus when they are infected than men. If women are infected with more versions of the HIV virus, this could mean that they would react differently to different drugs or to different vaccines. Women who are infected with the smaller number of the HIV virus became sick at the same rate as did men.

It has been reported recently by the American Civil Liberties Union that there are civil rights violations against individuals who have HIV and AIDS. The ACLU related that individuals are being fired, rental agreements are destroyed, and they receive inadequate care when they relate that they have HIV or AIDS. It is estimated that 900,000 people in the United States have AIDS or HIV. They are denied medical treatment and are discriminated against in their workplace. They have difficulty getting into nursing homes as well.

In New York, an AIDS mortality rate per 10,000 persons age 15 to 64 was studied. AIDS was among the five leading causes of death for men age 25 to 54 and the leading cause of death for men age 30 to 39. For women, AIDS was the fourth leading cause of death for women age 25 to 29 and the second-leading cause of death for women age 30 to 34. Premature mortality was noted to be 10 percent in men age 15 to 64 and 3.6 percent for women.

Condom use has been recommended as a method to prevent HIV transmission. A study published in 1989 revealed that 62 percent of men used condoms to prevent HIV virus transmission, whereas only 17 percent of women purchased or used condoms to prevent AIDS trans-mission. Public health professionals have been concerned about the devastation caused by HIV and AIDS in the developing world.

It is estimated that 10 percent of people in South Africa are infected with HIV. These rates are higher in other African countries. In Africa, for some reason, the HIV virus passes from women to men at a higher rate of efficiency than is observed in the West. In the year 2000, then-President Clinton declared the world AIDS epidemic a threat to U.S. national security.

It is estimated that if 1 million people in the United States now have HIV or AIDS, approximately 500,000 of them are either untreated or undiagnosed. Drugs for the treatment of AIDS are constantly being developed. Essentially, AIDS has gone from being an immediate sentence of death to a chronic manageable disease.

Currently, Russia has the fastest growing epidemic of AIDS, thought to be because of intravenous drug use. Epidemics are now beginning in China. The rate of AIDS cases and deaths did slowdown, which was attributed to successful antiretroviral therapy. The problem with some of the drug therapy is that some individuals either develop a resistance to the drugs, or they experience side effects from the drugs and stop taking them.

The aging population of people living with human immunodeficiency virus is exposed to a widening spectrum of non-AIDS-defining diseases. Coordinated health care throughout patients' lives is crucial, as health-care pathways evolve toward outpatient care as the patients get older.[10]

An effective vaccine against HIV infection continues to be researched. That one "magic bullet" remains to be developed. Some of the vaccines currently being studied provide protection for some individuals but not all. Two anti-HIV drugs have been shown to cause death in some pregnant women. These drugs are stavudine and didanosine. Between 1991 and 1995, there was a 63 percent increase in women diagnosed with AIDS. The increase in HIV infection in men was noted in younger women who date older men.

HIV infection increases the risk of non-communicable diseases common in the aged, including cardiovascular disease, neurocognitive decline, non-AIDS malignancies, osteoporosis, and frailty. These observations suggest that HIV accelerates immunological ageing, and there are many immunological similarities with the aged, including shortened telomeres.[11]

It has been shown that young women are less likely to insist that older men wear condoms during sexual intercourse. When HIV and AIDS was first made known in the 1980s, it was a disease of gay men as well as a disease of people who had received blood transfusions or individuals who shared needles for injecting drugs. An increasing number of women with AIDS have been reported, and the exposure to the HIV virus was through heterosexual sex.

The pain can be treated with narcotic drugs as well as antidepressants and anticonvulsant medications such as Neurontin. Mexiletine, an anticonvulsant medication, may also help to control the pain. Exercise therapy is sometimes beneficial for the management of the pain. It is believed that exercise can increase the body's endorphins, which in turns helps to manage pain. HIV-related pain becomes increasingly severe as the disease progresses.

Drugs used to treat the HIV infection can cause neuropathic pain. It is estimated that 30 percent of the neuropathic pain syndromes suffered by individuals who have the HIV disease are caused by drugs to attack the HIV virus. Neuropathic pain in the HIV-infected patient in most instances can be adequately controlled.

New therapies and increased knowledge about the causes of pain associated with the HIV virus has given HIV-infected individuals an increased quality and duration of life that several years ago would have been totally unimaginable. Overall, the AIDS incidence and mortality have continued to decline, probably because of new therapies, especially antiviral therapies.

However, for women, the benefits have been shown to be less than for men. It has been reported that there is gender-based discrimination in the treatment of women with HIV infections. It is also reported that there is insufficient attention to the medical community's response to women's HIV risks.

HIV Treatments include: Entry inhibitors, Integrase inhibitors, Nucleoside/nucleotide reverse transcriptase inhibitors, Non-nucleoside reverse transcriptase inhibitors, and Protease inhibitors.

HIV drugs are always used in combination to attack the virus at different points in its life cycle. This usually means using drugs from at least two classes. Highly active antiretroviral therapy has greatly reduced the morbidity and mortality of HIV/AIDS patients but has also been associated with increased metabolic complications and cardiovascular diseases.[12] The increased life expectancy of HIV-infected individuals due to improved treatment has revealed an unexpected increase in non-AIDS comorbidities that are typically associated with older age including cardiovascular disease, dementia and frailty.[13]

Combining HIV drugs is the best way to reduce the amount of HIV in the blood (viral load). Other important modalities include: Exercise therapy will help release endorphins that can help inhibit the pain. Prescriptions such as anticonvulsants, antidepressants, and narcotics should be taken to relieve the pain. New therapies are constantly evolving for HIV and the treatment of its pain.

References

1. Choi J, Fauce SR, Effros RB. Reduced telomerase activity in human T lymphocytes exposed to cortisol. Brain Behav Immun. 2008;22(4):600-605.
2. Effros RB. Telomere/telomerase dynamics within the human immune system: effect of chronic infection and stress. Exp Gerontol. 2011;46(2-3):135-140.
3. Hearps AC, Maisa A, Cheng WJ, et al. HIV infection induces age-related changes to monocytes and innate immune activation in young men that persist despite combination antiretroviral therapy. AIDS. 2012;26(7):843-853.
4. Hachfeld A, Ledergerber B, Darling K, et al. Reasons for late presentation to HIV care in Switzerland. J Int AIDS Soc. 2015;18:20317.
5. Chou JP, Effros RB. T cell replicative senescence in human aging. Curr Pharm Des. 2013;19(9):1680-1698.
6. Hirshfield S, Grov C, Parsons JT, Anderson I, Chiasson MA. Social media use and HIV transmission risk behavior among ethnically diverse HIV-positive gay men: results of an online study in three U.S. states. Arch Sex Behav. 2015;44(7):1969-1978.
7. Wejnert C, Hess KL, Rose CE, et al. Age-Specific Race and Ethnicity Disparities in HIV Infection and Awareness Among Men Who Have Sex With Men--20 US Cities, 2008-2014. J Infect Dis. 2016;213(5):776-783.
8. Hoots BE, Finlayson TJ, Wejnert C, Paz-Bailey G, Group NS. Early Linkage to HIV Care and Antiretroviral Treatment among Men Who Have Sex with Men--20 Cities, United States, 2008 and 2011. PLoS One. 2015;10(7):e0132962.
9. Martinez-Donate AP, Rangel MG, Zhang X, et al. HIV Prevention Among Mexican Migrants at Different Migration Phases: Exposure to Prevention Messages and Association With Testing Behaviors. AIDS Educ Prev. 2015;27(6):547-565.
10. Jacomet C, Berland P, Guiguet M, et al. Impact of age on care pathways of people living with HIV followed up in hospital. AIDS Care. 2016:1-7.

11. Hearps AC, Martin GE, Rajasuriar R, Crowe SM. Inflammatory co-morbidities in HIV+ individuals: learning lessons from healthy ageing. Curr HIV/AIDS Rep. 2014;11(1):20-34.

12. Dimala CA, Atashili J, Mbuagbaw JC, Wilfred A, Monekosso GL. Prevalence of Hypertension in HIV/AIDS Patients on Highly Active Antiretroviral Therapy (HAART) Compared with HAART-Naive Patients at the Limbe Regional Hospital, Cameroon. PLoS One. 2016;11(2):e0148100.

13. Bestilny LJ, Gill MJ, Mody CH, Riabowol KT. Accelerated replicative senescence of the peripheral immune system induced by HIV infection. AIDS. 2000;14(7):771-780.

35. Arthritis

Arthritis is the painful inflammation of the joints in the body and is common in older individuals. Arthritis can be defined as a degenerative inflammatory disorder affecting joints and muscles. Arthritis is painful inflammation of the joints caused by the wearing away of surface cartilage covering the bone. Eventually, small pieces of bone may break off and float freely in the joint causing greater pain and inflammation.

Telomeres are specialized nucleoproteic structures that cap and protect the ends of chromosomes. They can be elongated by the telomerase enzyme, but in telomerase negative cells, telomeres shorten after each cellular division because of the end replicating problem. This phenomenon leads ultimately to cellular senescence, conferring to the telomeres a role of biological clock. Oxidative stress, inflammation and increased cell renewal are supplementary environmental factors that accelerate age-related telomere shortening.[1]

The incidence of osteoarthritis (OA), the disease characterized by joint pain and loss of joint form and function due to articular cartilage degeneration, is directly correlated with age. The strong association between age and increasing incidence of osteoarthritis (OA) marks OA as an age related disease.[2] Osteoarthritis is the most common disease of joints caused by degradation of articular cartilage and subchondral bone. It is classified as primary form with unknown cause and as secondary form with known etiology. Genetic and epigenetic factors interact with environmental factors and contribute to the development of primary osteoarthritis. It also is called degenerative joint disease.

Osteoarthritis is the most common forms of arthritis, which largely affects the elderly. Osteoarthritis occurs in the joints of the body when the cartilage is worn down and damaged by overuse, sometimes allowing the rigid and brittle bone ends to come into direct contact with each other. The bones that compose the joint can then break down and develop irregular growths called osteophytes that can interfere with the proper movement of the joint and cause pain. In younger patients the joints provide range of motion and do support the body as well. To have normal and painless range of motion, the joints must have cartilage in between the bones.

During the last 10 years, studies on the telomere/telomerase system in autoimmune and/or systemic immune-mediated diseases have revealed its involvement in relevant physiopathological processes. Restoring defective telomerase activity emerges as a therapeutic target in resetting immune abnormalities in RA.3 Telomerase is a reverse transcriptase enzyme contributing to the maintenance of the telomeric structure by adding telomere repeat sequences to chromosomal ends, thus compensating for its shortening. Telomerase activity which is common in cancers and human germ line tissue, may also be increased, although to a lesser extent, in systemic autoimmune diseases.[4]

Bone spurs may also develop on the ends of the bone, which in addition contribute to pain and inflammation. Arthritis can be defined as a degenerative inflammatory disorder affecting the joints and muscles. There are various forms of arthritis, including inflammatory rheumatoid arthritis and non-inflammatory osteoarthritis. Arthritis is considered as the most common elderly related disease. The principal reason for arthritis among elderly patients has been attributed to lifestyle factors, including consumption of high-fat, high-cholesterol diet and sedentary behaviors.

Approximately, one out of seven people has some form of arthritis, and there are many different types a patient can have. More than 35 million people in the United States suffer from this disease, and every year treatment costs the United States billions of dollars. While arthritis is often thought of as an elderly patient disorder, and it is more common among seniors, arthritis can affect people of all ages.

Inflammation that occurs in the joints can cause pain as well as swelling of the joints. Joints in the arms and legs permit movement of the arms and legs. The bones of the joints are held together by a capsule that consists of a dense strong tissue; further, the joints are held by ligaments, which connect bones to each other. The joint is supported by muscles or tendons that lie over the joints. Tendons connect muscles to bones. On the inside of the joint, the surface of the joint is covered with a tissue called a synovium.

This tissue has special cells that exist within the lining of the synovial tissue. Some of these cells help to form some of the components that make the fluid in the synovial tissue thick. This thick fluid is like motor oil. A thick fluid will provide the joints with better lubricating properties than a watery fluid. The fluid that exists in the synovium lubricates the surfaces of the bones and cartilage that make up the joint. Cartilage is a tough, slippery layer of tissue that covers the surfaces where bones contact each other in joints.

Synovial tissues contain many blood vessels. The synovium also contains sympathetic fibers. This anatomical feature can be important if one develops an entity called reflex sympathetic dystrophy. There is also a joint in the body where the back bone meets the hip bone. This is called the sacroiliac joint. This joint is only slightly movable. Even though this joint does not move freely, it can cause significant pain. Other sites or cells exist in the joint that secretes chemicals that rebuild and degrade the joint. This process of rebuilding and degrading the joint keeps the joint anatomy in balance. If the joint becomes degraded, it will degenerate, and will develop arthritis in the degenerating joint.

Ultra-short telomeres caused by stress-induced telomere shortening are suggested to induce chondrocyte senescence in human osteoarthritic knees. There is a role of short telomeres in the development of arthritis in aging of articular cartilage.[5]

Weight loss and fatigue can be associated with rheumatoid arthritis. Scientists analyzed telomere length of individual chromosomes in peripheral blood lymphocytes of healthy individuals and patients with rheumatoid arthritis. Patients with rheumatoid arthritis had significantly shorter chromosome 4p telomeres, which can be essential for pathogenesis of this multifactorial disease.[6]

Normal joint fluid should be clear and straw colored. If a patient has osteoarthritis, the fluid can be straw colored. Other types of arthritis include rheumatoid arthritis or gout. The fluid may be yellow. The blood will be examined for any elevation in the white cells (a sign of inflammation), and a test for rheumatoid arthritis can be done at the same time.

A bone scan consists of injecting a very small and harmless dose of radioactive dye into the vein. After this has been done, a special camera takes a picture of the painful area. If a patient has arthritis, there will be an increased uptake of the radioactive material into the painful joint, showing that the joint is inflamed. Inflammation is the responses of the body's tissues to irritation or injury. The affected tissue can become warm swollen and/or red. The severity of inflammation depends on the cause, and the area affected.

Cartilage is a tissue that coats the ends of the bones. The synovium surrounds the bones as well as the cartilage. The cartilage does not have its own blood supply. This synovium is, therefore, filled with a liquid, and the synovial fluid supplies sugar and other nutrients as well as oxygen to the cartilage. The cartilage is also composed of collagen. Collagen gives the joint support as well as flexibility.

Osteoarthritis does not spread throughout the entire body and cause problems outside of the joints as may happen in other arthritic diseases such as rheumatoid arthritis. It is confined to the joints. Other arthritic diseases such as rheumatoid arthritis can affect the lungs and the heart. Pain in a joint in the arm or leg or the back or neck is usually the major symptom from osteoarthritis. Osteoarthritis can cause not only pain in the arms and legs, but also in the spine.

Osteoarthritis of the spine can occur in the neck, lower back, or even the mid back. Degenerative arthritis can become evident in the hips. Pain usually develops in the hips slowly. The pain in the hips can be referred to the buttocks or to the groin. Osteoarthritis also can become evident in the knees. The knee may become warm as well as swollen and may exhibit decreased range of motion in the knees over time.

Osteoarthritis also can affect the joints in the hands. Osteoarthritis can cause a painful range of motion around the fingers. In all of these bone structures affected by osteoarthritis, be aware that osteophytes can form in the joints. The osteophytes that form at the margins of the joints can be a source of pain.

The joint pain originates from nerves that transmit pain impulses located in the tendons, ligaments, periosteum of the bones, and the synovium of the joints. One chemical, substance P, is frequently released in joints. Capsaicin cream that depletes substance P from the nerve endings can be used to manage the joint pain.

Osteoarthritis usually occurs in older people. Approximately, 85 percent of people over 65 develop osteoarthritis. However, only half of these people experience any symptoms. Caucasians have a higher incidence of osteoarthritis than other ethnic groups. Before age 45, this disease occurs more frequently in men.

After age 55, osteoarthritis is seen more often in women. Osteoarthritis involving the knee is more prevalent in women than in men, perhaps a result of wearing high-heeled shoes. Obesity puts an increased pressure and stress on the joints in the legs. Any excess weight that a patient has may cause deterioration of the joints in the hips, knees, and ankles.

Women tend to report joint pain more often than men. If a patient has a weakness in the thigh muscles, called the quadriceps, he/she may be prone to develop osteoarthritis of the knees. Osteoarthritis can occur after trauma to a joint. Repetitive motions required in the job can also cause the onset of osteoarthritis.

The management of the osteoarthritic pain first involves correction of any abnormal biomechanics. One way of changing an irregular biomechanical factor is weight reduction. Obesity increases the incidence of osteoarthritis of the knees more in women than men. A cane or shoes that fit right and provide a cushion can decrease symptoms associated with osteoarthritis.

Telomere shortening is associated with a number of common age-related diseases. The quantification of ultra-short telomeres, stress a role of telomere shortening in human osteoarthritis.[7] The decreased telomere size and increased chromosome instability in chondrocytes from osteoarthritis affected joints may imply a local advanced senescence that could contribute to the pathogenesis or progression of the degenerative articular disease.[8] The presence of oxidative stress induces telomere genomic instability, replicative senescence and dysfunction of chondrocytes in OA cartilage, suggesting that oxidative stress, leading to chondrocyte senescence and cartilage ageing, might be responsible for the development of OA.[9]

Nonsteroidal anti-inflammatory medications are commonly used to treat osteoarthritis (for example, Celebrex, Mobic, and Day Pro). Be aware that nonsteroidal anti-inflammatory drugs may cause gastrointestinal complications. Steroid injections into the joints can also decrease the inflammation of the joints, which will decrease the pain. The doctor can also inject hyaluronic acid into the joints for pain modification. Glucosamine, which is available without a prescription, has been demonstrated to decrease pain associated with osteoarthritis.

Another form of arthritis is rheumatoid arthritis. This arthritis is characterized by redness, warmth, swelling, and painful joints. If a patient has rheumatoid arthritis, he/she will have decreased range of motion of some of the joints in the body. A patient also may complain of stiffness. The pathogenesis of RA, a disabling autoimmune disease, is incompletely understood. Early in the development of RA there appears to be loss of immune homeostasis and regulation, and premature immunosenescence.[10] This disease attacks the synovial linings of the joints as well as the tendons about the joints. Rheumatoid arthritis is a chronic inflammatory polyarthritis and is thought to be an autoimmune, multifactorial and polygenic disease.[11] The genetic predisposition to rheumatoid arthritis is confirmed by many family studies.

The exact cause of rheumatoid arthritis is unknown, but approximately 43 million people in the United States suffer from rheumatoid arthritis. Rheumatoid arthritis affects men and women, all races, and all ages. However, rheumatoid arthritis is three times more common in women than in men.

Family history plays an important role in the development of rheumatoid arthritis. Rheumatoid arthritis may result from an abnormality in the immune system. The antibodies may attack the joints to cause significant degeneration within the joints. It can usually have a slow onset. However, be aware that it can have an acute onset as well. The onset of rheumatoid arthritis occurs more often in the winter.

If patients are between the ages of 30 and 50, the chance of developing rheumatoid arthritis are increased. The rate of bone formation is largely determined by the number of osteoblasts, which in turn is determined by the rate of replication of progenitors and the life span of mature cells, reflecting the timing of death by apoptosis.[12] The accelerated WBC telomere shortening in RA occurs as a result of exposure to chronic inflammation.13

The treatment of rheumatoid arthritis is to relieve the pain and decrease the joint inflammation. In addition, the health-care provider will want to maintain as much range of motion about the joints as possible. Splinting, range of motion exercises and strengthening exercises can be extremely beneficial as well.

Elderly-onset rheumatoid arthritis is defined as RA starting after 60 years of age. Compared to RA in younger patients, it's characterized by a lower female/male ratio and frequently has an acute onset. Usually nonsteroidal anti-inflammatory drugs are prescribed for the management of the arthritic pain. As mentioned with regard to osteoarthritis, the COX-2 inhibitor, Celebrex is safer for the gastrointestinal system than the older nonsteroidal anti-inflammatory drugs.

Some doctors prescribe medications such as gold compounds, antimalarials, and sulfasalazine. However, each of these drugs has the potential to cause serious side effects. Steroids also may be necessary to decrease the inflammation of the joints. Steroids typically decrease pain and swelling.

If these methods do not relieve the pain, a patient may be a candidate for immunosuppressive therapy. Immunosuppressive therapy is the administration of a drug which eliminates or lessens an immune response. Methotrexate is used frequently for the treatment of the rheumatoid arthritis. Methotrexate can cause liver pathology. Surgery is the last resort for the treatment of rheumatoid arthritis and consists of total joint replacement. If the pain becomes intolerable, and if a patient has significant limitations in joint function, surgery can provide one with relief.

Joint replacements are now available for hips, knees, shoulders, elbows, and ankles. The American College of Rheumatology recommended, in their 2002 guidelines for the treatment of RA, early aggressive treatment with disease modifying anti-rheumatic drugs (DMARDs). Older patients receive lower doses of methotrexate. They're less likely to be treated with DMARD combinations, more likely to be taking prednisone, and are less often treated with new biologics. Both infliximab and etanercept are no less effective and no more toxic in RA patients over 65 than they are in the nger age group. Equal care must be provided in all age groups.

Be aware that sex hormones may play a role in the development of rheumatoid arthritis. Sex hormones can block some of the mechanisms involved in the development of rheumatoid arthritis. A premenopausal woman could develop rheumatoid arthritis if she has low levels of DHEA as well as testosterone. Both of these chemicals are called androgens. Apparently, androgens are of some benefit to a patient in preventing progression of this disease. On the other hand, men who have rheumatoid arthritis usually have low testosterone levels. Some medical scientists think that testosterone may decrease the incidence of rheumatoid arthritis. In addition, a history of smoking is associated with an increased risk for the development of rheumatoid arthritis in men but not in women.

Ankylosing spondylitis is a disease that predominantly affects men. Pain usually begins in the back and sacroiliac joint (the joint where the back and hip bones meet) early in life. An x-ray of the spine of a male with ankylosing spondylitis appears as bamboo and is called a bamboo spine. This pattern is also seen on MRI imaging studies. Ankylosing spondylitis usually affects men before the age of 40. Ankylosing spondylitis is present in 8 percent of Caucasians and 3 percent of African-American men A marker in the bloodstream called HLA-B27 is present in 90 percent of patients who have ankylosing spondylitis.

Usually ankylosing spondylitis will become manifest in a male around age 20. This arthritic disease does occur in women, but the symptoms are more prominent in men. The primary symptoms may be symptoms in the hip joints. A patient may have a progressive decrease of the back range of motion. may have some pain in the joints of the arms and legs as well. X-rays have shown arthritis in sacroiliac joints. Over time, the spine will continue to stiffen. The onset of ankylosing spondylitis is gradual. If the disease progresses, the lumbar spine symptoms will go upward toward the neck. The normal curve in the lower back will become straight. If the ankylosing spondylitis advances, the entire spine may become fused, which restricts the motion about the spine in all directions.

The earliest x-ray changes usually occur in the sacroiliac joints. Erosion of these joints becomes evident. The outer rings of the discs in the spine become calcified. Furthermore, calcification of the vertical ligaments that run in front and back of the vertebral bones occurs. When this happens, if one has an x-ray of the spine, it will appear as a bamboo stick. Remember that rheumatoid arthritis affects mostly small joints. Ankylosing spondylitis affects large joints. Osteoarthritis does not usually affect the sacroiliac joints.

If a patient has ankylosing spondylitis, physical therapy and non-steroidal anti-inflammatory drugs are important for the treatment of the pain associated with this disease. No treatment is currently available that will eradicate ankylosing spondylitis.

Occasionally stronger analgesics such as opioids are needed to control the pain. Sulfasalazine is sometimes useful for pain in arthritis in the arms and legs. The problem with ankylosing spondylitis is that one can have pain that is severe over decades of the life. The severity of the pain associated with this disease varies greatly. Approximately, 10 percent of patients have disability so severe that they are unable to return to work after 10 years.

Gout is the most common auto-inflammatory arthritis that leads to severe comorbidities such as cardiovascular diseases, renal impairment and metabolic disorders at an early age.[14] Gout results from crystals of uric acid that are deposited into joint spaces between the bones. These uric acid crystals deposited into the joints cause inflammation with swelling, redness, and warmth about the joint. Gout in the elderly differs from classical gout found in middle-aged men in several respects: it has a more equal gender distribution, frequent polyarticular presentation with involvement of the joints of the upper extremities, fewer acute gouty episodes, a more lethargic chronic clinical course, and an increased incidence of tophi.

In most people, uric acid is dissolved in the bloodstream and excreted through the kidneys. If the kidneys do not eliminate enough uric acid from the bloodstream, the uric acid will increase in the bloodstream. In many people, the uric acid deposits affect the joints in their great toes. The big toe is affected in approximately 75 percent of people suffering gout. The ankles, heels, knees, wrists, and fingers may also be affected by gouty arthritis.

Gout is more common in men than in women and is more prevalent in adults than in children. Obesity increases the risk of developing gout. An excess consumption of alcohol also interferes with the excretion of uric acid from the body. The increased uric acid that occurs can form crystals and deposit these crystals into the joints.

Adult men between the ages of 40 and 50 are most likely to develop gout. It is occasionally seen in women. It rarely occurs before menopause. Long term diuretic use in elderly patients with hypertension or congestive cardiac failure, renal insufficiency, prophylactic low-dose aspirin, and alcohol abuse are factors associated with the development of gout in the elderly.

A diagnosis of gout can be made by withdrawing fluid from the painful joints and analyzing the fluid for uric acid. When the gout attack is extreme, may be totally incapacitated. If the gout is not treated, may develop severe pathology of the affected joints. African-American men have a higher incidence of gout than Caucasian men.

The prevalence for men is nearly 14 cases per 1,000 men, whereas the prevalence in women is approximately 6 cases per 1,000 women. Estrogen hormones noted in women can help the body eliminate uric acid. For this reason, gout is rarely seen in premenopausal women.

When a gout attack occurs, the maximum pain associated with the gout usually occurs in approximately the first 10 hours. In general, attacks resolve in less than 14 days. Uric acid crystals can not only be deposited in the joints; they can also form in the soft tissues. A collection of uric acid crystals in the tissues can form a lump (called a tophi), often noted on the outer edges of the forearms. Tophi are nodules under the skin. Be aware that if a patient ha gout, he/she will have an increased risk of developing kidney stones. These stones are usually composed of uric acid.

Gout develops when there is an excessive amount of uric acid. Uric acid crystals are usually formed when the uric acid level exceeds 6.8 mg/dL. Sometimes overproduction of uric acid is related to a genetic disorder.

Excessive exercise can also increase uric acid, as can obesity. Starvation or dehydration can increase uric acid, too. Thyroid disease can also increase uric acid. Diuretics (medications that make one urinate), such as furosemide (Lasix) and hydrochlorothiazide (HCTZ), a common blood pressure medicine) and cyclosporine A (an immunosuppressive medicine) can increase the uric acid concentration in the bloodstream.

Approximately, 5 percent of the population has an elevated serum uric acid level. Only approximately 10 percent of these individuals develop gout. Therefore, an elevated uric acid level in the bloodstream does not mean that a patient has or will develop gouty arthritis. The diagnosis of gout is made by finding uric acid crystals in the fluid of the joints.

Colchicine is the medication that has been used extensively over the past two decades for the treatment of gout. It is most effective during the first 24 hours of an acute attack. Colchicine can cause a patient to have vomiting and nausea. If one has liver problems, the patient should not take colchicine.

Allopurinol is another drug that can decrease the uric acid levels. Allopurinol is usually used in people who produce excessive uric acid. Allopurinol should not be used during an acute gouty arthritis episode because allopurinol can prolong the attack. Probenecid is used by some rheumatologists because it has fewer side effects than Allopurinol.

If a patient has developed tophi (nodules under the skin) that are painful, he/she may need to have the uric acid crystals removed surgically. If a patient has significant destruction of one of the joints, an orthopedic surgeon may need to surgically correct any malformation that may be related to uric acid deposition in the joints and the resultant joint destruction.

Patients with systemic lupus erythematosus (SLE) have a higher rate of premature death compared to the general population, suggesting a phenotype of premature senescence in SLE.[15] Lupus is an autoimmune disease that can affect various parts of the body, including the skin, joints, heart, lungs, blood, kidneys, and brain. Normally, the body's immune system makes proteins called antibodies to protect the body against viruses, bacteria, and other foreign materials. The new ELISA for anti-telomere antibodies using standardized human dsDNA as antigen is a sensitive and highly specific test for SLE.[16]

Psoriatic arthritis occurs when the body's immune system begins to attack healthy cells and tissue. Psoriatic arthritis can affect joints on just one side or on both sides of the body. The signs and symptoms of psoriatic arthritis often resemble those of rheumatoid arthritis. Both diseases cause joints to become painful, swollen and warm to the touch. The age of psoriasis onset has an important impact on the clinical expression and heritability of psoriasis. Psoriasis characteristics according to the age at disease onset have been extensively studied. Clinical and genetic features of psoriasis may differ depending on the age at psoriasis onset.[17]

Drugs used to treat psoriatic arthritis as in other arthritic diseases include: Nonsteroidal anti-inflammatory drugs, disease-modifying anti rheumatic drugs, immune suppressants and tumor necrosis factor-alpha inhibitors.

Current research involves the study of new and safer medications for the treatment of all types of arthritis. Anti-inflammatory medications such as ibuprofen and acetaminophen will help reduce the swelling and pain sensations are experiencing. Physical therapy can help relieve the pain associated with the arthritis. Massage therapy can relax the muscles and often relieve swelling in the muscles and help the arthritis pain. Acupuncture can stimulate nerve fibers and help decrease the pain as well.

References

1. Georgin-Lavialle S, Aouba A, Mouthon L, et al. The telomere/telomerase system in autoimmune and systemic immune-mediated diseases. Autoimmun Rev. 2010;9(10):646-651.

2. Martin JA, Buckwalter JA. Aging, articular cartilage chondrocyte senescence and osteoarthritis. Biogerontology. 2002;3(5):257-264.

3. Fujii H, Shao L, Colmegna I, Goronzy JJ, Weyand CM. Telomerase insufficiency in rheumatoid arthritis. Proc Natl Acad Sci U S A. 2009;106(11):4360-4365.

4. Tarhan F, Vural F, Kosova B, et al. Telomerase activity in connective tissue diseases: elevated in rheumatoid arthritis, but markedly decreased in systemic sclerosis. Rheumatol Int. 2008;28(6):579-583.

5. Harbo M, Delaisse JM, Kjaersgaard-Andersen P, Soerensen FB, Koelvraa S, Bendix L. The relationship between ultra-short telomeres, aging of articular cartilage and the development of human hip osteoarthritis. Mech Ageing Dev. 2013;134(9):367-372.

6. Blinova EA, Zinnatova EV, Barkovskaya M, et al. Telomere Length of Individual Chromosomes in Patients with Rheumatoid Arthritis. Bull Exp Biol Med. 2016;160(6):779-782.

7. Harbo M, Bendix L, Bay-Jensen AC, et al. The distribution pattern of critically short telomeres in human osteoarthritic knees. Arthritis Res Ther. 2012;14(1):R12.

8. Tamayo M, Mosquera A, Rego I, Blanco FJ, Gosalvez J, Fernandez JL. Decreased length of telomeric DNA sequences and increased numerical chromosome aberrations in human osteoarthritic chondrocytes. Mutat Res. 2011;708(1-2):50-58.

9. Yudoh K, Nguyen v T, Nakamura H, Hongo-Masuko K, Kato T, Nishioka K. Potential involvement of oxidative stress in cartilage senescence and development of osteoarthritis: oxidative stress induces chondrocyte telomere instability and downregulation of chondrocyte function. Arthritis Res Ther. 2005;7(2):R380-391.

10. Costenbader KH, Prescott J, Zee RY, De Vivo I. Immunosenescence and rheumatoid arthritis: does telomere shortening predict impending disease? Autoimmun Rev. 2011;10(9):569-573.

11. Kawabata K, Yamamoto K. [Recent advances in the pathogenesis of rheumatoid arthritis]. Clin Calcium. 2009;19(3):303-309.

12. Yudoh K, Matsuno H. The role of telomerase in joint deterioration in rheumatoid arthritis. Drugs Today (Barc). 2001;37(9):595-606.

13. Steer SE, Williams FM, Kato B, et al. Reduced telomere length in rheumatoid arthritis is independent of disease activity and duration. Ann Rheum Dis. 2007;66(4):476-480.

14. Vazirpanah N, Radstake TR, Broen JC. Inflamm-ageing and Senescence in Gout: The Tale of an Old King's Disease. Curr Aging Sci. 2015;8(2):186-201.

15. Haque S, Rakieh C, Marriage F, et al. Shortened telomere length in patients with systemic lupus erythematosus. Arthritis Rheum. 2013;65(5):1319-1323.

16. Salonen EM, Miettinen A, Walle TK, Koskenmies S, Kere J, Julkunen H. Anti-telomere antibodies in systemic lupus erythematosus

(SLE): a comparison with five antinuclear antibody assays in 430 patients with SLE and other rheumatic diseases. Ann Rheum Dis. 2004;63(10):1250-1254.

17. Queiro R, Alperi M, Alonso-Castro S, et al. Patients with psoriatic arthritis may show differences in their clinical and genetic profiles depending on their age at psoriasis onset. Clin Exp Rheumatol. 2012;30(4):476-480.

36. Abdominal Pain

Pain in the abdomen can be disabling and can be severe. Abdominal pain in general occurs more often in women than in men. The incidence of abdominal pain decreases with age. On the other hand, many elderly patients with serious abdominal pathology initially are misdiagnosed with benign conditions such as gastroenteritis or constipation. Many elderly patients with abdominal pain will have a functional disorder such as an irritable bowel syndrome.

Even though abdominal pain among the elderly is reported to be decreased in aging individuals, the irritable bowel syndrome (IBS) in people over the age of 65 is under recognized. IBS is a highly prevalent and frequently lifelong gastrointestinal disorder. Epidemiological studies suggest that the prevalence of IBS declines with age.

IBS is frequently associated with non-colonic symptoms, including lethargy, backache and chest pains, which can result in inappropriate referral of elderly patients to different specialties with the condition remaining unrecognized. IBS is the most common functional disorder of the gastrointestinal tract. A study is currently being done to attempt to find out what physiological or psychological change associated with aging may protect you against continuation of the abdominal pain.

Cramping and intermittent pain is easily caused by disorders of the bowel, gallbladder, ureter, or fallopian tubes. This chapter includes information about an irritable bowel syndrome that can be associated with bloating. Irritable bowel syndrome is under-recognized in elderly care.

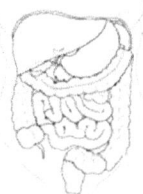

Figure 1. The abdomen has many organs that can cause chronic pain.

A common syndrome in adults is the irritable bowel syndrome (IBS), which is frequently diagnosed in the general population. Approximately 30 percent of patients seen by gastroenterologists suffer from IBS. It is more common in women and may even be seen in adolescents. This disease has begun to become more closely studied, and the pharmaceutical industry has begun marketing new drugs to decrease the symptoms of IBS.

The exact cause of IBS remains to be discovered. IBS has become a defined clinical entity. IBS can be caused by physiological, psychological, and behavioral factors. Sometimes you may have severe symptoms without any physical findings. A diagnosis of IBS is determined by the symptoms. There is increased prevalence of diverticulosis and intra-abdominal surgeries like hysterectomies and cholecystectomies in the elderly, and these entities have the potential to cause and/or contribute to symptoms that mimic IBS.

This pain is not confined in one area of the gut, but it is global over the stomach. Usually this abdominal pain is relieved followed a bowel movement. A patient may suffer diarrhea alternating with constipation. Some investigators believe that the colon is the cause of IBS. A patient can have symptoms daily, or may have symptoms once a week or once a month. IBS can involve the central nervous system (the brain and spinal cord) as well. If a patient suffers from psychological distress, he/she can have a negative effect on the central nervous system that may send signals to the peripheral nervous system and cause one to have hypersensitivity with respect to the gastrointestinal (mouth to rectum) system. IBS can coexist with ulcerative colitis or Crohn's disease.

Pain associated with IBS can be a result of depression or other illness. Stress and diet are currently being investigated as causes of abdominal pain in general. The gastrointestinal pain will decline after age 40. The pattern of declining abdominal pain is consistent in both sexes. However, overall, the incidence of abdominal pain is higher in women than in men from childhood years to old age. These findings of various abdominal pains include pain in the upper, mid, or lower abdomen.

A diagnostic criterion for the diagnosis of IBS is hard to establish because of the variety of physical complaints associated with IBS. In other words, the pattern of the pain as well as the location and severity differ among patients. To be diagnosed with IBS, a patient needs to have abdominal pain first of all. The pain must be relieved with a bowel movement. The onset of the pain must be associated with a change in the frequency of the stool habits. The onset of the pain must be associated with a change in the appearance of the stool.

Approximately, 70 percent of individuals with IBS have only mild symptoms. On the other hand, 25 percent of patients have symptoms that can interfere with work, school, or social functions. Approximately, 5 percent of individuals have severe symptoms that severely limit their activities of daily living and their quality of life. If one has mild or moderate symptoms, these symptoms can be managed by the primary-care doctor. A patient may only need a dietary or lifestyle change.

Upper abdominal pain not associated with ulcers can be present in 50 percent of the IBS population and nausea and vomiting can also be present in 50 percent of the IBS population. Increased urination among women is also associated with IBS. Women who have IBS can also have chronic pelvic pain and other gynecological symptoms. If a patient has a history of physical or sexual abuse or has suffered the loss of a parent or other important person during childhood, he/she is more prone to develop IBS. A patient can have sexual dysfunction if he/she has IBS. Decreased sexual drive has been seen in both men and women who suffer from IBS. Current studies reveal that symptoms associated with IBS are not imagined but are real and have a neurological basis.

It is estimated that more than 50 percent of patients with IBS who were seen at a gastroenterologist clinic had psychiatric problems. The possibility of developing IBS is extremely high in individuals who suffer panic disorders. Greater sympathetic nervous system responses to abdominal pain have been reported in men when compared to women. Studies have demonstrated that men have heightened sympathetic nervous system activation. The gut function can decline precipitously in the face of minor insults, especially in older patients. The presence of systemic medical conditions like diabetes mellitus, postsurgical adhesions, polypharmacy, and alterations in pain perception as well as poor pain localization frequently clouds the usual classic clinical presentation seen in younger patients.

In 1917, a German scientist determined that in the wall of the gut was a self-contained nervous system that could function on its own without impulses from either the brain or the spinal cord. In other words, the gut has a brain of its own. Small nerves are in the lining of the esophagus, stomach, small intestine, and the colon. Because of new findings associated with IBS, a pharmaceutical company has developed a drug called Lotronex. This new drug can help manage the symptoms associated with IBS. Be aware; however, that the gastrointestinal system is closely connected to the brain.

Prozac can work on serotonin in the brain and spinal cord, but also cause a patient to have abdominal cramping and diarrhea. Anti-anxiety drugs are currently being studied to determine whether they can decrease the symptoms associated with the IBS. Imitrex, which is used to treat migraine headaches, is being studied for the treatment of the IBS symptoms. Lotronex is an anxiety type of drug. This drug is becoming increasingly popular in the treatment of IBS.

IBS has become the most diagnosed but the least understood medical ailment. The new drug Lotronex is used to treat abdominal pain and discomfort as well as any diarrhea. More individuals suffer from IBS than asthma or diabetes. Lotronex is the first drug approved by the FDA to be used for IBS treatment. Lotronex should be used with caution in elderly patients, patients with mild or moderate hepatic impairment, and patients taking medications that decrease gastrointestinal motility such as narcotics. As people age, the incidences of women suffering from IBS outnumber men by three to one.

A newer drug now available is called Zelnorm. It is a drug that is in a class of medications called gastrointestinal serotonin agonists. This drug is used in the treatment of constipation, bloating, and abdominal pain. In the United Kingdom, another drug called renzapride is being studied in the treatment of IBS. Preliminary studies that are being done with respect to this drug for the treatment of IBS symptoms are extremely promising. The use of this drug in elderly patients is not recommended and should be restricted to women below the age of 55. Research continues with the development of new drugs in the treatment of IBS because this disease costs the health-care system approximately $30 billion per year.

Sometimes anti-anxiety drugs can be used for the treatment of the IBS. Sex steroids may work to modulate abdominal pain associated with IBS. They can have direct effects on the gastrointestinal motility and inhibit the emptying of the stomach. Studies have shown that post-menopausal women who are taking hormones had slower stomach-emptying times with solids when compared with men and when compared with postmenopausal women who were not taking hormones.

Testosterone has no influence on the gastric emptying in men. However, estrogen and progesterone will slow down the gastric emptying time in men. A study has demonstrated that a male's complaint of discomfort with distention of a balloon in the male's rectum was higher if the male had a low testosterone level.

Inflammatory (in contrast to irritable) bowel disease (IBD) is another entity that can also cause a patient to have significant pain. Both IBS and inflammatory bowel diseases have similar symptoms. The IBS is characterized by pathology within the intestine. Both IBS as well as inflammatory bowel disease can be affected by stress. They both can be affected by the central nervous system as well as the immune system within the gastrointestinal system. Antibiotics and anti-inflammatory agents are used in inflammatory bowel syndromes. There has been some suggestion that these pharmacologic methods can be useful also in IBS.

Inflammatory bowel disease is believed to be a disease of the immune system. IBS can respond to diet. However, the inflammatory bowel disease rarely responds to changes to the diet. Inflammatory bowel disease includes ulcerative colitis and Crohn's disease. Ulcerative colitis and Crohn's disease both may occur among the elderly. In many populations, a second peak in the incidence of inflammatory bowel disease occurs near age 70. Clinical manifestations of inflammatory bowel disease in the elderly are generally similar to those seen in younger patients, although there is a tendency for both ulcerative colitis and Crohn's disease to involve more distal segments of the gut in older patients.

Inflammatory bowel disease is more common in Caucasians and more common in Jewish men and women. The incidence is almost equal in men and women. The incidence of ulcerative colitis and Crohn's disease is similar. Usually inflammatory bowel disease begins in early adult life. However, there are cases reported among the elderly. Genetic factors can make one prone to inflammatory bowel disease. It is possible that the immune system may attack the lining of the gastrointestinal system.

Emotional stress can worsen the symptoms of inflammatory bowel disease. Ulcerative colitis is most common during young adulthood and middle life, but it can occur at any age. It affects both men and women. Ulcerative colitis is especially dangerous in the elderly. A systemic process of telomere uncapping which could represent a biomarker for inflammatory bowel disease associated cancer risk.[1]

Ulcerative colitis is a chronic disease and a recurrent disease. It involves inflammation of the lining of the colon. It can also involve the rectum. Crohn's disease can involve any part of the gastrointestinal tract, including the mouth all the way to the anus. The cause of Crohn's disease and ulcerative colitis are unknown. Ulcerative colitis and Crohn's disease both may occur among the elderly. In many populations, a second peak in the incidence of inflammatory bowel disease occurs near age 70. Clinical manifestations of inflammatory bowel disease in the elderly are generally similar to those seen in younger patients, although there is a tendency for both ulcerative colitis and Crohn's disease to involve more distal segments of the gut in older patients. Older patients with IBD-related hospitalizations have substantial morbidity and higher mortality than younger patients.

A study explored the hypothesis in ulcerative colitis (UC), a chronic inflammatory disease that predisposes to colorectal cancer and in which shorter telomeres have been associated with chromosomal instability and tumor progression. Colonocytes of UC patients show premature shortening of telomeres, which might explain the increased and earlier risk of cancer in this disease.2 Shorter leukocyte telomeres and increased gammaH2AX in colonocytes might reflect oxidative damage secondary to inflammation. Inflammation plays a role in the progression to cancer and it is linked to the presence of senescent cells.[3] Ulcerative colitis is a chronic inflammatory disease that predisposes to colorectal cancer.

While Crohn's disease is often thought of as a disease among the young, about 25% of new cases are diagnosed in individuals over age 60. Crohn's disease usually involves the lower ileum (the lowest part of the small intestine). The rectum can be involved. Approximately one-third of Crohn's disease patients have their pathology in the colon, whereas one-third of patients have their pathology in the ileum and one-third have their pathology in both the ileum and colon. The inflammation of the gastrointestinal system can go from the inside of the bowel to the outside. The inner lining of the gastrointestinal system can develop ulcers. An ulcer is a break in the lining of the wall of the gut. This break in the gut lining can fail to heal and can be accompanied by inflammation. A fistula from the inside of the bowel to the outside can develop. A fistula is an abnormal communication between a hollow organ and the exterior.

With Crohn's disease, the inner aspect of the intestine or colon can decrease in diameter, which is called a stricture. The bile salts are not absorbed properly through the ileum. The thickened loop of inflamed bowel can be tender to deep palpation. A chronic inflammation of the gastrointestinal system can cause anemia. The gastrointestinal system may not be able to absorb protein. A barium enema and a colonoscopy may be necessary. Crohn's disease patients have shorter telomeric lengths than intestinal intraepithelial lymphocytes from control patients, suggesting that they have been chronically stimulated. Such perturbation of the intestinal intraepithelial lymphocytes population within the ileac mucosa could contribute to the inflammation in Crohn disease.[4]

A barium enema is an enema with opaque contrast liquid that outlines the intestines on x-ray images. This test helps the doctor look for abnormalities in the bowel. To examine the lower bowel, the doctor may also use air with the barium to distend the bowel. Through the colonoscope (a flexible fiber optic instrument), a doctor can obtain biopsies of the colon and ilium. White blood cells protect the body against foreign substances. If the white cells are elevated and the abdomen is tender, this will necessitate a CT of the abdomen. A patient may be given antibiotics and will be given nutritional supplements. Occasionally, surgery is required to drain an abscess.

If the gastrointestinal system develops an obstruction somewhere in the system, the food cannot pass through this obstruction. Steroids can be necessary to treat the inflammation caused by Crohn's disease. Be aware that chronic cramping, abdominal pain, and diarrhea are noted in both IBS and Crohn's disease.

Patients with chronic inflammatory bowel disease, such as ulcerative colitis and Crohn's disease, have an increased risk of colorectal cancer. Lifelong colonoscopy surveillance is performed to detect the presence of dysplasia, but this approach is expensive and time-consuming. Thus, there is intensive research to identify molecular factors with prognostic value. Improved understanding of the molecular biology of cancer progression in inflammatory bowel disease will hopefully lead to the identification of useful prognostic biomarkers.[5]

Sulfasalazine is effective in reducing the symptoms of Crohn's disease. Drugs that can affect the immune system such as azathioprine and mercaptopurine are useful in the treatment of the disease if it is unresponsive to the other methods that we mentioned. Smoking can cause you to have a recurrence of Crohn's symptoms. If conservative treatments fail, a patient may require surgery. Elderly patients can use the same medications that younger adults use. Some find, however, that they can only tolerate reduced doses.

Ulcerative colitis involves the inner lining of the colon. Crohn's disease can go through the entire lining of the gastrointestinal system. Organs that are part of the gastrointestinal system are usually the cause of the abdominal pain. If a patient has pain in the upper abdomen on the right side, he/she may have an inflamed gallbladder or an ulcer. Hepatitis can cause one to have abdominal pain. Pancreatitis, a painful inflammation of the pancreas, can cause pain in the mid abdomen that radiates to the back. Renal stones and kidney stones on occasion can cause abdominal pain in addition to pain in the flanks as well.

Ulcerative colitis, a chronic inflammatory disease of the colon, is associated with a high risk of colorectal carcinoma that is thought to develop through genomic instability.[6] Ulcerative colitis is a bowel disease which may lead to dysplasia and adenocarcinoma in patients when long-lasting. Short telomeres have been reported in mucosal cells of UC patients.[7]

Interstitial cystitis is an inflammatory disease of the bladder that can cause a patient to have lower abdominal pain. Interstitial cystitis is an inflammation of the urinary bladder in which the bladder becomes small, scarred, and less able to expand. The bladder wall experiences pinpoint areas of bleeding (hemorrhages). Resulting scar tissue may cause the bladder to stiffen and contract, reducing its capacity from twelve ounces to two ounces.

Ovarian cysts can cause one to have pain in the lower abdomen. A patient should be aware that pain in the abdomen can originate from the chest or the pelvis. The symptoms of interstitial cystitis often mimic the symptoms of a urinary tract infection.

An aneurysm is a weakness in the wall of the aorta. This weak area could rupture, which could be fatal. The appendix, if it is inflamed, can cause a patient to have abdominal pain as well. The appendix is part of the gastrointestinal system. A viral infection in the intestine or gas can cause significant abdominal pain. Causes of abdominal pain include gas, constipation, milk intolerance, stomach flu, an irritable bowel syndrome, indigestion, esophageal reflux, ulcers, gallstones, and diverticular disease.

Sulfasalazine can be prescribed to treat the symptoms. Mesalamine can also be used. For some reason, the use of a nicotine patch has been shown to be effective in some patients suffering from this disease. The reason for this finding remains unknown. Steroid enemas can be used to treat the symptoms. Oral steroids can be used as well. Approximately, 15 percent of individuals with ulcerative colitis develop symptoms that are severe.

Parasites as well as Helicobacter pylori can cause abdominal pain. This bacterium is called in microbiological terms gram-negative bacteria and can be found in the moist membrane lining of the stomach. The doctor will help the body eradicate these bacteria with antibiotics and other drugs.

If the abdomen distends and becomes increasingly tender, a patient runs the risk of perforation of the bowel. The colon can become excessively dilated. This finding is in less than two percent of cases of ulcerative colitis. This expansion of the bowel can cause a decrease in the blood flow to the bowel tissue. This is called toxic megacolon. If the symptoms remain severe, a patient may require surgery. Severe bleeding as well as the perforation of the bowel are indications for surgery.

Abdominal aortic aneurysm (AAA) has a complex pathophysiology; in which both environmental and genetic factors play important roles, the most important being smoking.[8] Abdominal aortic aneurysms (AAA) are an age-related vascular disease and an important cause of morbidity and mortality. Patients with AAA have shorter leukocyte telomere length compared to controls. This suggests that vascular biological aging may have a role in the pathogenesis of AAA.[9]

Telomere and telomerase activity's detection might be used as predictor biomarkers of sporadic Thoracic aneurysms as well. Their impairment also further suggests a strong role of vascular ageing in sporadic aneurysms, evocated by both environmental and genetic inflammatory factors.[10] Abdominal aortic aneurysm is a complex multi-factorial disease with life-threatening complications. AAA is typically asymptomatic and its rupture is associated with high mortality rate. Both environmental and genetic risk factors are involved in AAA pathogenesis. Telomeres were found to be significantly shortened in AAA patients.[11] Patients with AAAs have attenuated telomerase endothelial expression compared to controls, implying a protective role of telomerase against AAA formation.[12]

Ascending aortic aneurysm is a connective tissue disorder. On the other hand, significant differences in the mean length of blood leukocyte telomeres in ascending aortic aneurysm and controls have been noted. Mean relative telomere length was significantly longer in ascending aortic aneurysm blood samples compared with controls.[13]

Pancreatitis can cause severe abdominal pain as Telomere shortening is a cell-intrinsic mechanism that limits cell proliferation by induction of DNA damage responses resulting either in apoptosis or cellular senescence. Shortening of telomeres has been shown to occur during human aging and in chronic diseases that accelerate cell turnover, such as chronic hepatitis. Telomere shortening can limit organ homeostasis and regeneration in response to injury.

Pancreatic regeneration is limited in the context of telomere dysfunction.[14] Telomeres may be an essential gatekeeper for maintaining chromosomal integrity, and thus, normal cellular physiology in pancreatic ductal epithelium. A critical shortening of telomere length may predispose these noninvasive ductal lesions to accumulate progressive chromosomal abnormalities and to develop toward the stage of invasive carcinoma.[5] Telomerase activity is detected in pancreatic cancer but not in benign tumors.[16]

References

1. Da-Silva N, Arasaradnam R, Getliffe K, Sung E, Oo Y, Nwokolo C. Altered mRNA expression of telomere binding proteins (TPP1, POT1, RAP1, TRF1 and TRF2) in ulcerative colitis and Crohn's disease. Dig Liver Dis. 2010;42(8):544-548.

2. Risques RA, Lai LA, Brentnall TA, et al. Ulcerative colitis is a disease of accelerated colon aging: evidence from telomere attrition and DNA damage. Gastroenterology. 2008;135(2):410-418.

3. Risques RA, Lai LA, Himmetoglu C, et al. Ulcerative colitis-associated colorectal cancer arises in a field of short telomeres, senescence, and inflammation. Cancer Res. 2011;71(5):1669-1679.

4. Meresse B, Dubucquoi S, Tourvieille B, Desreumaux P, Colombel JF, Dessaint JP. CD28+ intraepithelial lymphocytes with long telomeres are recruited within the inflamed ileal mucosa in Crohn disease. Hum Immunol. 2001;62(7):694-700.

5. Risques RA, Rabinovitch PS, Brentnall TA. Cancer surveillance in inflammatory bowel disease: new molecular approaches. Curr Opin Gastroenterol. 2006;22(4):382-390.

6. O'Sullivan JN, Bronner MP, Brentnall TA, et al. Chromosomal instability in ulcerative colitis is related to telomere shortening. Nat Genet. 2002;32(2):280-284.

7. Friis-Ottessen M, Bendix L, Kolvraa S, Norheim-Andersen S, De Angelis PM, Clausen OP. Telomere shortening correlates to dysplasia but not to DNA aneuploidy in longstanding ulcerative colitis. BMC Gastroenterol. 2014;14:8.

8. Bjorck M, Wanhainen A. Pathophysiology of AAA: heredity vs environment. Prog Cardiovasc Dis. 2013;56(1):2-6.

9. Atturu G, Brouilette S, Samani NJ, London NJ, Sayers RD, Bown MJ. Short leukocyte telomere length is associated with abdominal aortic aneurysm (AAA). Eur J Vasc Endovasc Surg. 2010;39(5):559-564.

10. Balistreri CR, Pisano C, Martorana A, et al. Are the leukocyte telomere length attrition and telomerase activity alteration potential predictor biomarkers for sporadic TAA in aged individuals? Age (Dordr). 2014;36(5):9700.

11. Cafueri G, Parodi F, Pistorio A, et al. Endothelial and smooth muscle cells from abdominal aortic aneurysm have increased oxidative stress and telomere attrition. PLoS One. 2012;7(4):e35312.

12. Dimitroulis D, Katsargyris A, Klonaris C, et al. Telomerase expression on aortic wall endothelial cells is attenuated in abdominal aortic aneurysms compared to healthy nonaneurysmal aortas. J Vasc Surg. 2011;54(6):1778-1783.

13. Huusko TJ, Santaniemi M, Kakko S, et al. Long telomeres in blood leukocytes are associated with a high risk of ascending aortic aneurysm. PLoS One. 2012;7(11):e50828.

14. von Figura G, Wagner M, Nalapareddy K, et al. Regeneration of the exocrine pancreas is delayed in telomere-dysfunctional mice. PLoS One. 2011;6(2):e17122.

15. van Heek NT, Meeker AK, Kern SE, et al. Telomere shortening is nearly universal in pancreatic intraepithelial neoplasia. Am J Pathol. 2002;161(5):1541-1547.

16. Hiyama E, Kodama T, Shinbara K, et al. Telomerase activity is detected in pancreatic cancer but not in benign tumors. Cancer Res. 1997;57(2):326-331.

37. Diagnostic tests

Laboratory tests check a sample of the blood, urine or body tissues. A doctor analyzes the test samples to see if the test results fall within a normal range. The tests use a range because what is normal differs from person to person. Some laboratory tests are precise, reliable indicators of specific health problems. Others provide more general information that simply gives doctors clues to possible health problems. Information obtained from laboratory tests may help doctors decide whether other tests or procedures are needed to make a diagnosis. The information may also help the doctor develop or revise a patient's treatment plan.

All laboratory tests are generally used along with other exams or test such as MRIs, X rays, EMGs etc. The doctor who is familiar with their patient's medical history and current condition is in the best position to order and to explain test results and their implications. Patients are encouraged to discuss questions or concerns about laboratory test results with the doctor. Two common tests that one should be familiar with are the complete blood count and the blood chemistry tests. A complete blood count measures the levels of different types of blood cells. By determining if there are too many or not enough of each blood cell type, a CBC can help to detect a wide variety of illnesses or signs of infection. A blood chemistry test measures the levels of certain electrolytes, such as sodium and potassium, in the blood. A C reactive protein and erythrocyte sedimentation rate teat may be useful in the diagnosis of rheumatoid arthritis or other inflammatory disease.

Doctors order urine tests to make sure that the kidneys are normal or when they suspect an infection in the kidneys or bladder. This is important if one is taking a medication like an anti-inflammatory medication that can affect the kidneys. A urine test can be done in the doctor's office or even at home. It's easy for one to give a urine sample since one can urinate in a cup. In other cases a catheter (a narrow, soft tube) can be inserted through the urinary tract opening into the bladder to get the urine sample.

Tylenol (acetaminophen) can cause liver damage if one takes too much (more than 4000 mg per day). Liver function tests ascertain how the liver is working and helps diagnose any sort liver damage or inflammation. The doctor may order one when looking for signs of a viral infection or liver damage from other health problems. On occasion, blood tests may be done to determine that one do not have a bleeding problem such as hemophilia.

Aspirin can cause bleeding by decreasing the ability of the blood to clot. Before doing a nerve block it is prudent to know if the blood will clot in a normal time. Otherwise a needle can result in significant bleeding.

Plain X rays can be done in a physician's office . X rays can assess bone-joint arthritis. X rays can diagnose degeneration of the discs. The bone alignment (do the bones line up with each other?) can be assessed as well. Bone fractures can also be identified. One should be aware that one is subject to radiation exposure with this diagnostic test. If one has the possibility of having osteoporosis, the physician may order a DEXA (dual energy x-ray absorptiometry) that is a specific test for the diagnosis of osteoporosis. A Computed Tomography (CT scan) allows a physician to assess a disc in the back as well as arthritic changes affecting the bones in the neck and back.

A CT scan of the head can be useful for the diagnosis of a bleeding injury to the brain following trauma to the head. Patients receive radiation exposure with this test. Myelography or a myelogram is primarily of use when surgical therapy is planned. A dye is placed in the fluid that surrounds the spinal cord. An image is formed which tells a physician that a nerve coming off the spinal cord is compressed or not compressed by a disc herniation.

An image does not identify painful areas of the body. An image demonstrates abnormal anatomy that could be an area of pain generation. Degenerative disc disease noted on an X ray for example does not imply that one have a disease or are supposed to have pain. This entity is a normal aspect of aging. Therefore, one should not be alarmed if the doctor tells one that one have degenerative disc disease.

The same is true if one are told that one have a disc herniation. Not every disc herniation causes pain and not every disc herniation requires surgery. People have had disc herniations documented years ago. It was not until the 1930's that doctors began operating on herniated discs. The United States has a higher incidence of spine surgeries when compared to other countries.

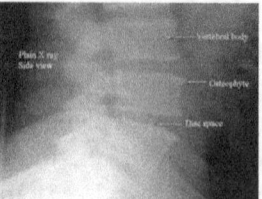

Figure 1. Plain X ray of the low back taken from the patient's side.

Ultrasound is another valuable diagnostic tool. For example, an ultrasound test can be used to look for collections of fluid in the body, or for problems with the kidneys. An ultrasound is painless and uses high-frequency sound waves to bounce off organs and create a picture. A special jelly is applied to the skin, and a handheld device is moved over the skin. The sound waves that come back produce an image on a screen.

Computerized axial tomography is a specialized x ray. CAT scans are a kind of X-ray, and typically are ordered to examine for pathologies such as appendicitis, internal bleeding, or abnormal organ growths. Tomography in which computer analysis of a series of cross-sectional scans made along a single axis of a bodily structure or tissue is used to construct a three-dimensional image of that structure. The technique is used in diagnostic studies of internal bodily structures, as in the detection of tumors or brain aneurysms. A scan is not painful.

A scan may require the use of a contrast material (a dye or other substance) to improve the visibility of certain tissues or blood vessels. The contrast material may be swallowed or given through an IV. CAT scans consist of a highly sensitive x-ray beam that is focused on a specific plane of the body. As this beam passes through the body, it is identified by a detector, which feeds the information that it receives into a computer. The computer then analyzes the information on the basis of tissue density.

Generally a CT is preferred where bone details necessary (long bones like the arm or leg, spine, skull), while a MRI produces much better soft tissue details (brain, spinal cord etc.) CT scans are useful for examining body cavities (thorax, abdomen, pelvis) for calcium deposits, cysts, and abscesses.

With some diseases, either a CT scan or MRI is commonly ordered. Spinal stenosis, for example which is a bone growth around the spinal cord or around the holes in the bones of the low back and neck where the nerves from the spinal cord exit to the extremities and is usually seen in individuals over 50 years old.

Stenosis can compress the nerves resulting in pain and numbness in the extremities. Because of numbness on the bottom of the feet, one may have difficulty with balance. A CT scan or MRI can identify this pathology. Magnetic Resonance Imaging (MRI) is done by utilization of a magnetic field that is applied around the body. MRIs use radio waves and magnetic fields to produce an image.

MRI's are often used to look at bones, joints, and the brain. Contrast material is sometimes given through an IV in order to get a better picture of certain structures. Nuclei within the body cells with an odd number of protons orient themselves with the magnetic field.

The MRI scanner applies a certain amount of energy and the nuclei assume a new orientation with respect to the magnetic field. This energy is removed and the nuclei emit energy as they reorient in the magnetic field. The energy emitted is detected and displayed as an image. The MRI involves no radiation.

Magnetic resonance imaging provides a picture of the soft tissue that may be better than the CT scan. A MRI cannot be done if one has certain metals in the body or a heart pacemaker or a defibrillator. Magnetic resonance imaging allows visualization of the discs, spinal cord and cerebrospinal fluid. A MRI can be used with a contrast dye to identify an extruded disc, infection or tumor.

Plain X rays give physicians images in a front to back plane. A side-to-side plane and a oblique view are helpful in diagnosing the possible causes of the pain. On the other hand, a CT and MRI image shows slices of the body as well as a three hundred and sixty degree image of a defined section of the body. Images only show pathology. They do not show pain.

Pain is a subjective experience. If one views a photograph of an old scratched and dented telephone, one has no idea if it is ringing or not by the picture. The same is true with an X ray image. An abnormal X ray does not mean that one hurts.

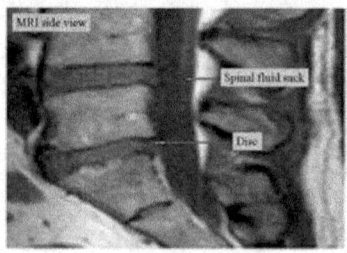

Figure 2. MRI from a side view. Note that when compared to a plain X ray that one can see more anatomic structures.

Bone scanning is done using a technetium isotope tracer injected into a vein. This tracer is distributed according to the bone blood flow. A greater blood flow to the bone from trauma such as a fracture or arthritis is compatible with greater bone absorption of the tracer. Total body radiation occurs but is low following a bone scan.

The three-phase bone scan consists of the administration of a radioactive tracer followed by scanned images on three occasions. The first image is phase 1 Phase one measures blood flow on the first pass of the tracer. The second phase assesses the blood vessel system while the third phase assesses the turnover of bone, which can be seen in fractures or tumors. Bone scans are frequently used to diagnose RSD.

Electromyography (EMG) and the Nerve Conduction Velocity Tests (NCV) are two diagnostic tools that are helpful to the. These two tests allow the assessment of the location, the pathogenesis, and the prognosis of neuromuscular lesions. Loss of the outside wrapper (myelin) of a nerve or nerves is assessed by the nerve conduction velocity test. Abnormalities of a nerve take 3-5 days to develop. An EMG is a needle test to determine if the muscle is diseased or injured.

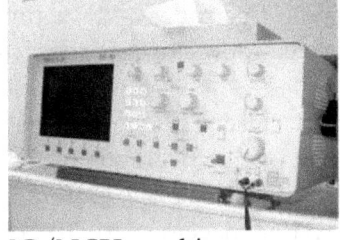

Figure 3. EMG/NCV machine.

Abnormalities in the painful nerve or muscle can take five to six weeks to become evident. Muscles that are closer to the brain manifest electrophysiological abnormalities sooner than more distal muscles. Focal defects in the nerve may cause NCV slowing across the defect. A NCV measures how fast the nerve sends and impulse. Stimulation of the nerve is done at one end of the nerve and the velocity is measured at another end of the nerve. Generalized nerve pathology results in a reduced nerve conduction velocity. In other words the nerve impulses are slower than normal.

Electromyography (EMG) measures the response of muscles and nerves to electrical activity. It's used to help determine muscle conditions that might be causing muscle weakness, including muscular dystrophy and nerve disorders. A needle electrode is inserted into the muscle (the insertion might feel similar to a pinch) and the signal from the muscle is transmitted from the electrode through a wire to a receiver/amplifier, which is connected to a device that displays readout. EMGs can be uncomfortable and scary to children, but aren't usually painful. Occasion-ally kids are sedated while they're done.

Distal latency is the assessment of the distal conduction velocity of the painful nerve that can be affected by the neuromuscular junction that is the location where the nerve and muscle join. Some muscle diseases may have normal NCV studies but electromyographic (EMG) abnormalities usually occur in these situations. EMG measures muscle electrical activity. A reduction in the size of the waves on an oscilloscope (a screen with waves that move across the screen) is proportional to the nerve loss to the muscle. It should be noted when a muscle is penetrated by an EMG needle, the normal muscle is quiet when it is at rest.

Muscle fiber firing at the time of needle insertion can give the doctor an indication of any muscle disease. The NCV assesses the speed at which the peripheral nerves transmit electrical signals. The nerve is stimulated, usually with surface electrodes, which are electrodes placed on the skin over the nerve at various locations. One electrode stimulates the nerve with a very mild electrical impulse. The other electrode records the resulting electrical activity. The distance between electrodes and the time it takes for electrical impulses to travel between electrodes are used to calculate the nerve conduction velocity.

A needle electrode is inserted through the skin into the muscle. There should be a short burst of electrical activity at this time. The electrical activity detected by this electrode is displayed on an oscilloscope, and may be heard through a speaker. After placement of the electrodes, one may be asked to contract certain muscles. The presence, size, and shape of the waveform make up an action potential. This waveform provides information about the ability of the muscle to respond to electrical stimulation. These tests are useful for investigating nerve and muscle function in diseases such as peripheral neuropathy, compresion neuropathy etc.

Ultrasound imaging involves exposing part of the body to high-frequency sound waves to produce pictures of the inside of the body. Ultrasound can show the structure and movement of the body's internal organs, as well as blood flowing through blood vessels. Doppler ultra-sound is a special ultrasound technique that evaluates blood flow through a blood vessel, including the body's major arteries and veins in the abdomen, arms, legs and neck.

Ultrasound is a useful way of examining many of the internal organs: heart and blood vessels, abdominal organs, the scrotum, the thyroid gland as well as the uterus and ovaries. Doppler ultrasound permits viewing of blood flow which aids in the evaluation of the major arteries and veins of the body.

A new blood telomere length test could potentially offer some proof that many people really are physiologically older than they look. Research on telomeres is an expanding and important scientific area, as evidenced by the awarding of the 2009 Nobel Prize in medicine to three American geneticists who studied these small DNA segments.[1] The test can provide people with valuable information that can encourage them to adopt healthier lifestyles. If a patient's telomeres are much shorter than most people their age that could be a red flag that perhaps a patient needs to do something to try and reverse the conditions that led to that observation. The telomere length is a biomarker of overall well-being that is predictive of disability of older individuals in the U.S. population.[2]

References

1. Falus A, Marton I, Borbenyi E, et al. [The 2009 Nobel Prize in Medicine and its surprising message: lifestyle is associated with telomerase activity]. Orv Hetil. 2010;151(24):965-970.
2. Risques RA, Arbeev KG, Yashin AI, et al. Leukocyte telomere length is associated with disability in older u.s. Population. J Am Geriatr Soc. 2010;58(7):1289-1298.

38. Telomere length and health outcomes

Chronic pain conditions are characterized by significant individual variability complicating the identification of pathophysiological markers. Leukocyte telomere length (TL), a measure of cellular aging, is associated with age-related disease onset, psychosocial stress, and health-related functional decline. Psychosocial stress has been associated with the onset of chronic pain and chronic pain is experienced as a physical and psychosocial stressor.

Recent studies have found a correlation between psychological stress, telomere length, and health outcome in humans. Possible cellular mechanisms by which low telomerase may link stress and traditional risk factors to CVD are discussed. These findings may implicate telomerase as a novel and important mediator of the effects of psychological stress on physical health and disease.[1]

Chronic pain conditions are characterized by significant individual variability complicating the identification of pathophysiological markers. cellular aging may be more pronounced in older adults experiencing high levels of perceived stress and chronic pain.[2]

Chronic psychological distress has been linked to shorter telomeres, an indication of accelerated aging.[3] High phobic anxiety was associated with shorter telomeres. Although telomere shortening occurs as a natural part of aging, there is now a robust body of research that suggests that there is a relationship between psychosocial, environmental, and behavioral factors and changes in telomere length.[4] Chronic mood disorders have been associated with a shortened telomere, a marker of increased mortality rate and aging, and impaired cellular immunity.

Cellular aging may be more pronounced in older adults experiencing high levels of perceived stress and chronic pain. For these reasons behavioral and psychological pathologies must be addressed.[2] Poor sleep quality and short sleep duration are associated with increased incidence and progression of a number of chronic health conditions observed at greater frequency among the obese and those experiencing high levels of stress. Accelerated cellular aging, as indexed by telomere attrition in immune cells, is a plausible pathway linking sleep and disease risk.

More recently, shorter telomeres have been demonstrated in several psychiatric conditions, particularly depression. Sustained psychosocial stress of a variety of types in adulthood appears to be associated with shorter telomeres. Now, emerging work suggests a robust, and perhaps dose-dependent, relationship with early-life stress. These findings present new opportunities to reconceptualize the complex relationships between experience, physical and psychiatric disease, and aging.[5]

Accelerated telomere shortening may reflect stress-related oxidative damage to cells and accelerated aging, and severe psychosocial stress has been linked to telomere shortening. We propose that chronic stress associated with mood disorders may contribute to excess vulnerability for diseases of aging such as cardiovascular disease and possibly some cancers through accelerated organismal aging.[6] Although current perceived stress was only modestly associated with shorter telomeres in this broad sample of women, our findings suggest the effect of stress on telomere length may vary depending on neuroendocrine responsiveness, external stressors, and age.

It is unknown whether psychological well-being is associated with telomere length in patients with the somatic condition of chronic heart failure. Decreased perceived mental health is associated with shorter leukocyte telomere length in patients with heart failure.[7] Future work should determine whether psychological stress accelerates biological ageing.

The association in adults of psychosocial stress or stress biomarkers with lower telomere length suggests telomere biology may represent a possible underlying mechanism linking stress and health outcomes. There is empirical evidence linking stress and mental illnesses at various times across the lifespan with telomere erosion.[8]

Older pain patients need to have his/her sleep patterns addressed as well. Evidence has demonstrated that poor sleep quality explains significant variation in telomere length which is a marker a marker of cellular aging. Reduced telomere length is also associated with chronic psychological stress and mood disorders. Telomerase, which prevents telomere shortening, can be upregulated in T lymphocytes in concert with activation, thereby retarding telomere shortening.

Telomeres are protective DNA-protein complexes at the end of linear chromosomes that promote chromosomal stability. Telomere shortness in human beings is emerging as a prognostic marker of disease risk, progression, and premature mortality in many types of cancer, including breast, prostate, colorectal, bladder, head and neck, lung, and renal cell.[9]

In modern society, patients are faced with excessive psychological stress, as well as an epidemic of overeating, and the two together appear to have synergistic effects. Chronic stress can lead to overeating, co-elevation of cortisol and insulin, and suppression of certain anabolic hormones. This state of metabolic stress in turn promotes abdominal adiposity. Both the direct stress response and the accumulation of visceral fat can promote a milieu of systemic inflammation and oxidative stress.

This biochemical environment appears to be conducive to several cell aging mechanisms, mainly dampening telomerase and leading to telomere length shortening and cell senescence. Immune cell telomere shortness is linked with many chronic disease states and earlier mortality.[10] Dispositional pessimism may increase IL-6 and accelerate rate of telomere shortening and should be addressed in older patients.

It should be mentioned that older adults with higher income or being married have longer telomeres when other socio demographics, physical diseases, mental status and neighborhood experience are adjusted.[11] The major depressive disorder is associated with a high rate of developing serious medical comorbidities such as cardiovascular disease, stroke, dementia, osteoporosis, diabetes, and the metabolic syndrome.[12] Depression and other psychological pathologies in older pain patients must be addressed as part of their pain treatment.

Telomere attrition, causing accelerated aging, might be one of the mechanisms through which neuroticism leads to somatic disease and increased all-cause mortality. High neuroticism is significantly and prospectively associated with telomere attrition independent of lifestyle and other risk factors.[13]

Early life stress poses a risk for mental disorders and aging-related diseases.[14] Women with the highest levels of perceived stress have telomeres shorter on average by the equivalent of at least one decade of additional aging compared to low stress women.[15] These findings have implications for understanding how, at the cellular level, stress may promote earlier onset of age-related diseases.

To adequately treat pain, there are relationships of dynamic telomerase activity with exposure to an acute stressor or stressors, and with aspects of the stress responses with perceived psychological stress and neuroendocrine (cortisol) responses to the stressors.[16] Strategies for activating telomerase may help maintain telomere length and, thus, may lead to improved health during aging. A natural product telomerase activator is advertised that this product TA-65 lengthens telomeres in humans. TA-65 is a dietary supplement based on an improved formulation of a small molecule telomerase activator that was discovered in a systematic screening of natural product extracts from traditional Chinese medicines.[17]

Scientific findings suggest that TA-65 can lengthen telomeres in a statistically and possibly clinically significant manner. After more than 3 years of research and development, TA Sciences in conjunction with experts in Canada, Hong Kong, and the U.S. has perfected an exclusive method for extracting the naturally-occurring TA-65 molecule from the Astragalus root.

TA-65 treatment results in telomerase-dependent elongation of short telomeres and rescue of associated DNA damage, thus demonstrated that TA-65 mechanism of action is through the telomerase pathway.[18] In addition, it was demonstrate that TA-65 is capable of increasing mouse telomerase reverse transcriptase levels in some mouse tissues and elongating critically short telomeres when supplemented as part of a standard diet in mice. Finally, TA-65 dietary supplementation in female mice leads to an improvement of certain health-span indicators including glucose tolerance, osteoporosis and skin fitness, without significantly increasing global cancer incidence.

Other natural substances have also been reported to increase telomere length in a study.19 The tested single compounds were (1) alpha-lipoic acid, (1) green tea extract, (2) dimethylaminoethanol L-bitartrate, (3) N-acetyl-L-cysteine hydrochloride (HCL), (4) chlorella powder, (5) L-carnosine, (6) vitamin D3, (7) rhodiola PE 3%/1%, (8) glycine, (9) French red wine extract, (10) chia seed extract, (11) broccoli seed extract, and (12) Astragalus (TA-65). The compounds were tested singly and as blends.

Results have confirmed that many naturally occurring compounds hold the potential to activate telomerase and that those compounds have demonstrated synergistic effects to produce more potent blends. Given the relationship between telomere shortening, aging, and the decline of tissue function, it is reasonable to hypothesize that such telomerase-activating blends may have health-promoting benefits, particularly in relation to aging-associated conditions. However, the safety of these substances needs to be determined. Further investigation of such blends in human studies that are designed to evaluate safety and the effects on telomere length are thus warranted.[19]

References

1. Epel ES, Lin J, Wilhelm FH, et al. Cell aging in relation to stress arousal and cardiovascular disease risk factors. Psychoneuroendocrinology. 2006;31(3):277-287.

2. Sibille KT, Langaee T, Burkley B, et al. Chronic pain, perceived stress, and cellular aging: an exploratory study. Mol Pain. 2012;8:12.

3. Okereke OI, Prescott J, Wong JY, Han J, Rexrode KM, De Vivo I. High phobic anxiety is related to lower leukocyte telomere length in women. PLoS One. 2012;7(7):e40516.

4. Starkweather AR, Alhaeeri AA, Montpetit A, et al. An integrative review of factors associated with telomere length and implications for biobehavioral research. Nurs Res. 2014;63(1):36-50.

5. Price LH, Kao HT, Burgers DE, Carpenter LL, Tyrka AR. Telomeres and early-life stress: an overview. Biol Psychiatry. 2013;73(1):15-23.

6. Simon NM, Smoller JW, McNamara KL, et al. Telomere shortening and mood disorders: preliminary support for a chronic stress model of accelerated aging. Biol Psychiatry. 2006;60(5):432-435.

7. Huzen J, van der Harst P, de Boer RA, et al. Telomere length and psychological well-being in patients with chronic heart failure. Age Ageing. 2010;39(2):223-227.

8. Shalev I, Entringer S, Wadhwa PD, et al. Stress and telomere biology: a lifespan perspective. Psychoneuroendocrinology. 2013;38(9):1835-1842.

9. Ornish D, Lin J, Daubenmier J, et al. Increased telomerase activity and comprehensive lifestyle changes: a pilot study. Lancet Oncol. 2008;9(11):1048-1057.

10. Epel ES. Psychological and metabolic stress: a recipe for accelerated cellular aging? Hormones (Athens). 2009;8(1):7-22.

11. Yen YC, Lung FW. Older adults with higher income or marriage have longer telomeres. Age Ageing. 2013;42(2):234-239.

12. Wolkowitz OM, Reus VI, Mellon SH. Of sound mind and body: depression, disease, and accelerated aging. Dialogues Clin Neurosci. 2011;13(1):25-39.

13. van Ockenburg SL, de Jonge P, van der Harst P, Ormel J, Rosmalen JG. Does neuroticism make you old? Prospective associations between neuroticism and leukocyte telomere length. Psychol Med. 2014;44(4):723-729.

14. Savolainen K, Eriksson JG, Kananen L, et al. Associations between early life stress, self-reported traumatic experiences across the lifespan and leukocyte telomere length in elderly adults. Biol Psychol. 2014;97:35-42.

15. Epel ES, Blackburn EH, Lin J, et al. Accelerated telomere shortening in response to life stress. Proc Natl Acad Sci U S A. 2004;101(49):17312-17315.

16. Epel ES, Lin J, Dhabhar FS, et al. Dynamics of telomerase activity in response to acute psychological stress. Brain Behav Immun. 2010;24(4):531-539.

17. Salvador L, Singaravelu G, Harley CB, Flom P, Suram A, Raffaele JM. A Natural Product Telomerase Activator Lengthens Telomeres in Humans: A Randomized, Double Blind, and Placebo Controlled Study. Rejuvenation Res. 2016.

18. Bernardes de Jesus B, Schneeberger K, Vera E, Tejera A, Harley CB, Blasco MA. The telomerase activator TA-65 elongates short telomeres and increases health span of adult/old mice without increasing cancer incidence. Aging Cell. 2011;10(4):604-621.

19. Ait-Ghezala G, Hassan S, Tweed M, et al. Identification of Telomerase-activating Blends From Naturally Occurring Compounds. Altern Ther Health Med. 2016;22 Suppl 2:6-14.

39. Palliative care

Some elderly patients may require palliative care. Palliative Care is a relatively new medical specialty. The goal of palliative care is to improve the quality of life for patients as well as their families. Palliative care is appropriate at any point in an illness. Palliative care can be provided at the same time as conventional treatment that is meant to cure you.

Palliative care is dedicated to maximizing a person's comfort, independence, and quality of life when the prolongation of life is no longer a realistic goal. Palliative care optimizes the quality of life. When an elderly person is comfortable, they eat more, sleep better, not as fatigued, not as depressed and at least have the possibility of enjoying their day.

Leukocyte telomere length is related to both dementia and mortality and may be a marker of biological aging.[12] Telomere erosion, cellular senescence, and death characterize aged diseased hearts and the development of cardiac failure in humans.[13] However, this testing may not be covered by one's health insurance. It is speculated that patients requiring palliative care will have short telomeres.

Unscheduled acute hospital admissions and subsequent deaths in hospitals of patients considered palliative are increasing, despite many patients' preference to die at home. A large proportion of these patients are admitted via acute medical units or emergency departments. Unscheduled admission for patients with palliative care needs remains prevalent.[1] Physicians appear more willing to accommodate requests to continue life-sustaining treatment when those requests are based on particular religious communities or traditions, but not when based on expectations of divine healing.[2]

Recently, after completing hospital treatment, 3 elderly female patients were introduced to a home care department for end-of-life care at home. However, these patients recovered almost by themselves and now spend quiet days.[3]

Palliative care is the active total care of patients whose disease is not amenable to curative treatment. Control of a patient's pain and other symptoms, and of psychological, social, and spiritual problems is mandatory. The goal is the achievement of the best possible quality of life for patients and their families.

Palliative care aims to relieve symptoms such as pain, shortness of breath, fatigue, constipation, nausea, loss of appetite and difficulty sleeping.

It helps patients gain the strength to carry on with daily life. It improves their ability to tolerate medical treatments. And it helps them better understand their choices for care. The goal of palliative care is to offer patients the best possible quality of life during their illness.

Palliative care is not the same as hospice care. Palliative care may be provided at any time during a person's illness, even from the time of diagnosis. And, it may be given at the same time as curative treatment. Hospice care always includes palliative care. However, it is focused on terminally ill patients-people who no longer seek treatments to cure them and who are expected to live for about six months or less.

Palliative care affirms life and regards dying as a normal natural process. It neither hastens nor postpones death. Palliative care provides relief from pain and cognitive symptoms. Its goal is to integrate the psycho-logical and spiritual aspects of a patient's care. It offers a support system to help patients live as actively as possible until their death. It offers a support system to help families cope during the patient's illness.

Prescription of long-acting opioids for chronic noncancerous pain, compared with anticonvulsants or cyclic antidepressants, was associated with a significantly increased risk of all-cause mortality, including deaths from causes other than overdose, with a modest absolute risk difference. These findings should be considered when evaluating harms and benefits of treatment.[4]

Patients with glioblastoma have a limited life expectancy and an impaired quality of life and they should be offered palliative care soon after the diagnosis is established. Still, only a quarter of patients aged over 65 return home or medical institution after completing treatments.[5] Home care must be promoted by coordinating assistance and care, combining disciplines such as physiotherapy and ergotherapy, medical and nursing care and psychosocial support. Palliative care is infrequently delivered particularly in community settings and to non-cancer patients and occurs close to death.[6]

Palliative care is not provided by one physician but by a team of experts, including palliative care doctors, nurses and social workers. Chaplains, naturopaths, massage therapists, pharmacists, nutritionists and others are also a part of the team. Palliative care can be provided when you are at home, in an assisted-living facility, nursing facility or hospital.

Historically, palliative care and hospice care were developed for of cancer care. Palliative care in contrast to hospice care is not just for patients who are very close to death. Palliative care is increasingly recognized, however, as an appropriate approach for a wider range of patients, in terms of both primary diagnosis and estimated survival.

Palliative care is therefore, more than health care just for dying persons. Palliative care is a health care philosophy aimed at improving the essence of life when a cure is no longer possible. Palliative care is a health care discipline with its own research knowledge base, and a specific set of skills aimed at pain and other forms of suffering, which become the major focus of treatment.

The American Board of Anesthesiology has subspecialty certification in palliative care. Palliative care is not totally defined by a prognosis but by what it inspires, offers, and achieves. A patient does not have to be dying to have palliative care. Palliative care is in addition to providing medical care, is also a provider of paramedical support services. Palliative care ensures that informed choices be offered to patients.

African-Americans and Hispanics receive disproportionately less aggressive non-critical treatment for chronic diseases than their Caucasian counterparts. However, when it comes to end-of-life care, minority races are purportedly treated more aggressively in Medical Intensive Care Units (MICU) and are more likely to die there.[7]

The management of pain is an important aspect of palliative care. The major goals of palliative care are maintenance of a full connection with the dying person. The patient must be regarded as a living person and therefore, the full human experiences; physical, emotional, and spiritual, must be addressed. A patient must not die with severe pain. The patient must be comfortable. Most important, a patient must be able to live out his or hers last moment as fully and consciously as possible. In fact, palliative care should make dying to be a patient's finest hour. A dying patient is unique and should be treated as someone special.

Despite increased use of analgesics, pain is still prevalent in people with dementia. Validated pain tools are available but not implemented and not fully tested on responsiveness to treatment. Official guidelines for pain assessment and treatment addressing people with dementia living in a nursing home are lacking.[8]

For chronically critically ill elderly patients on mechanical ventilation, prognosis for significant recovery may be minimal. These individuals, or their surrogates, may decide for "palliative extubation."[9] Palliative extubation at end of life was an option selected by an ethnically diverse elderly population. Approximately three-fourths of subjects died in hospital, and one-fourth was discharged alive. Over 50% who died did so within 24 hours, making this useful information for counseling and anticipatory planning.

Palliative care is any form of medical care or treatment that concentrates on reducing the severity of disease symptoms rather than trying to seek a cure. The goal is to prevent and relieve suffering and to improve quality of life for people facing serious, complex illnesses. Palliative care should not be confused with hospice care, which delivers palliative care to those at the end of life. In essence, palliative care provides care to those with life limiting illness at any stage of their disease.

The challenges of providing end of life care to prisoners and may inspire nurses to consider steps they can take individually or within nursing organizations to improve this care and address the unique challenges faced by dying inmates. By being aware of these issues and advocating for best practices, nurses can help inmates at the end of life to have a dignified death.[10]

There is limited available evidence concerning the clinical, physical, psychological or emotional effectiveness of end-of-life care pathways.[11]

References

1. Mason E, Jenkins D, Williams M, Davies J. Unscheduled care admissions at end-of-life - what are the patient characteristics? Acute Med. 2016;15(2):68-72.
2. Ayeh DD, Tak HJ, Yoon JD, Curlin FA. U.S. Physicians' Opinions About Accommodating Religiously Based Requests for Continued Life-Sustaining Treatment. J Pain Symptom Manage. 2016;51(6):971-978.
3. Ohara H, Sato M. [Three Elderly Female Patients Who Experienced Self-Recovery during End-of-Life Care at Home]. Gan To Kagaku Ryoho. 2015;42 Suppl 1:63-65.
4. Ray WA, Chung CP, Murray KT, Hall K, Stein CM. Prescription of Long-Acting Opioids and Mortality in Patients With Chronic Noncancer Pain. JAMA. 2016;315(22):2415-2423.
5. Dieudonne N, De Micheli R, Hottinger A. [Palliative care for glioblastoma]. Rev Med Suisse. 2016;12(516):853-856.
6. Tanuseputro P, Budhwani S, Bai YQ, Wodchis WP. Palliative care delivery across health sectors: A population-level observational study. Palliat Med. 2016.
7. Chima-Melton C, Murphy TE, Araujo KL, Pisani MA. The Impact of Race on Intensity of Care Provided to Older Adults in the Medical Intensive Care Unit. J Racial Ethn Health Disparities. 2016;3(2):365-372.
8. Husebo BS, Achterberg W, Flo E. Identifying and Managing Pain in People with Alzheimer's Disease and Other Types of Dementia: A Systematic Review. CNS Drugs. 2016;30(6):481-497.
9. Pan CX, Platis D, Maw MM, Morris J, Pollack S, Kawai F. How Long Does (S)He Have? Retrospective Analysis of Outcomes After

Palliative Extubation in Elderly, Chronically Critically Ill Patients. Crit Care Med. 2016;44(6):1138-1144.

10. Wion RK, Loeb SJ. CE: Original Research: End-of-Life Care Behind Bars: A Systematic Review. Am J Nurs. 2016;116(3):24-36; quiz 37.

11. Chan RJ, Webster J, Bowers A. End-of-life care pathways for improving outcomes in caring for the dying. Cochrane Database Syst Rev. 2016;2:CD008006.

40. Who pays for elderly care?

Pain management is becoming more expensive for elderly patients each year. Elderly patients must realize that Medicare health insurance is for the most part, not free. Furthermore, provider reimbursement for services may be decreased by Medicare (the primary health care provider for the elderly) making access to pain treatments less. A problem is emerging with respect to provider reimbursement for pain treatments performed. Medicare, furthermore will not test fore telomere length analysis.

Approximately, forty-eight million Americans suffer from chronic pain. Over one-third of all adult Americans suffer from prolonged pain. Over the counter annual analgesic costs amount to three billion dollars. Chronic pain is a prevalent and a costly problem. One must assess the clinical effectiveness and cost-effectiveness of the most common treatments for patients with prolonged pain. A problem exists in that there are 10,000 persons a day who turn 65 in the United States. This number will increase to 12,000 in the near future.

Most primary care physicians are not adequately treating elderly patient pain, primarily because they are not trained to do so, and because they are afraid of litigation and regulatory drug prescribing restrictions. Chronic pain with conservative care such as medications, physical therapy, chiropractic, etc. costs North American adults an estimated $10,000 to $15,000 per person per annum. Furthermore, estimates of the cost of pain do not include the nearly 30,000 people that die in North America each year due to non-steroidal anti-inflammatory drug-induced gastric lesions. Economically, the management of pain costs more than the treatment for heart disease and cancer combined.

Pain in the absence of disease is not a normal part of aging, yet it is experienced daily by a majority of elderly adults in the United States. Older adults are at high risk for under treatment of pain due to a variety of barriers. These include lack of adequate education of health care professionals, cost concerns and other obstacles related to the health care system, and patient related barriers, such as reluctance to report pain or take analgesics.

The incidence of pain more than doubles once individuals surpass the age of 60 with pain frequency increasing with each decade. Unrelieved pain in the older adult has significant functional, cognitive, emotional, and societal consequences.

Because patients may have to pay a portion of their bills for fees charged for procedures done on them as well as for medications pre-scribed (copayments), representative published studies that evaluate the clinical effectiveness of pharmacological treatments, conservative (standard) care, surgery, nerve blocks and pain rehabilitation programs must be examined and compared. When you're in pain, the last thing you want to think about is the cost of getting the relief you need. However, you do want a procedure or medication that may benefit you. The cost-effectiveness of various treatment approaches must also be considered. Outcome criteria of a particular treatment should include the incidence of pain reduction.

Patients prior to consenting to any treatment modality should evaluate medication use and health care consumption. In addition to clinical effectiveness, the cost-effectiveness of conservative care, surgery and nerve blocks must be compared.

There are limitations to the success of all available treatments. Chronic pain programs are in many instances in need of rehabilitation. Although hard statistics regarding such programs are difficult to obtain, one frequently hears of programs closing down or modifying their treatment protocols to meet their own survival needs rather than meeting the needs of the patients they serve.

After rapid growth during the 1980s and through the mid-1990s, the number of inpatient chronic pain management programs actually declined. Concurrent with the decline in intensive programs is the rise of procedural interventions and medications, which receive a great deal of support from hospitals and pharmaceutical companies. The use of muscle relaxants for patients appears to be increasingly prevalent when compared with teaching relaxation techniques, and implanting a device is more lucrative than giving patient's guidance or advice.

Healthcare specialists have to determine whether this apparent shift in treatment emphasis away from rehabilitation is a healthy development for the patients they serve. Many hospitals encourage physicians with minimal or no training to open pain clinics in their facilities. They can charge facility fees of $1000.00 or more for a procedure like an epidural steroid injection. Your physician who is doing the procedure may own shares in a surgery center or hospital. As a result, every time that a physician schedules a procedure in the hospital he or she has ownership in makes a share of the profit. The sad fact is that this behavior is legal.

Medical procedures, such as trigger point injections, sympathetic nerve blocks, and epidural steroid injections, are rated as significantly less helpful, fewer invasive modalities than surgery, despite their considerably higher average costs. Research is needed to identify which patients are most likely to benefit from the available treatments and to study combinations of the present treatments since none of them appears capable of eliminating pain or substantially improving functional outcomes for all treated. The cost of chronic benign (non-cancer pain) spinal pain is large and is increasing.

The costs of interventional treatments for spinal pain, for example, were at a minimum of $13 billion (U.S. dollars) in 1990, and the costs are growing at least 7% per year. The interventional medical treatment of chronic pain costs $9000 to $19,000 per person per year. It should be understood that only a small percentage of patients receive long-term relief with these procedures. You should inquire about the cost of any treatment before agreeing to have the procedure done. You also need to contact your insurance carrier and ascertain if your treatment is covered under your insurance plan.

Before consenting to a potential expensive therapy do research. Check the Internet for a description of the procedure and if it is effective. Ask a physician what the cost is for the treatment in question. Is there a surgery center charge in addition to the physician fee? A patient should ask the physician if there is an extra fee for sedation if a patient has to have a nerve block. Some centers bundle this fee with the facility charge while others charge separately for these charges.

Medicare may pay for some pain treatments, but one needs to be aware of the total cost to treat the pain. Medicare usually does not pay all of the medical expenses. The treatment for back pain may only cost $3.00 for a bottle of aspirin. However, a patient needs to calculate and add the chiropractor fees or the costs of a massage. What about the housekeeper to do the housework that a patient can't do while he/she was disabled? What about the heating pad? Most elderly patients have Medicare health insurance that at least pays part of an elderly patient's medical expenses.

Medicare is a health insurance program for people age 65 or older. Medicare is partially financed by payroll taxes imposed by the Federal Insurance Contributions Act (FICA) and the Self-Employment Contributions Act of 1954. Medicare has Two Parts: Part A (Hospital Insurance) and Part B (Medical Insurance). Part A pays for care in hospitals as an inpatient, skilled nursing facilities, hospice care, and some home-health care. Part B pays for doctors' services, outpatient hospital care, and some other medical services that Part A doesn't cover, such as the services of physical and occupational therapists, and some home-health care.

The Medicare Website indicates in general, that all persons 65 years of age or older who have been legal residents of the United States for at least

5 years are eligible for Medicare. Medicare Part D covers pre-scription drugs. Medicare Advantage plans, also known as Medicare Part C, are another way for beneficiaries to receive their Part A, B and D benefits. All Medicare benefits are subject to medical necessity. This means if the Medicare administration feels that you do not need a certain procedure, you will have to pay for it out of pocket. Most people do not pay a monthly Part A premium because they or a spouse has 40 or more quarters of Medicare-covered employment.

The Part A premium is $248.00 per month for people having 30-39 quarters of Medicare-covered employment. The Part A premium is $450.00 per month for people who are not otherwise eligible for premium-free hospital insurance and have less than 30 quarters of Medicare-covered employment. The Medicare Part B premium is increasing in 2011 due to possible increases in Part B costs.

If one's income is above $85,000 (single) or $170,000 (married couple), then the Medicare Part B premium may be higher than $115.40 per month. Part A coverage is for each benefit period Medicare pays all covered costs except the Medicare Part A deductible (2011 = $1, 132) during the first 60 days and coinsurance amounts for hospital stays that last beyond 60 days and no more than 150 days. For Part B, you pay $162.00 per annum. (Note: You pay 20% of the Medicare-approved amount for services after you meet the $162.00 deductible).

For people who choose to enroll in a Medicare Advantage health plan, Medicare pays the private health plan a fixed amount every month. Members typically also pay a monthly premium in addition to the Medicare Part B premium to cover items not covered by traditional Medicare (Parts A & B), such as prescription drugs, dental care, vision care and gym or health club memberships. In exchange for these extra benefits; a patient may be limited in the providers whom one may receive services from providers without paying extra. Neither Part A nor Part B pays for all of a covered person's medical costs. The program contains premiums, deductibles and coinsurance, which the covered individual must pay out-of-pocket.

The Parts of Medicare are: Part A – Hospital Insurance, Part B – Medical Insurance, Part C – Medicare Advantage and Part D – Prescription Coverage. Everyone who is eligible for Medicare receive Medicare Part A benefits automatically. Part A initially covered inpatient hospital care and skilled nursing facility care. Today, home health care and hospice facility care are also included. Most people do not have to pay a premium to get Part A.

There was a short coming in the original Medicare plan. It only covered the hospital costs. It did not cover medically necessary services like doctor's services, diagnostic tests and outpatient care. Medicare Part B added coverage for medically necessary services. Physical therapy and some preventive screenings are also covered. Part B is optional and a patient must pay a premium. If a patient is still working, the employer's insurance may cover this part. Otherwise, one will have to pay a premium to receive this coverage.

Medicare part A B C D does not cover everything. There are holes or "gaps" in the Medicare part A and B coverage. This is the reason for Medicare Supplement Insurance. The MediGap plans are standardized by the government. They are not sold or administered by the government. You must go to a private insurance company to receive this coverage. Medicare Supplemental Insurance is only available if you are receiving benefits from Part A and B.

A patient now have the option to enroll in Medicare part C. Part C allows one to have Medicare benefits administered through private health insurance plans. A patient pays the premium to private insurer. The insurer provides the benefits and not the government. Part D is the Medicare program which covers prescription drugs.

Before the Affordable Care Act (ACA), many surveys showed majority support for national health insurance (NHI), also known as single payer; however, little is currently known about views of the ACA's targeted population.[1]

Beginning January 1st, 2011 in the United States the Affordable Care Act enhanced Medicare coverage for preventive services by eliminating patient cost-sharing under Part B and by introducing an "Annual Wellness Visit," also free-of-charge.[2] Educating and incentivizing physicians about the need to refer/recommend screenings, and enhancing knowledge among seniors about the importance of preventive care are two steps that would likely go a long way towards increasing utilization.

Elderly people (aged 65 years or more) are at increased risk of polypharmacy (five or more medications), inappropriate medication use, and associated increased health care costs. The use of clinical decision support (CDS) within an electronic medical record (EMR) could improve medication safety.[3]

The majority of developed countries are currently experiencing demographic aging. The most frequently expressed concerns related to the changing age structure are the increased costs of social and medical care, a lack of labor force in the job market, and financial sustainability of the pension system.[4] Medicare Part D improved medication adherence among the elderly, but to date, its effect on disparities in adherence remains unknown. Increasing access and improving quality of medication use among disadvantaged seniors should remain a policy priority.[5]

For people with low and moderate incomes, the Affordable Care Act's tax credits have made premium costs roughly comparable to those paid by people with job-based health insurance. For those with higher incomes, the tax credits phase out, meaning that adults in marketplace plans on average have higher premium costs than those in employer plans. The law's cost-sharing reductions are reducing deductibles.[6]

References

1. Saluja S, Zallman L, Nardin R, et al. Support for National Health Insurance Seven Years Into Massachusetts Healthcare Reform: Views of Populations Targeted by the Reform. Int J Health Serv. 2016;46(1):185-200.

2. Jensen GA, Salloum RG, Hu J, Ferdows NB, Tarraf W. A slow start: Use of preventive services among seniors following the Affordable Care Act's enhancement of Medicare benefits in the U.S. Prev Med. 2015;76:37-42.

3. Alagiakrishnan K, Wilson P, Sadowski CA, et al. Physicians' use of computerized clinical decision supports to improve medication management in the elderly - the Seniors Medication Alert and Review Technology intervention. Clin Interv Aging. 2016;11:73-81.

4. Kacetl J, Maresova P. Legislative and ethical aspects of introducing new technologies in medical care for senior citizens in developed countries. Clin Interv Aging. 2016;11:977-984.

5. Hussein M, Waters TM, Chang CF, Bailey JE, Brown LM, Solomon DK. Impact of Medicare Part D on Racial Disparities in Adherence to Cardiovascular Medications Among the Elderly. Med Care Res Rev. 2016;73(4):410-436.

6. Gunja MZ, Collins SR, Doty MM, Beutel S. Americans' Experiences with ACA Marketplace Coverage: Affordability and Provider Network Satisfaction: Findings from the Commonwealth Fund Affordable Care Act Tracking Survey, February--April 2016. Issue Brief (Commonw Fund). 2016;17:1-20.

Index

accelerated aging 361

Action potentials 19

Acute pain 13, 17, 151, 152

Addiction 101

Age-related bone loss 187

Aging 1

AIDS, 322

alternative medicine 61

ankylosing spondylitis 336

Aspirin 107

Axons 20

biological clock 14

Bone spurs 330

capsaicin 141

carpal tunnel syndrome 256

CAT scans 355

chiropractic 71

cluster headache 209

conversion disorder 48

CRPS 231

Cytokine inhibitors 68

dendrite 20

Diabetic neuropathy 259

DNA 1

Dynorphins 21

electroencephalography 23

Electrostimulation 130

EMG 357

Enkephalins 21

Entrapment neuropathies 256

GABA 21

genetic makeup 9

headache 207

hip fracture 301

HIV virus 322

Hypochondriasis 49

internuncial fibers 21

irritable bowel syndrome 341

Kaposi's sarcoma 322

Massage 31, 76, 226, 338

Medicare 375

migraine headache 207

morphine pump 133

myofascial pain syndrome 195

NCV 357

Neck pain 167

Neurons 18

neuropathic pain 118

neuropathy 10, 13, 19, 26, 119, 120, 121, 141, 195, 255, 256, 258, 259, 260, 261, 262, 263, 287, 321, 358

non-Hodgkin lymphoma 322

NSAIDs 27, 107, 108, 109, 110, 111, 112, 113, 114, 115, 135, 139, 141, 144, 148, 249

Nutrition 9, 7, 81, 88

opioid drugs 91

pain assessment 36

painful inflammation 329

palliative care 367

PET studies 22

physiologic changes 11

poena 17

post-herpetic neuralgia 247

Prostaglandin inhibition 110

Prostaglandins 20

provider reimbursement 373

Psoriatic arthritis 338

Psychological assessments 50

Psychological treatment 43

replicative senescence 14, 16, 147, 187, 251, 315, 326, 327, 333 sleep deprivation 25

Somatization 48, 175

Spinal deterioration 213

spinal infusion pump 133

Steroid creams 144

steroid injections 158

substance P 141

telomerase 1, 6, 7, 14, 15, 16, 81, 88, 147, 148, 149, 189, 192, 193, 218, 219, 253, 265, 271, 273, 275, 277, 285, 286, 311, 312, 326, 329, 338, 339, 348, 350, 359, 361, 363, 364, 365, 366

telomere 7, 9, 1, 4, 5, 6, 7, 14, 16, 24, 35, 53, 54, 55, 57, 81, 82, 83, 84, 86, 87, 88, 89, 98, 100, 102, 105, 106, 109, 110, 115, 117, 124, 130, 136, 147, 148, 189, 192, 195, 196, 199, 200, 203, 205, 206, 207, 208, 209, 211, 212, 216, 217, 218, 219, 221, 228, 231, 243, 252, 261, 263, 265, 270, 271, 274, 275, 277, 282, 285, 286, 295, 296, 299, 305, 306, 309, 312, 315, 329, 331, 332, 334, 338, 339, 345, 348, 349, 350, 358, 359, 361, 362, 363, 364, 365, 367

Telomere length 10, 4, 5, 6, 15, 54, 88, 115, 117, 189, 203, 221, 273, 281, 297, 309, 312, 313, 361, 365

TENS 127

topical analgesics 137

Trigeminal neuralgia 288

Ultrasound 355

Vertebral compression fractures 56

vitamins 81, 84, 87, 261

whiplash injury 177

www.ingramcontent.com/pod-product-compliance
Lightning Source LLC
Chambersburg PA
CBHW070220190526
45169CB00001B/24

About the Author

Dr. William Ackerman is a pain management specialist, author and researcher. He is double-board certified in both Anesthesiology and Pain Medicine. Dr. Ackerman was the former medical director of pain management and was an associate professor at a university hospital. He has authored over 135 scientific articles in prestigious journals such as Anesthesia Analgesia, Canadian Journal of Anesthesia, Regional Anesthesia and Pain Management etc. He was on the editorial Board of two medical journals.

Dr. Ackerman maintains an active private practice. His practice consists of interventional and medical treatment of chronic pain and is considered an expert in Reflex Sympathetic Dystrophy. He has published chapters in multiple medical textbooks and has published twelve books including coauthoring and editing the AMA best seller book the **AMA Guides to Injury and Disease Causation** (First and Second Editions).

Dr. Ackerman has expertise in the treatment of a variety of chronic painful conditions including neck and low back pain, intractable neuropathic pain, shingles, joint pain, myofascial pain, complex regional pain syndrome (CRPS), cancer-related pain etc., with a multi-modal Evidence Based Medicine approach.

Dr. Ackerman has been a Lt. Col. in the U.S. Army and Chief of Anesthesiology at two Army medical centers. He has been an Associate Professor of three academic, universities, pain management departments and has been on the academy faculty at three medical schools. He has been on the Editorial Board of two peer reviewed medical journals. He was nominated previously for the Southern Medical Society Medical Research Award and the Bristol-Meyers Squibb award for distinguished achievement in Pain Research.

He was a past recipient of the prestigious Karl Koeller research grant from the American Society of Regional Anesthesia and Pain Medicine and was selected to "Who's Who in International Medicine". He has a strong interest in diversity and the appropriate pain management in different gender, age, race and ethnic groups. He analyzes the effectiveness of a pain management intervention in certain subsets of the population, such as in people sharing particular genetic features, as well as compared to the whole population.